THE EDINBURGH CITY HOSPITAL

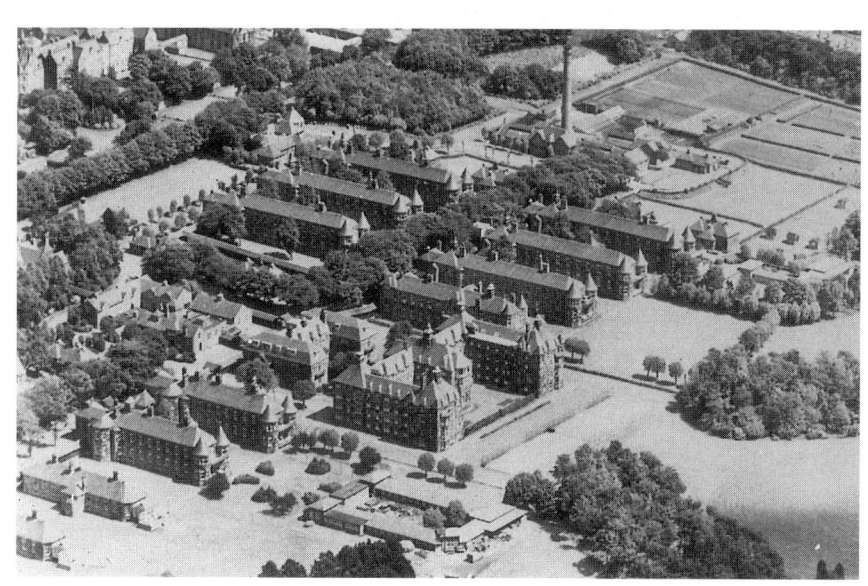

Aerial view of the City Hospital from the south west (ca. 1960). The wooden TB wards occupy the central foreground and behind them are the nurses' home and to its left the servants' home. Cottage 12 is at the right of the picture. The tall chimney locates the laundry, boiler house, and incinerator. Part of Greenlea (formerly the Craiglockhart Poorhouse and now The Steils) is in the top left corner. (Photo: Aero Pictorial Ltd, London)

THE EDINBURGH CITY HOSPITAL

James A. Gray

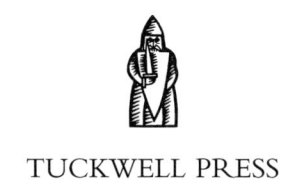

TUCKWELL PRESS

First published in 1999 by
Tuckwell Press Ltd
The Mill House
Phantassie
East Linton
East Lothian
EH40 3DG
Scotland

Text copyright © James A. Gray 1999

All rights reserved

ISBN 1 86232 096 9

A catalogue record for this book is available
on request from the British Library

Typeset by Carnegie Publishing, Lancaster
Printed and bound by Redwood Books, Trowbridge, Wiltshire

To
Jennifer for her loving support
and in memory of
my father, Dr J. D. Allan Gray
and
my school teacher Mr Philip D. Whitting,
both of whom imbued in me a love of history

Contents

	Foreword by Dr Helen Zealley	xi
	Preface and Acknowledgements	xiii
1	Setting the Scene	1

PART ONE Infectious Diseases and the Development of Public Health Services in Edinburgh up to the Nineteenth Century

2	Early Measures for the Control of Infectious Disease and for the Care of Fever Patients	7
3	Edinburgh's Problems with Overcrowding and Defects in Housing, Water Supply and Sanitation	19
4	Something has to be Done: The Public Health Movement in Edinburgh under Sir Henry Littlejohn	25

PART TWO Early Hospital Provision for Edinburgh's Fever Patients

5	The Royal Infirmary	37
6	Queensberry House Fever Hospital, 1818–35	41
7	The First City Fever Hospital: The Canongate Poorhouse	48
8	Who Should Care For Fever Patients? The Second City Fever Hospital at Infirmary Street	53
9	The Reorganisation and Expansion of the Old Infirmary Site	61
10	The Smallpox Outbreak 1892–5 and a Change of Plans	74

PART THREE The Planning, Building and Opening of the Third City Fever Hospital, 1894–1903

11	Choosing a Site for the Third City Fever Hospital	85
12	The Bailie, the Architect and the Builder	91
13	Planning the Hospital	97
14	Building the Hospital: The Town Council v. John Lownie	108
15	A Description of the Third City Hospital	120
16	The Royal Opening, 13 May 1903	132

PART FOUR Dr C. B. Ker's Superintendentship 1903–25, The City Hospital and Tuberculosis, and Dr W. T. Benson's Superintendentship 1925–36

17 Dr Ker's Early Years and the Temporary Smallpox Hospital 141
18 Dr Ker's Later Years: The Nursing Staff; Scarlet Fever, Meningitis, Influenza; The First World War 154
19 The Contribution of the City Hospital to the Control of Tuberculosis: Sir Robert Philip, Sir John Crofton and some Notable Chest Physicians 167
20 Dr W. T. Benson's Superintendentship, 1925–36: Serotherapy for Scarlet Fever; Immunisation for Nurses 183

PART FIVE Dr Alec Joe's Superintendentship 1937–60

21 1937–41: The Advent of Sulphonamides; Poliomyelitis, Dysentery and Meningitis 197
22 1939–42: The Second World War and Edinburgh's Last Outbreak of Smallpox 204
23 1943–47: The End of the War; The Nursing and Domestic Staff; Penicillin; Anxieties about the Coming NHS 216
24 The Early Years of the NHS; The Bacteriology Laboratory; Thoracic Surgery Unit; and the Half Centenary Celebrations 235
25 1954–60: Changing Patterns of Disease 253

PART SIX Dr N. W. Horne's Superintendentship 1960–74, Two Decades of Change, 1974–94, and the Closure

26 1960–74: The Building Boom Years; Infectious Diseases, Pyelonephritis, and Tropical Medicine 269
27 1960–74: The Surgical Units, Care of the Elderly Unit and New Laboratories; A Continuing Nursing Shortage; The Tea Room; The Bus Service 286
28 1974–94: A Reorganised Health Service; Infectious Diseases and AIDS; the Fire in the Nurses' Home; Milestone House 310
29 1974–94: Respiratory and Chest Medicine; the Rayne Laboratory; Thoracic, ENT and Maxillofacial Surgery; Care of the Elderly Unit; the X-ray Department 333
30 Changes in Nursing Management and Practice; Nurses' Medals and Badges 351
31 The Pharmacy; the Professions Allied to Medicine; the Dietetic and Social Work Departments 359

32 Records and Secretarial Services; Catering, Laundry, Area
   Sterilising Service; Domestic and Portering Services; Buildings,
   Grounds and Gardens   376
33 The Chaplains' Department, the Patients' Library and the
   League of Friends   389
34 The Future   398

   Abbreviated References and Selected Abbreviations   404
   Notes and References   419
   Index   449

Foreword

The story of a hospital has many parallels with the life history of a family. Its historical roots are important and it provides the common purpose for an evolving set of key players who reflect both their own individuality and the mores of their time. Some have a more dominant role than others and countless thousands of other people have transient contact which, for some, becomes a critical turning point in their lives. One of the longest serving characters in the story of Edinburgh's third 'City Hospital' was Dr Alec Joe. In his 1953 speech for the hospital's half-centenary he hoped that '... some day a chronicler may appear among us to relate all these things ...'. That chronicler is James Gray, another 'fever doctor' whose professional life has been linked closely to the City Hospital for almost thirty years.

For this fascinating story of the hospital, James Gray has painstakingly reviewed the annual reports of all the superintendents of the hospital, as well as those of the city's health department. The chronicle begins with a resumé of the city's history of infectious diseases – the fevers that were feared by all. It traces their links with poverty, overcrowding, illiteracy and lack of water and sanitation; and leads the reader to imagine life on, say, the sixth floor of a High Street tenement with no running water or sanitation. As it grew upwards before expansion to the New Town, no wonder the Old Town of Edinburgh became one of the filthiest cities in Europe.

Efforts to reduce the resulting ill health came, as they do now, from a combination of action to improve the environment and living conditions, active measures to protect the public's health, and better organised services to identify and treat those who were sick. A critical adjunct to the treatment of fevers was the effective isolation of patients – and indeed of those with different fevers from each other. As the story unfolds, we learn of the need for expanded isolation facilities for the citizens of Edinburgh at the end of the nineteenth century. What we would now call an 'option appraisal' favoured transfer from the second city hospital in Drummond Street to the vacated site of the 'old' Royal Infirmary close by. But a major smallpox epidemic in 1894 resulted in a change of plan. The result – an impressive purpose-built fever hospital on the green-field site at Colinton Mains which has served the city so well for almost a century.

Since its opening by the King and Queen in 1903, the City Hospital has seen the virtual disappearance of poliomyelitis. It has been at the forefront of international developments in the treatment of tuberculosis and heroin related HIV. As many of the infectious diseases came under control through the impact of immunisation and antibiotics, the hospital has evolved to serve the needs of a wider range of patients. The staff – initially doctors, nurses and a dispenser but gradually expanding as new professional groups added their skills – have provided loyal service within a hospital which provided them in turn with friendship and camaraderie. That they continued to do so through a succession of organisational structures owes a great deal to the spirit of the hospital itself which is so well captured in this authoritative and fascinating account.

Dr Helen Zealley OBE QHP MD FRCPE FFPHM
Director of Public Heath, Lothian Health

Preface and Acknowledgements

On a sunny August afternoon in 1969, to my great surprise and delight, I was informed by an Advisory Appointments Committee of the South-Eastern Regional Hospital Board, Scotland, that I had been the successful applicant for the newly created consultant post in communicable diseases at the Edinburgh City Hospital. After the interview in Drumsheugh Gardens, I walked back triumphantly to Morningside via Bruntsfield. Having been unbearably tetchy in the run up to my interview, I decided to make amends and send some flowers to my wife, then in London.

Flushed with pride and smug self-satisfaction that, for the first time in my life, I would command a salary of over £3,000 per annum, I imperiously ordered the flower shop assistant to send off a dozen red roses. I well remember that she was a rather sweet, middle-aged lady wearing spectacles and she had her grey hair scraped back into a bun. She wore the traditional green pinafore over her dress. As we finalised the arrangements, she smiled politely and enquired in her best Morningside accent 'Maybe a wee celebration then?' To which I pompously replied 'Well yes, actually, I've just been appointed as a consultant physician to the City Hospital.' On hearing this the lady looked startled, quickly distancing herself from me to retreat behind the big mahogany counter saying 'Oh dear! Oh dear! I'm so very sorry for you!'

Over the years since, and particularly after my research for this book, I have come to appreciate why the lady in the flower shop reacted as she did. The City Hospital was not always a happy place for patients, relatives and staff. Who knows which of her family or friends may have succumbed there to one of the infections that all too often had a fatal outcome. I had not then realised that patients with advanced tuberculosis were at one time sent to the City Hospital to die, that outbreaks of smallpox, diphtheria, typhus and typhoid could carry such a high mortality and that 'routine' infections like scarlet fever, erysipelas, measles, whooping cough and poliomyelitis also took a heavy toll. With so many epidemic infections tamed or conquered today, we often forget how fortunate we are – until new diseases like HIV infection, E. coli 0157 or new variant Creutzfeldt-Jakob Disease (CJD) come to replace the old ones, and bacteria like tubercle bacilli and staphylococci became multiply resistant to modern drugs.

In 1995, knowing the City Hospital would close within the foreseeable future, my colleague Dr Ray Brettle asked me if I would like to document the history of the Regional Infectious Diseases Unit (RIDU). Having always been interested in history, I accepted but was certainly unprepared, when a few days later, Mike Pearson, the Business Manager, thanked me for agreeing to write, not simply an account of the RIDU, which would have been reasonably straight forward, but a history of the whole of the City Hospital. As I was about to retire I agreed, wisely or unwisely. I have to acknowledge the support and encouragement Mike Pearson has given me since.

Although the hospital was built between 1897 and 1903 purely for the management of communicable diseases, by the early 1960s, infectious disease patients occupied only one quarter of the wards, and other disciplines were already playing a major role in the work of the hospital. Chronologically, units concerned with tuberculosis and respiratory medicine, thoracic surgery, ear, nose and throat (ENT) surgery, geriatric medicine and lastly maxillofacial surgery arrived and contributed to the hospital's research, teaching and clinical commitment. I gratefully acknowledge the help given to me by many of those who work, or have worked, in these areas and in the hospital's laboratories. The nursing staff, the X-ray staff, those in the pharmacy and professions allied to medicine and those in administration and the service units, some now retired, others still working, have willingly contributed valuable information. Some have given up hours of their time over a meal or cups of coffee, providing me with insight to their departments with which I was previously unfamiliar. This book could not have been written without their help.

I apologise now to anyone from whom I have received assistance if I have accidentally omitted to mention him or her or if I have by oversight misrepresented personalities or events. Any errors in this book are mine and certainly not to be laid at the door of those who have been so helpful to me. I must stress also that this book represents only one man's view of a long history which becomes increasingly complex in modern times. I reiterate the wise words in *Toxophilus* written by Roger Ascham in 1545:

> YF I HAUE SAYED A MISSE, I AM CONTENT THAT ANY MAN AMENDE IT, OR YF I HAUV SAYD TO LYTLE ANY MAN WYL TO ADDE WHAT HYM PLEASETH TO IT.

Dr Helen Zealley worked as a virologist at the City Hospital before embarking on a successful career in Public Health Medicine. I thank her for writing the foreword, for allowing me to reproduce illustrations from the Annual Reports of her Department and for kindly putting me in touch with Miss Rachel A. Hedderwick, a granddaughter of Sir Henry Littlejohn, Edinburgh's first Medical Officer of Health.

For continuous encouragement and for the finding of funds, I am indebted to Mike Pearson. His secretary, Mrs Anne Knowles, has bravely coped with the enormous task of converting tapes and manuscript onto hard discs, and then revising many drafts. I wish to take this opportunity to thank also the Trustees of the Douglas Guthrie Trust for their very generous financial assistance in awarding me a substantial grant. After covering my own expenses, I intend that any surplus royalties received will be devoted to the work of Tansen Hospital in rural Nepal where my late son worked for four years as a medical missionary.

I am particularly indebted to the Hon. Lord Gill who not only steered me through the long and complex legal dispute between the Town Council and the builder of the hospital (1897–1904), but has also given me valuable advice and constructive criticism after reading drafts of the whole book. Ms Mairi Sutherland's editorial suggestions have been particularly helpful. Mrs Hilary Flenley also deserves my thanks for bravely undertaking the task of indexing the work. My publishers, John and Val Tuckwell, have shown great patience as several deadlines came and went. Their kind encouragement is acknowledged.

Much of the source material has come from Edinburgh libraries. In particular I thank Dr Mike Barfoot and Mrs Julie Hutton of the Lothian Health Services Archive and Special Collections Department in the University Library; Ms Alison Scott, Richard Hunter and Ms Stefanie Davidson of the Edinburgh City Archive; Andrew Bethune and Ian Nelson of the Edinburgh Room in the Central Library; Richard Phillips, Newington Branch, Edinburgh City Libraries; Miss Joan Ferguson and the present Librarian, Iain Milne, of the Royal College of Physicians of Edinburgh; Ian Gow of the Library of the National Monuments Record of Scotland; the Trustees and staff of the National Library of Scotland, including the Map Library; John Simmons, Supervisor, West Search Room and the staff of the Scottish Record Office; Ingval Maxwell and John Hume of Historic Scotland and Professor David Walker, recently retired from Historic Scotland; Miss M. M. Stewart, Dumfries and Galloway Archive Centre; and finally the staff of the Erskine Medical Library of the University. They have all helped in different ways and have shown me unfailing courtesy. Access has been given to original documents as required and permission kindly granted for the reproduction of several of the illustrations in this book. I thank them all.

Several fellow authors and local historians have kindly imparted their knowledge and given me encouragement. I thank Charles J. Smith, Malcolm Cant and Drs David Boyd and Martin Eastwood. Permission from Thames and Hudson to quote extracts from Professor David Daiches' book *Was – A Pastime from Time Past* is acknowledged.

In trying to find out the route taken from the Caledonian Railway to the building site by the Dumfriesshire quarried stone used to build the hospital, I have bothered many experts, several of whom are mentioned elsewhere in these acknowledgements. In addition I wish to thank Alan Brotchie, Dr R. N. Crockett, Leigh Crowther, Andrew Hajducki, QC, David M. E. Lindsay, A. McLean, A. J. Mullay, William Munro, Neil D. G. MacKenzie, Angus M. Peterson, Donald Shaw, Alan Simpson, Dr Graham Smith, Michael Smith, Ms Elspeth Third and Douglas Yuill.

Perhaps the most enjoyable aspect of the research for this book has been the opportunity it has given me to meet so many new and former friends and colleagues. Miss Rachel A. Hedderwick enlightened me about Sir Henry Littlejohn. Mrs Rankine, formerly Director of Nursing Services at Queensberry House, showed me over the building and provided me with a copy of the history. Miss P. A. Morham, granddaughter of the City Hospital's architect, Robert Morham, and the Hon. Judge Ralph Lownie, grandson of the builder, John Lownie, both provided me with much useful information about their forebears. As mentioned above, the Hon. Lord Gill explained the tortuous litigation surrounding the building of the hospital and the dispute between Robert Morham and John Lownie which is described in Chapter 14.

Lay administrators and managers have assisted me throughout the writing of this book. I particularly wish to thank Alec G. Welstead, William J. Farquhar, Don Nicolson, Jack Burton, Mike Pearson and Jim Smith. Some medical administrators and managers who helped were Drs Ian Campbell and Sheena Parker, and in the laboratories Drs Sheila Burns, Nancy Conn, Ross McHardy and Brian Watt. I have drawn heavily on their knowledge. It is unlikely that I could have completed the book without the unfailingly kind assistance of Dr Norman W. Horne, chest physician and, between 1960 and 1974, the hospital's Physician Superintendent. He gave me much encouragement and information from his rich fund of clinical and administrative experience.

In the story of infectious diseases, Mrs Rosemary Koelliker and Mrs Maureen Ward (daughters of Dr W. J. Benson), Mrs Florrie Sangster (widow of Dr George Sangster) and Mrs Irene Murdoch (widow of Dr James McC Murdoch), Drs Philip D. Welsby, Ray P. Brettle and Mike E. Jones have all kindly supplied information or photographs. Dr Judy Greenwood assisted with details of the Community Drug Problem Service.

Shortly before he died in 1996, Dr Fred J. Wright generously supplied me with a written account of the Tropical Diseases Unit.

For information about the hospital's role in tuberculosis, chest medicine and respiratory function assessment I am indebted to Dr Christopher Clayson, Sir John Crofton, Dr Andrew C. Douglas, Professor Neil J. Douglas, Mrs Hilary Flenley (widow of Professor David C. Flenley), Drs Norman Horne and Ross McHardy, Professor Bill McNee, Miss Sylvia Merchant, Drs Michael Sudlow and Pat Warren and Professor James Williamson. For advice about the anaesthetic service, I thank Dr Archie C. Milne. Both Mr Andrew Logan and Mr Evan Cameron have kindly informed me about cardio-thoracic surgery, Professor Arnold Maran about ENT surgery and Mr Glenn Lello about maxillofacial surgery. Professor James Williamson, Dr Colin T. Currie and Professor Bill MacLennan kindly assisted me regarding the Care of the Elderly Unit.

The nursing staff have been very helpful and I wish to thank Mrs Mina Begg, Miss Marion Buchanan, Miss A. E. Christie, Mrs Jean Day, Miss Isobel Duncan, Mrs Pat Hunter, Miss Margaret Kerr, Mrs Maureen Lees, Mrs Isobel Lorimer, Mrs Isobel McFarlane, Mr Ron Munro, Mr Robert Purves and especially Miss J. K. Taylor for her fund of information and photographs of hospital life. I am also grateful to Nurse Fiona Scott for giving me photocopies of the architect's designs which assisted my early researches.

Mr Andrew Hunter kindly supplied a summary of the activities of the pharmacy and Mr Jimmy Rawlings an account of the X-ray department. In the professions allied to medicine I acknowledge the assistance of Mrs Angela Lindsay (Physiotherapy), Mrs Nola Meikle (Occupational Therapy), Ms Sandra Anderson (Speech and Language Therapy) and in dietetics Miss Enid Henery. Three former social workers have helped me greatly, Mrs Elizabeth Dunbar, Mrs Kim Shandley and Mrs Pam Leaver.

I am also indebted to Ernie Whiteoak (Records), Tom Ferguson and Martin Henry (Catering), George Nixon and Gordon Rawson (Laundry), Mark Lavery and Ian Robertson (Area Sterilising Service), Mrs Mary Kelly and Jim Smith (domestic services and portering), David Pithie (Senior Foreman), Willie Maben (estates offices) and Barrie Liston (fire officer).

Rev. Dr Bob Mathers and Rev. Harry Telfer have assisted me with the story of the chaplaincy and Dr Mathers put me in touch with Mr J. K. Thomson, Chaplaincies Administrator, who kindly consulted records from the Edinburgh Presbytery for me. Mrs Christine Craig explained the patients' library service. Both Mr Frank Snell and Mrs Pat Macleod kindly reported on the work of the League of Friends.

For the future development of the hospital site I have been helped by Mr Alan Ezzi, Project Manager of the new Royal Infirmary, Mr Derick Reid, Morrison Homes, and Mrs Gillian Gray, Cala Homes (Scotland) Ltd.

Acknowledgements for the illustrations accompany the figures and I am most grateful to everyone who supplied me with photographs or gave permission for their publication. Both the University Department of Medical Illustration and the Medical Photography Unit of the Royal Infirmary have been very helpful.

Many friends, colleagues and members of my family, especially my daughters Emma and Lucy, have shown a kindly interest throughout. My late mother-in-law, Mrs Elizabeth Hunter, generously provided me with some difficult-to-obtain books from her library to help my early researches.

Last, but by no means least, I wish to thank my wife Jennifer for her encouragement and support and also her patient forbearance over several years while I commandeered our dining room as my study during the writing of this book.

Jim Gray, Edinburgh, 1999

CHAPTER ONE

Setting the Scene

Today it is difficult to imagine what it was like to live and work in Edinburgh at the end of the nineteenth century when the present City Fever Hospital had its origins. To find out why such hospitals were needed, the pattern of health and disease over the previous centuries will be reviewed in Chapters 2–4; this does not always make palatable reading.

Illiteracy, poverty, and overcrowded buildings with inadequate water supplies and sanitation, combined with keeping and slaughtering animals in or close to the dwellings, made Edinburgh a fertile breeding ground for infection. In the eighteenth and nineteenth centuries, it was reputedly one of the filthiest cities in the country. James Boswell, strolling home up the High Street arm in arm with Dr Samuel Johnson one night in August 1773, 'could not prevent his being assailed by the evening effluvia of Edinburgh'.[1] Boswell also quoted a late baronet who observed that 'walking the streets of Edinburgh at night was pretty perilous, and a good deal odoriferous'.[2]

Despite progress in public health legislation, in which Edinburgh was a forerunner, outbreaks of typhus, typhoid, cholera and smallpox occurred throughout the nineteenth century. These necessitated major rethinking when the Public Health Committee of the City of Edinburgh became responsible for isolation accommodation for its infected citizens all year round as well as during epidemics. A new model City Fever Hospital was therefore built on a green-field site on the south west outskirts of the city; it was opened by King Edward VII in 1903.

This City Hospital has served the citizens of Edinburgh very well for nearly a century. Most of the patients in the early years had scarlet fever, diphtheria, typhoid, cerebro-spinal meningitis or poliomyelitis. Improvements in housing, nutrition and social services, immunisation and the advent of antibiotics reduced, but never quite eliminated, the need for 'fever beds'. Tuberculosis, however, remained a major scourge until the 1950s and many beds were occupied by patients with 'phthisis'. Thereafter, a chest X-ray campaign screening the population and the institution of modern antimycobacterial treatment caused the number of patients affected by tuberculosis to plummet.

Thoracic surgery, ear nose and throat surgery and more recently maxillofacial surgery units then used the wards that had previously accommodated patients with infectious diseases. The Chest Unit and Professorial Departments of Respiratory Medicine and the Care of the Elderly made further contributions in academic research and teaching as well as providing clinical services at the hospital. In the late 1960s intravenous heroin abuse in disadvantaged areas of Edinburgh led to increasing numbers of patients being admitted with virus hepatitis type B and staphylococcal endocarditis. In the mid-1980s needle sharing among drug misusers became common and unfortunately coincided with the introduction of HIV infection. This necessitated further out-patient and in-patient services and a counselling clinic for HIV infected patients. The first purpose-built AIDS hospice in the United Kingdom was built in the grounds of the City Hospital.

The hospital was originally funded by the City of Edinburgh, as the local authority responsible for infectious disease management. With the inception of the National Health Service in 1948 it came under the aegis of the South-Eastern Regional Hospital Board, Scotland. When Scottish Health Care was divided into 15 Health Boards, the City Hospital became the responsibility of the Lothian Health Board. In 1994, the hospital joined the Royal Infirmary of Edinburgh NHS Trust, providing services to the 'Purchaser' which was still the Lothian Health Board.

In the 1990s the Secretary of State for Scotland and the Scottish Office finally decided to provide Edinburgh with a new Royal Infirmary. It would be built on a green-field site at Little France, just as the present Edinburgh City Hospital had been built in the late 1890s on the greenfield site at Colinton Mains Farm. To provide resources for this long awaited development, smaller hospitals including the Princess Margaret Rose Orthopaedic Hospital and the City Hospital have had to close. Accommodation for the clinical and academic disciplines represented in the City Hospital is being found in the Western General Hospital, the new Royal Infirmary of Edinburgh, the Royal Hospital for Sick Children and St John's Hospital at Howden.

The City Hospital fulfilled its role as a model fever hospital for its first half century and, as health requirements changed, it adapted itself admirably to new purposes whilst still coping with infectious disease, albeit in a different guise from that envisaged by the Town Council and their medical advisers at the end of the nineteenth century. Sadly, therefore, the City Hospital will not achieve its centenary in 2003.

Those who have been privileged to have associations with the City Hospital mourn its passing. It has always been a friendly hospital, small enough for its staff to provide that truly personal service so often lacking in bigger institutions, yet at the same time big enough to be largely self-sufficient. Its contribution to clinical services, research and teaching equals if not surpasses that of other Edinburgh hospitals. Its attractive buildings, and spacious wooded grounds, the haunt of birds, squirrels, rabbits, foxes and in a hard winter even deer, have been envied by patients and staff in hospitals elsewhere. They will be sorely missed. The spirit of the hospital affects all who work in it. Past and present members of staff will remember this great hospital with affection. Many patients who owe their lives and the restoration of their health to the City Hospital will remember it too. It has served Edinburgh well.

PART ONE

Infectious Diseases and the Development of Public Health Services in Edinburgh up to the Nineteenth Century

CHAPTER TWO

Early Measures for the Control of Infectious Disease and for the Care of Fever Patients

Today the diagnosis of infectious diseases is made clinically but it can be quickly confirmed by modern microbiological laboratories. Contagious illness in past centuries, particularly during outbreaks, was often simply labelled 'epidemic fever', making retrospective diagnosis difficult. Some infections, however, such as leprosy, syphilis, smallpox and bubonic plague (the Black Death), produced outward signs like spots and rashes that were only too obvious to the terrified layman.

Long before the germ theory of infection was understood, there was some appreciation of the transmissibility of disease from infected persons and from items contaminated by them such as bedding and clothes (fomites). The high death toll in epidemics caused justifiable alarm. The civic authorities would insist on the isolation and quarantine of those infected, the burning of fomites and the fumigation of the houses of 'fever' victims. The movement of travellers, especially vagrants, from one town to another was prohibited. Punishments for disobedience were often draconian; but, simultaneously, the hospices and houses of charity, often run by monastic orders, offered fever victims and their families shelter, support and treatment.

Although sensible legislation was enforced during epidemics, little was done to relieve overcrowding and improve water supplies and sanitation until the eighteenth and nineteenth centuries.

Dr John D. Comrie described at length the early public health regulations concerning leprosy, syphilis and the plague.[1] Even in the twelfth century, Scottish burghs, including Edinburgh, decreed that a leper with his own funds should be isolated in hospital. Those without funds were forbidden to beg from door to door, but were permitted to sit on the main highways in the town and ask for alms from passersby. The forest laws of Scotland provided for flesh from wounded and dead animals found in the forests to be sent to leper houses. The south Edinburgh suburb Liberton – originally Leper Toun – may have had a leprosy hospital as early as the twelfth century. The still surviving Balm Well at Gracemount was popular for the alleged healing properties of its oily water to people suffering from leprosy and other skin disorders.[2]

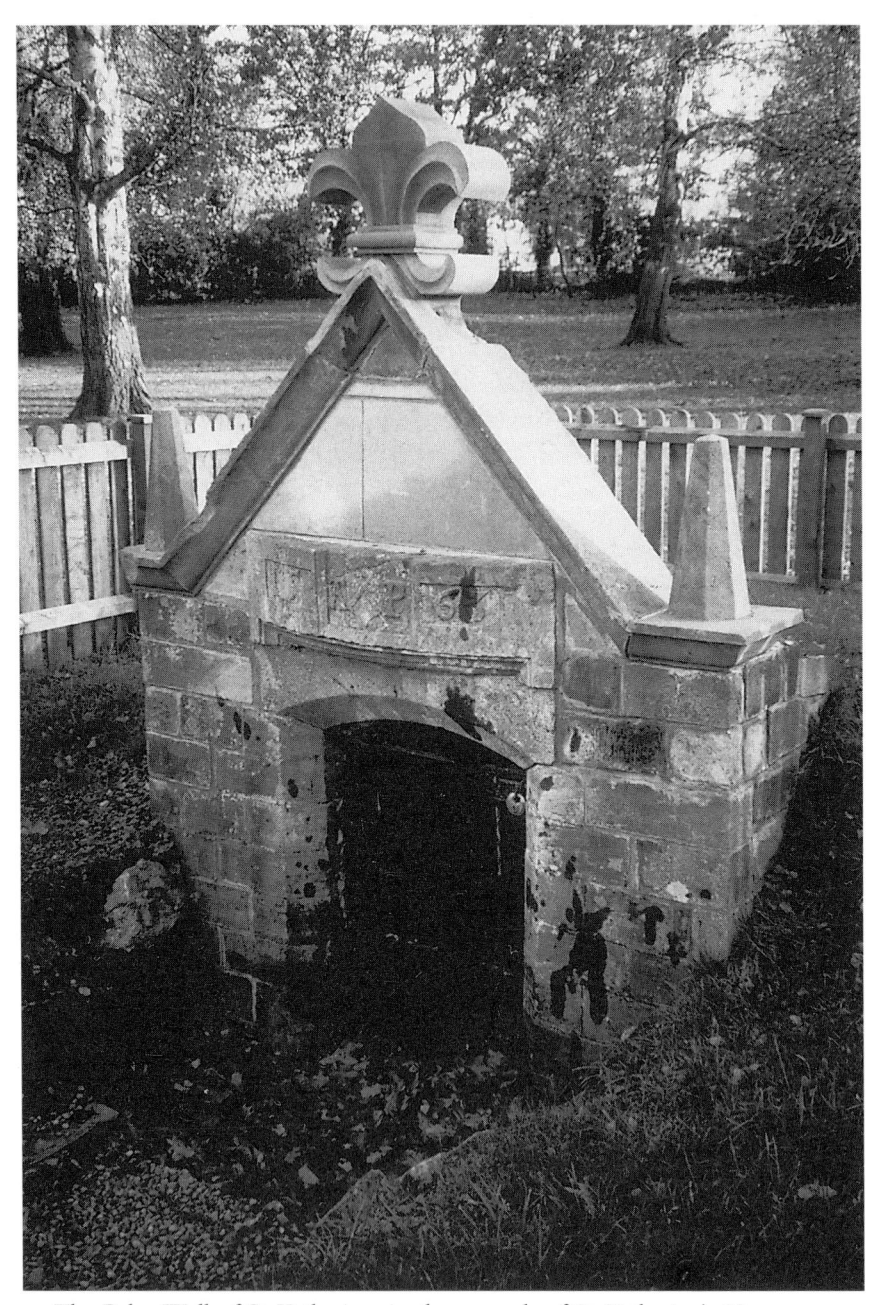

The Balm Well of St Katherine, in the grounds of St Katherine's Home, Gracemount. Its oily water was reputed to improve skin disorders, including leprosy. (Photo: J. A. Gray)

An edict of Edinburgh Town Council in 1528 insisted that lepers caught conversing with 'clene folkis' would be banished from the town. In 1584, a leprosy hospital was founded by the Town Council but it quickly fell into disrepair and was resited at Greenside. Five male lepers were incarcerated there, two with their wives. They were ordered to stay within the hospital at all times under pain of death, to which end, a gallows was erected on the gable end, of the hospital to remind the occupants that the bailies really meant what they said.

Syphilis, possibly introduced from the New World by those who sailed with Christopher Columbus, spread rapidly in Scotland as elsewhere in Europe at the end of the fifteenth century. It was then known variously as the French sickness, the sickness of Naples or the grand gore. Edinburgh Town Council banished those infected and transported them to the tiny island of Inchkeith in the Firth of Forth, together with those professing to cure them. In 1509 any failure to cure the grand gore, which resulted in the patient's death, attracted a fine from the carers.

As early as the seventh century, bubonic plague ravaged the district now known as the Lothians; and Scotland did not escape the Black Death sweeping through Europe in the 1360s. To combat plague, in 1498 the Provost, Bailies and Council in Edinburgh forbade citizens from harbouring or receiving any traveller without first obtaining permission. The penalty for contravention was banishment and confiscation of goods. Children under the age of 15 caught wandering the streets were to be put in the stocks and scourged. The next year stray animals found roaming in the town were ordered to be slaughtered. The official cleaners of houses of infected persons were given a generous 'danger money' wage. Infected furniture was to be washed in the running waters of the Water of Leith at Drumsheugh, but not in any of the town's stagnant lochs. Those burying the dead were not allowed to mingle with the population. Penalties for disobeying included branding on the cheek and even amputation.

By 1505, cases of plague had to be notified to officers of the town within 24 hours, a time limit later reduced to 12 hours. The duty of notification fell on the head of the household, who could be branded and banished for not complying. An official was paid to clean the High Street from Castle Hill to the head of Leith Wynd. The sum of 4d was to be contributed by every inhabitant and 16d from butchers and fishmongers who were considered to cause much more filth than ordinary citizens.

When plague revisited Edinburgh in 1512–13 the previous regulations were revived together with a 40 day quarantine period for everyone infected. In 1514 Bailies were appointed for the four quarters of the city to supervise and implement these orders. The importation of infected goods was made a capital offence. In 1530, ships bound for Leith or Newhaven from countries known to be infected were unloaded on one of the islands in the Forth. Only after appropriate quarantine were their cargoes allowed to be transferred into port. Ritchie describes how vessels to be disinfected were bored and then immersed in sea water with their decks awash for several tides to eliminate rats and fleas.[3] Clothing had to be boiled. Some cargoes were subject to 'cleaning by fyre and wattir' done first by burning with heather and then immersion in sea water'.

Infected persons or their relatives who attended mass or went visiting were guilty of a serious offence and could be sentenced to death. In the 1520s the Burgh Muir to the south west of the city was used to isolate infected people and the vagrants and beggars who had also been excluded from the town. The Burgh Muir was used again in the 1560s when wooden huts were built there to receive infected and suspect cases of the plague. A gallows erected on the Muir reminded town folk to obey the Council's regulations. Stray animals were captured and slaughtered by the local hangman. Official cleaners wore a grey gown with a white St Andrews Cross front and back and a staff with a warning white cloth attached to it.[4] They were forbidden to carry corpses on their backs and had to use instead a black bier carrying a bell.

Plague victims and their contacts were often isolated in wooden accommodation at the Chapel of St Roque or Roche at the west of the Burgh Muir in the grounds of the present Astley Ainslie Hospital. St Roque, patron saint of plague victims, was born at Narbonne and died at Montpelier in 1327. Chapels dedicated to him were also founded in Glasgow, Paisley, Stirling and Dundee.[5] Edinburgh's chapel was probably built about 1507 with support from King James IV who is reputed to have prayed there on his way to Flodden Field in September 1513. The chapel fell into disrepair and was pulled down in the mid eighteenth century. It had largely disappeared by 1791. The carved stones still to be seen at the Astley Ainslie Hospital, however, probably did not come from the Chapel of St Roque. They were more likely transported there from the fifteenth-century Trinity Church, demolished in 1848, which once stood near the present Waverley Centre.[6]

The nuns at the little Convent of St Catherine of Sienna (later corrupted to Sciennes) at the east end of the Burgh Muir may also have tended plague victims. In the sixteenth century some were probably buried in the grounds of the convent building which had by then been all but destroyed by fire.[7] A plaque in the garden of No. 16 St Catherine's Place marks the site of the former convent.

Although the rectangular tree lined lawn in the middle of Greenhill

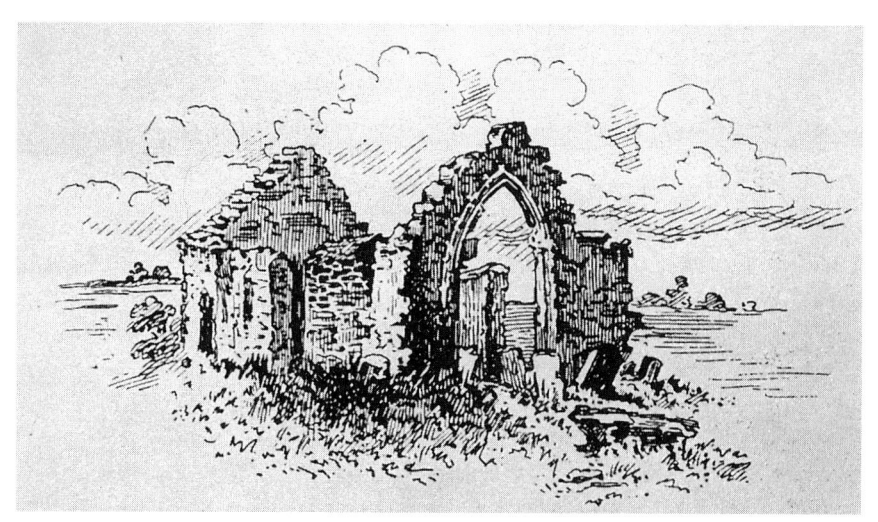

Ruins of St Roque's Chapel, near where plague victims were cared for in the sixteenth and seventeenth centuries. (From J. Stewart Smith's *The Grange of St. Giles,* p. 9)

Gardens in Bruntsfield has been called a plague pit there is no evidence to support this hypothesis. Nearby, however, in the little walled mausoleum at Ashfield Nursing Home in Chamberlain Road there stands a carved grave slab commemorating an Edinburgh apothecary, John Livingstone, who died in Edinburgh's last plague epidemic in 1645.[8]

In 1585 a surgeon, James Henryson, was given a paid appointment to look after plague victims. He received free medicaments for their treatment. Sadly his wife died of plague, which he also contracted himself but survived. In 1645, a Dr John Paulit was appointed at the town's expense to care for plague victims as had Dr Henryson 60 years before.[9] This last outbreak in 1645 was particularly severe with 2,746 deaths in Leith. In Edinburgh Maitland wrote that 'there were scarce sixty Men left capable of assisting in Defence of the Town in case of Attack'.[10] The plague also hit the public purse. Edinburgh was asked to raise 1,200 men for the army:

> But the City being still thin of Inhabitants, occasioned by the late dreadful Ravages committed by this Plague, the Town Council agreed to give Forty thousand Pounds *Scottish* money in lieu thereof.[11]

Smallpox was known in Scotland from the sixteenth century onwards, causing much mortality, particularly in young children. T. C. Smout quotes from an anonymous author writing about 1760 who stated:

> there may be born annually in Scotland about fifty thousand souls of which

ANE BREVE DESCRIPTIOUN OF THE PEST

QVHAIR IN THE CAVSIS, SIGNIS
and sum speciall preseruatioun and
cure thairof ar contenit.

Set furth be MAISTER GILBERT SKEYNE, Doctoure in Medicine.

IMPRENTIT AT EDINBVRGH
BE ROBERT LEKPREVIK.
ANNO DO. 1568.

Gilbert Skeyne's *Ane Breve Descriptioun of the Pest*, 1568, one of the earliest medical books to be printed in Scotland. For Pest, now read: bubonic plague. (By kind permission of the Trustees of the National Library of Scotland – NLS:H. 33. d. 41) two thousand may escape the disease (small pox): of the remaining forty eight thousand by reckoning one of six to die the nation loses eight thousand yearly and their posterity.[12]

Inoculation, or the introduction of material from a smallpox pock, was practised in Edinburgh by 1745. Although it carried a significant mortality it was recommended by the Royal College of Physicians.[13] The relatively safe Jennerian vaccination with cowpox was strongly advocated by Sir Henry Littlejohn in the later nineteenth century.

Smallpox epidemics occurred in Edinburgh in 1817–18 and 1830–40. Between 1855 and 1865, there were 10,548 smallpox deaths in Scotland. Nearly two thirds of these were in children, under 5 years of age. As late as 1894 a smallpox outbreak demanded the use of unsatisfactory temporary wooden isolation facilities in the Queen's Park near St Leonards. This finally persuaded the Town Council to build the present day City Hospital at Greenbank.

'Epidemic fever' caused much morbidity and mortality during the eighteenth and nineteenth centuries. This was probably typhus spread by ticks, much in the same way as plague had been spread by rat fleas in previous centuries. The contagious nature of 'epidemic fever' was well recognised, as were the benefits of instant isolation, the cleansing and fumigation of houses, the white washing of walls and the washing of the clothes of the infected. For the destitute, clean straw was exchanged for contaminated bedding. When houses were lime washed, the poorest were given a free coal supply to heat and dry out their homes afterwards. Records of hospital admissions show there was a shortage of beds during epidemics, for example from March 1838 to January 1839, when 2,242 cases were admitted and 408 houses cleansed.[14]

As an offshoot of the Destitute Sick Society, the Edinburgh Fever Board probably came into being early in the nineteenth century. It was responsible for arranging urgent hospital admission of fever patients and the disinfection of their contacts and homes. The Board's Officer acting under the guidance of medical men had considerable authority. Compared with Glasgow where a similar Board spent much smaller sums per capita on the infected poor, Edinburgh's Board prided itself on spending £10 weekly, and contributed greatly to hospital funds, this money coming largely from public subscription.[15]

During epidemics the Edinburgh Fever Board had to fund additional isolation facilities. They persuaded the Lord Provost, the Council and the Lord Advocate to raise enough money, again by public subscription, to convert the old Surgeons' Hall off Drummond Street into 60 beds for fever patients.[16]

The common 'epidemic fever', spotted or relapsing fever, or typhus, became less of a problem as housing, hygiene and sanitation improved. Other illnesses, like typhoid, a bacterial infection, were often confused with typhus, a rickettsial infection, before the microbiological distinction could be made. Even malaria was sometimes quoted as a cause of 'the ague' or 'epidemic fever' but it is unlikely that the life cycle of malaria parasites in mosquitoes could be completed in the relatively low atmospheric temperatures in Scotland.

Mortality from tuberculosis in the late nineteenth century was far greater in Scotland than in England and Ireland.[17] Much of this was bovine tuberculosis spread from dairy produce directly to man. The research laboratory of the Royal College of Physicians of Edinburgh was the first to demonstrate that human disease could be acquired from infected milk. A combination of poverty, malnutrition, overcrowding and the insanitary conditions of humans and cows kept in the town as well as in the country made Edinburgh a prime target for tuberculosis. Later Sir Robert Philip of Edinburgh, who held the first Chair of Tuberculosis in the world, was to revolutionise the management and prevention of tuberculosis. In the mid twentieth century, Sir John Crofton and colleagues at the Edinburgh City Hospital introduced modern antimycobacterial therapy. With better detection through mass miniature radiography, followed by BCG vaccination, this chemotherapy made tuberculosis, or 'The White Death', into a more manageable disease.

In 'The Cholera Board of Health, Edinburgh, 1831–34',[18] Dr Tait highlighted the other main infectious scourge of the nineteenth century. Cholera spreads quickly in overcrowded, insanitary conditions and dramatically when water supplies are contaminated with sewage. The whole of Europe was affected by epidemics of Asiatic cholera. Mortality was very high because of the profound dehydration brought on by diarrhoea.

Intravenous fluids were not then generally available and many people perished. The pioneering work of Dr Thomas Latta of Leith[19] sadly did not gain acceptance for many years. As Dr David Boyd[20] explains in *Leith Hospital 1848–1988*, Dr Latta and colleagues at the Drummond Street Cholera Hospital were the first to administer intravenous saline injections for 'malignant cholera'. Another famous physician Dr John Abercrombie advised the Board of Health on cholera management.[21] He wrote that neither blood letting nor warming the body with a calorifier were effective in severe cases of 'cholera asphyxia'. However, appreciating the absorptive capacity of the rectum and colon for fluids, Dr Abercrombie found that the 'frequent injection into the bowels of two or three pounds of very hot water, with the addition of six or eight ounces of spirits'

Handwritten cholera notification from early in the 1832 outbreak. The rapid progress of this illness is remarkable. (By courtesy of the Royal College of Physicians of Edinburgh. W. P. Alison MS and Papers) was highly beneficial or better still 'large injections of warm port wine and water".[22]

From 27 January 1832 to mid December 1832, 1,886 people with cholera were reported in Edinburgh, of whom 1,065 died. In response, the Cholera Board of Health was established in association with the Royal College of Physicians of Edinburgh. The Board consisted initially of 35 members later reduced to 27, including 14 doctors.[23]

Action undertaken by the Board included street cleaning, removal of animal nuisances, especially pigs, and the closing of a tannery. An open sewer in the Old Town was redirected but unfortunately not replaced. The poor were fed and clothed, soup kitchens set up and blankets supplied. Police forbade vagrants from known infected areas to enter the city. Vagrants already within the city were collected and comfortably confined in a house of refuge, where they were well fed and their children educated, all at the Board's expense.[24] Patients were to be admitted to hospital quickly. Cere cloth and tar impregnated sacks were provided for the dead who were to be buried within 24 hours. Edinburgh was divided into 30 districts and the 11 stations for reporting new cases

CHOLERA REPORT for the TOWN of LEITH, and VILLAGES under the Charge of the LEITH BOARD.

8 o'clock, PM 23 May 1832.

	LEITH.	NEWHAVES.	Newhaven field		
Remaining at last Report,	6	~	0		
New Cases,	0	~	0		
Total,	6	—	0		
Recovered,	0	~	0		
Died,	0	~	0		
Remaining,	6	~	0		
Total Cases from commencement,	65	6	4		
Total Deaths,	37	4	3		
Total Recoveries,	22	2	1		

Villau Scarth
Secretary to the Board.

Printed cholera notification from later in the 1832 outbreak. Between January and May the system of reporting became streamlined. (By courtesy of the Royal College of Physicians of Edinburgh. W. P. Alison MS and Papers)

Early Measures to Control Infectious Disease

were manned night and day. Daily notification slips were sent in to the Cholera Board.[25] Rudimentary education on hygiene was disseminated to the public. All this was made possible by the raising of £7,914 from voluntary contributions, church collections and subscriptions from private individuals, the banks and insurance companies.

In 1854, Dr W. D. Adams, a district surgeon in the City Parish of Edinburgh, reported an excessive case load during cholera outbreaks.[26] There was only one cholera doctor for 22,244 persons in Edinburgh, compared with one for every 12,343 in Glasgow, and Dr Adams moaned, perhaps justifiably, that the term 'Cholera Doctor' necessarily implied the sacrifice of his private practice. From 28 August to 30 November 1854, he reported to the Sanitary Committee of the Parochial Board that 23 had died of cholera and 96 had survived in their own homes in his Parish but, of the 25 admitted to hospital, 15 had died. He felt that voluntary assistance was essential. A stop should be made to the malingerers who abused the system and called out cholera doctors on trivial pretexts at night. (Perhaps times have not changed all that much.) He also advocated thorough cleansing of infected premises and the setting up of temporary houses of refuge for entire families in which cholera deaths had occurred.

One has only to imagine the frustration of this compassionate Dr Adams describing a scene in the City Parish of Edinburgh in 1854:

> Let the reader visit with me, if but in imagination, one of the many hovels comprised in my epitome of cases, say No. 99. In a small dingy apartment, devoid of furniture, except some dirty straw, a bit of ragged carpet, and some potato peelings and cinders scattered on the floor, is seen a pale, ill clad, and miserable looking mother, crouched before a fireless hearth; across her lap is stretched a stricken boy, whose sunken and upturned eye, leaden features, and pulseless wrist, too surely indicate nature's expiring struggle with a mortal malady. She is gazing upon him in silence and despairing agony, and with such feeling of intense affection as mothers can only realize. She is deserted by neighbours and friends, without food, fire, bedding, and all the other necessaries and comforts of life; her husband is absent somewhere seeking employment; she has rejected the offer of the Hospital, and will not be separated from her dying child. It is not my province to inquire whether the wretched condition of this and other such families, be that of blameless poverty, or the result of improvidence and vicious habits; the danger of fostering and propagating a deadly pestilence is the same in either case; and the destitution from whatever cause, is too closely interlaced with the interests and well-being of society to be lightly estimated or passed by without relief; but with the limited resources of the District Surgeon, what

is he to do? How is he to deal with the patient, the mother, the apartment in which they are domiciled?

Expediency and humanity dictate what *should* be done; the Surgeon can only use the means placed at his disposal, or draw upon his own private resources, from the impulses of the benevolence and Christian charity.[27]

Why Edinburgh was so much affected by contagious disease will become more apparent in the next chapter.

CHAPTER THREE

Edinburgh's Problems with Overcrowding and Defects in Housing, Water Supply and Sanitation

Much of the congestion in Edinburgh's Old Town resulted from the building of the city walls.[1] King James II authorised the Magistrates to strengthen the town's defences against 'ore enemies in England' and the King's Wall went up between 1450 and 1475. After the disaster at Flodden Field in 1513 there was a levy by the Town Council to finance the building of new walls and to strengthen existing walls. Finally the 'Telfer Wall' (after John Tailefer, its builder) was constructed in 1628–36.

These walls were relatively ineffective military defences and were sometimes breached, as in 1544 when the English detonated Netherbow Port. Lord Cullen comments that the walls 'were perhaps more effective in peace time for preventing the spread of disease, securing payment of customs dues and controlling crime'.[2] Unfortunately, as building outside the walls was considered unsafe, the tenements or 'lands' of Edinburgh's Old Town became confined and grew upwards sometimes reaching a height of 14 storeys. In 1698 the Dean of Guild was unsuccessful in enforcing an Act limiting houses to 'five storeys above the causeways'.[3] The house construction was often poor and the upper wooden balconies overhung the narrow streets excluding light and fresh air.

Fire was a continual hazard as heather, whin and brush wood were often stored in the basements. Examples of the highly inflammable interior wooden panelling and the roof shingles are exhibited in Huntly House museum. Disastrous fires occurred in 1700 and twice again in 1824. The first fire of 1824 broke out in Royal Bank Close on 24 June on the same site as the fire of 1700. It destroyed five houses six storeys high. One of the town's officers died after trying to rescue valuable papers. The second fire of 1824 started on 15 November in a seven-storey house and continued sporadically for three days. Except for one tenement left standing, all the property from the Old Assembly Close to the Exchequer Buildings (now the City Chambers) was destroyed. The next day sparks ignited the steeple of the Tron Church fusing its two ton bell of 1673 with the heat. That evening the fire spread again and demolished an

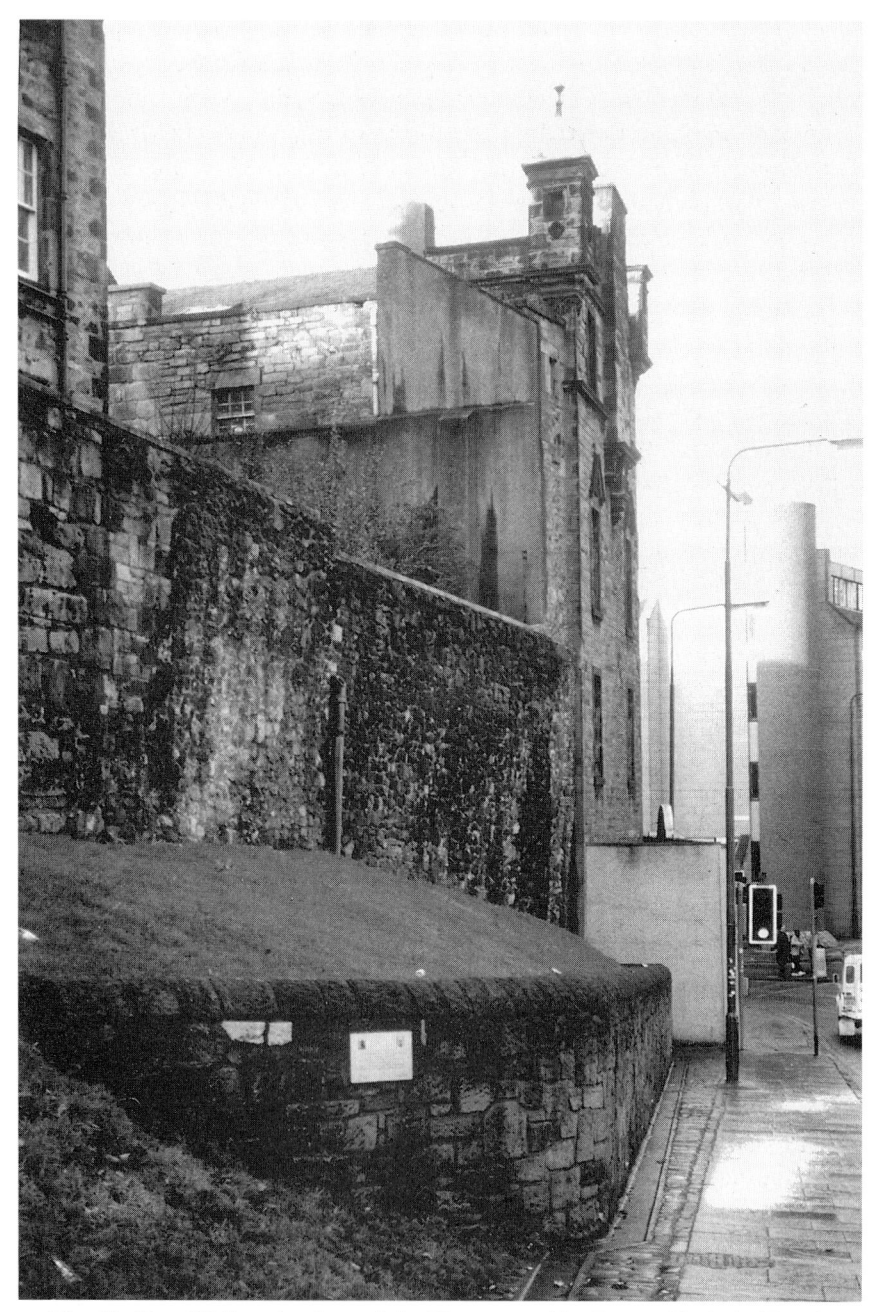

The Flodden Wall at the foot of the Pleasance with George Heriot's (Trust) School of 1840 towering above. Unless a bridge was built over the Pleasance, this was to be the eastern boundary of the second City Fever Hospital site about 1884. (Photo: J. A. Gray)

eleven-storey tenement south of Parliament Square. Eight people were killed or died of their injuries. Nearly 400 homeless families were found temporary shelter in Queensberry House on the south side of the Canongate and an estimated £200,000 worth of property was destroyed.[4] The ensuing public outcry was immense and resulted in Edinburgh having the first Municipal Fire Brigade in the United Kingdom rather than relying haphazardly on the fire engines of insurance companies as before.

Sanitation and piped water supplies were scarce in much of the Old Town. As late as 1865 in the notorious Middle Mealmarket Stair, 248 people, including 51 children under the age of 5, shared 59 rooms with no sink or water closet in the whole tenement.[5] Water had to be carried up the tenement stairs from the public wells or bought for a penny a barrel from the water carriers. Water shortage was a major disincentive to personal hygiene and must have encouraged the lice and ticks that were vectors of diseases such as typhus.

All household waste and excrement not discharged illegally into a public street had of course to be carried out again. Human nature being what it is, however, at 10 p.m. on the chiming of St Giles' Cathedral bell, waste was flung from the windows into the street or back courts, with or without the shouted warning of 'Gardy-Loo' (from the French 'Gardez-l'eau!'). 'How long' complained John Wesley visiting the City in 1761, 'shall the capital of Scotland, Yea, and the chief street of it, stink worse than a common sewer?'[6]

Lodging houses, too, were insalubrious and contributed to the drunkenness, much frowned upon by respectable Victorians. The workman had:

> on his way homeward to run the gauntlet of a dozen gin-palaces, and be tempted to delay his return. Were he near his household, the attractions of his house might prove stronger than the call of pleasure.[7]

Despite the overcrowded and insanitary conditions of the Royal Mile, this was where many of the gentry lived in the eighteenth century, close by the labourers and the destitute, often occupying accommodation in the same wynds and closes. Robert Chambers[8] records that in 1769 there lived in the Canongate the Dukes of Hamilton and Queensberry, the Countesses of Tweeddale and Lothian, 16 Earls, 7 Lords and 7 Lords of Session, 13 Baronets, 14 Commanders in Chief and sundry eminent men, a banker and the mistress in charge of a ladies' boarding school. Craig[9] claimed this proximity between the classes encouraged a mutual understanding and preparedness of neighbours to help each other irrespective of their income and social standing.

It might have been expected that after the building of the New Town, whose foundation stone was laid in 1761, many of the public health problems of the Old Town would be resolved. It seems, however, that gentry were slow to leave the overcrowded, insanitary closes of the High Street and Canongate. Even when they did go, their vacated accommodation was often sub-divided and taken by itinerant Irish labourers who sought employment building the Union Canal, the New Town, and later the railways. Conditions may have temporarily worsened with this influx of poor people and their families. Besides, diversion of water supplies to the New Town deprived the Old Town of some of its own precarious supply. Even in the New Town, conditions were barely hygienic. It was not until some time after 1824 that water closets replaced cess pits and the nefarious collection of 'night soil' in carts.[10] From 1819 when the Edinburgh Joint Stock Water Company was set up to provide water from Glencorse there was some improvement. It eventually supplemented the by then inadequate water supply that had originally been piped from Comiston Springs to the city between 1681 and 1704.[11]

The names still visible today on various closes, wynds and streets in the Old Town, such as FleshMarket Close, FishMarket Close, New Skinners' Close, and Candlemakers' Row, denote sites that previously caused a particular nuisance from the accumulation of animal waste in addition to human waste. Pigs often slept comfortably with their owners who were loath to remove them, even when ordered to do so, as in the cholera outbreak of 1832.[12] There were 171 byres housing 2,085 cows in the municipal area in 1865.[13] Many byres below dwellinghouses

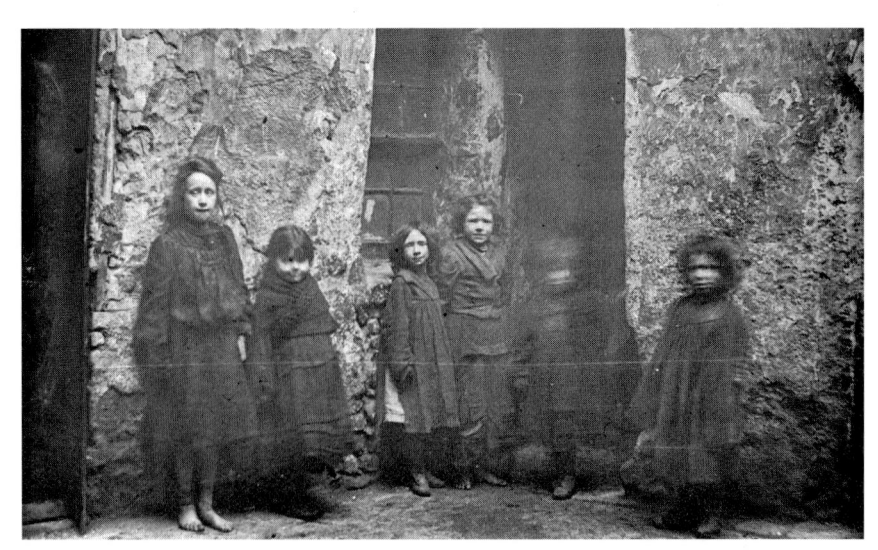

Slum Children, late nineteenth century, two bare-footed. (By courtesy of Lothian Health Services Archive, Edinburgh University Library)

Defects in Housing, Water Supply and Sanitation

were unflagged. In some of the unpaved back courts, regulations concerning the removal of offal were repeatedly ignored. The drains were purposely blocked to improve the quality of the manure, or fulzie, which was later sold as fertiliser when sufficiently ripe.[14]

In his report of 1847 on the *Nuisances in Edinburgh*[15] Alexander Murray, Inspector of Lighting and Cleaning, pointed out the more obvious defects in the series of Police Acts, which had been passed since 1771. These concerned slaughterhouses, the killing of horses and dealing in carrion, offensive manufactories, feeding and breeding of pigs, imperfect drainage, a want of 'public necessaries', ruinous and waste property, the disgusting practice of throwing 'nuisance' from windows and the appalling state of the causeways and pavements in back courts and closes. In particular, the General Commissioner of Police lacked the powers to make regulations in keeping with the changing condition of the property and population.

Murray explained in his report how, at Livingston's Yards, slaughterhouse refuse was purposely mixed with the contents of cess pools in the West Port and then sold to a dealer in manure. Without adequate drainage from the slaughterhouses in Causewayside, fulzie was allowed to lie there before it was taken away. By an Act of William IV, fulzie should not lie for more than four days between 1 April and 1 November or for more than seven days from 1 November to 1 April. Failure to comply meant the fulzie would become the property of the General Commissioners. However, penalties were unusual. The Inspector on his own could not remove the fulzie that had lain longer than the 4-7 day period prescribed by the Police Act. He had first to cite the parties and prove his allegation to the judge of police. In the meantime, the butcher, who was called before a magistrate, would first remove the offensive matter and immediately start a new midden, knowing that it could not be seized until he was called again and the charge proved.

Murray[16] recommended that there be only three killing grounds and that these be well regulated. He drew attention to the 352 pigs in 180 pigsties within the city bounds and the inadequate drainage in the High Street, Canongate and Nicolson Street. He insisted that every house must have a water closet to discourage people from throwing waste out of the windows. He suggested in the meantime that scavengers should be employed to carry waste matter down from the houses and that householders be charged for this service. He also proposed new regulations about dung hills and deplored the keeping of animals within dwellings.

Although men like Alexander Murray had long been pressing for the proper implementation of Public Health legislation, it needed someone of the calibre and persuasion of Sir Henry Littlejohn to ensure that something major was done.

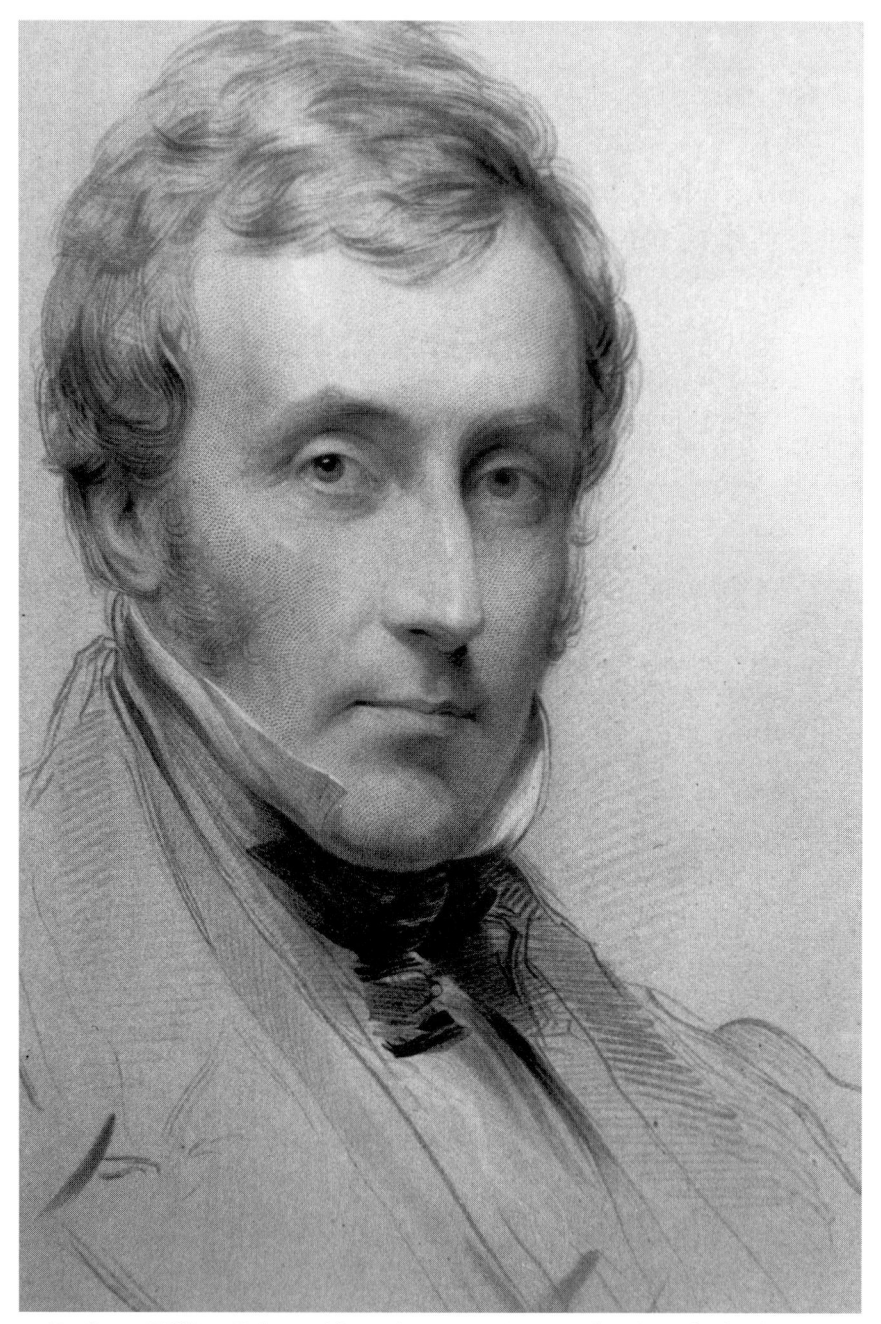

Professor William Pultney Alison (1790–1859), a social and medical reformer and Member of the Cholera Board of Health. (From J. D. Comrie's *History of Scottish Medicine*, Vol. II, p. 631 by kind permission of the Wellcome Institute Library, London)

CHAPTER FOUR

Something has to be Done: The Public Health Movement in Edinburgh under Sir Henry Littlejohn

Although leprosy and plague were no longer problems in the eighteenth century, other communicable diseases like typhus and smallpox still had to be reckoned with and Asiatic cholera was yet to come. The 'Rules' for coping with infection which William Maitland proposed in *The History of Edinburgh*, 1753,[1] included the setting up of an office in each City district 'where certain of the most judicious citizens might attend and give directions in respective disorders'. Physicians were also obliged to inspect any patient who might be infectious. If found so, the illness was to be compulsorily notified by the householder, the patient instantly removed to a 'lazaretto' and the household quarantined. All combustible fomites were to be burned, infected houses fumigated with brimstone, then the windows kept open whilst the house was left unoccupied for one month. During epidemics night-time travellers had to carry a light, to help detect anyone illegally removing infected materials. Provost George Drummond appreciated the need for these provisions but, sadly, no one could persuade the Council to implement them.[2] This had, however, been a real attempt to improve health in the long term and not, as previously, simply a knee-jerk response to each epidemic as it came along.

Robert Deuchar, Secretary to the Edinburgh Fever Board, wrote in 1844 that it was:

> many years since the medical men of the Edinburgh Fever Board saw the necessity and importance of effecting a complete separation betwixt the healthy and the sick portions of the poor in times of epidemic fever; as well as the benefits which would arise from cleaning and fumigating the homes of fever patients, and washing their bed clothes when necessary.[3]

The Cholera Board in the 1830s also made recommendations to help the sick and poor.[4]

In 1840 Dr W. P. Alison, who had worked with cholera patients in the New Town Dispensary and appreciated the connection between poverty and disease, wrote his influential work *Observations on the Management of the Poor in Scotland and its Effects on the Health of the Great Towns*. He felt that the poor should not have to rely on charity alone, but should be properly protected by Poor Law legislation.

In 1844 The Royal Commission on The Poor Laws of Scotland, much influenced by Dr Alison's work, showed how inadequate the provision for the sick poor was. The amended Poor Law Act passed in 1845 made the Parochial Boards responsible for poor relief. Unfortunately much of the Act was couched in terms of supervision and recommendation rather than compulsory enforcement. Indeed the Act attempted to address the results of poverty, destitution and disease rather than tackle the causes of these evils. Things did not change greatly as a result.[5]

Following the Poor Law (Amendment) Act, dilapidated cottages were sometimes pulled down rather than have them become lodgings for poor people who would then be a financial liability on the parish. Overcrowding inevitably got worse and was exacerbated by the increase in population after 1820. The numbers in Edinburgh were swelled by vagrants, unemployed workers and the destitute. As conditions for the poor were even worse in Ireland, the Edinburgh population was supplemented by Irish labourers and their families, seeking employment on new building projects. Sadly this combination of overcrowding of poor people in dilapidated tenements and lodging houses and the defects in fresh water supply and sanitation caused even more infectious disease with a continuing high or even rising death rate in the first half of the nineteenth century.[6]

It required a further catastrophe before something was done. At 1 a.m. on Sunday 24 November 1861 near Paisley's Close, 99–103 High Street, Edinburgh, a tall, rickety, overcrowded tenement housing 100 people suddenly collapsed storey by storey into the street.[7] Thirty-five people were killed and many seriously injured. A boy trapped beneath the rubble encouraged his rescuers by shouting 'Heave awa' lads, I'm no deid yet'. This event is commemorated over the archway at Paisley's Close by John Rhind's sculptured head of the boy and his plea misquoted as 'Heave awa' chaps, I'm no dead yet'.

It was not the first time an Edinburgh house had collapsed. In 1751 a six-storey tenement on the High Street near the Mercat Cross sank from top to bottom again causing loss of life.[8] But it was the tragedy of 24 November 1861 at Paisley's Close that so horrified Edinburgh citizens and accelerated the movement towards the establishment of a permanent Public Health Service. It was hoped that this would lead to improvements in maintenance of buildings, water supplies and sanitation and above all reduce overcrowding. The professional, clerical and public outcry following the 1861 tenement collapse further

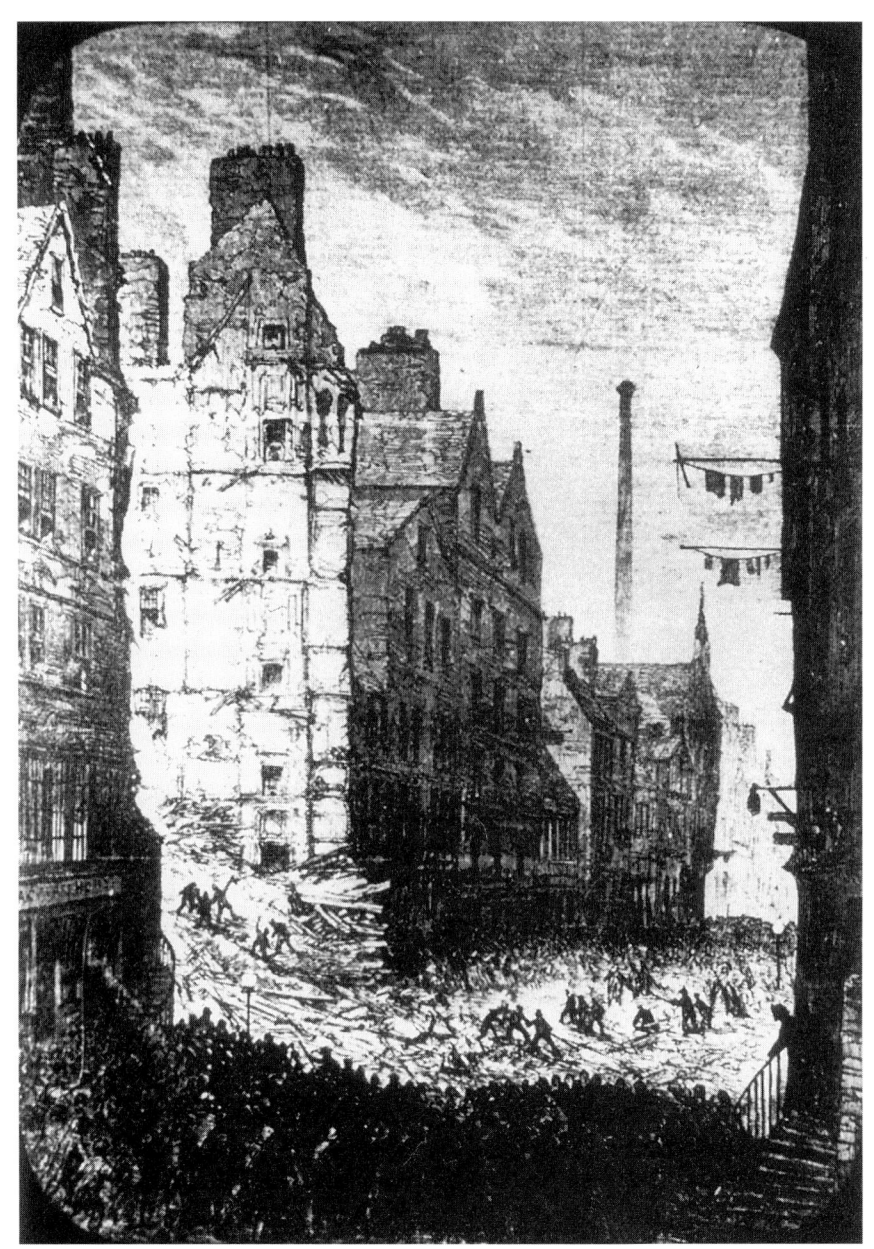

The collapsed High Street tenement, Heave awa' land, 24 November, 1861. (From *Illustrated News*, 1861. By courtesy of Edinburgh City Libraries)

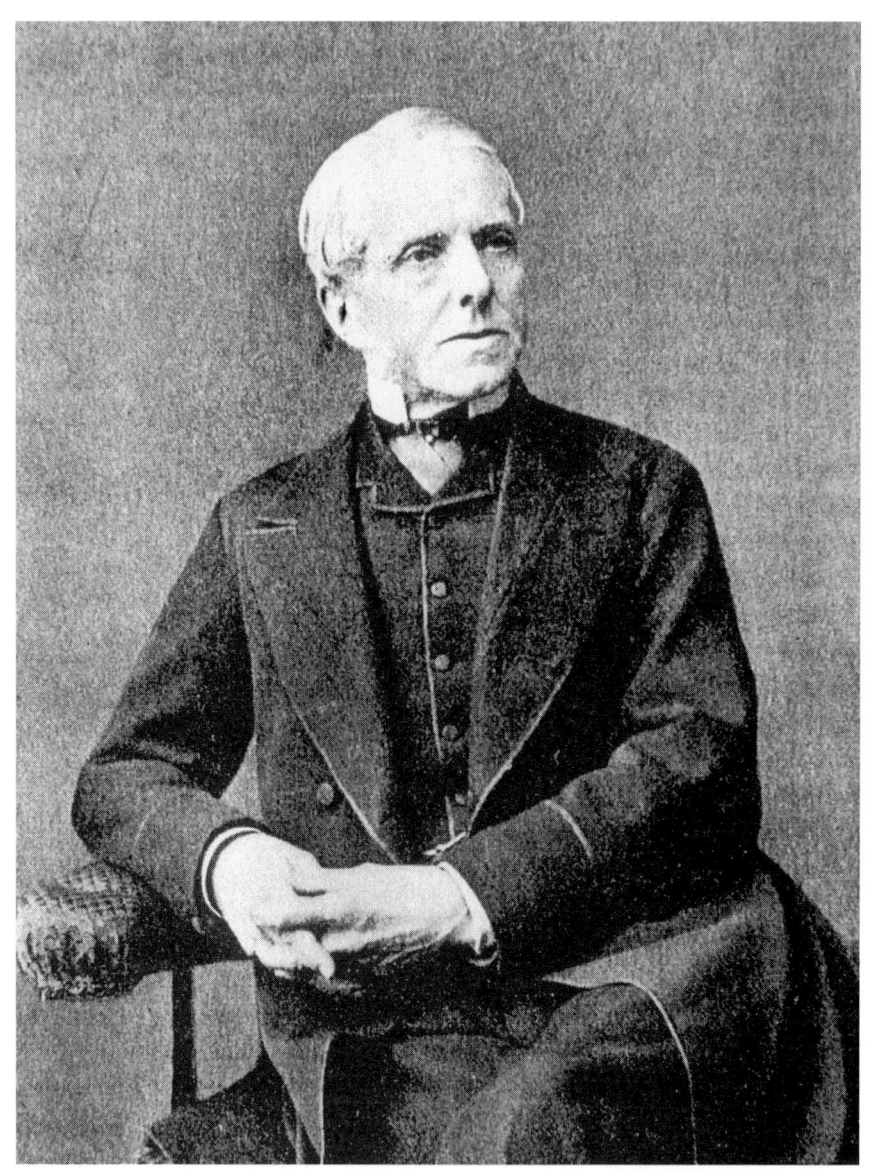

Sir Henry Duncan Littlejohn, appointed as Edinburgh's first Medical Officer of Health in 1862. (From J. D. Comrie's *History of Scottish Medicine*, Vol. II, p. 705. By kind permission of the Wellcome Institute Library, London)

increased the pressure on the Town Council. This soon brought about the appointment in Edinburgh of an Officer of Health as had taken place as early as 1847 in Liverpool and a year later in London. In 1862, therefore, began the illustrious 46 year long career of the talented Dr Henry Duncan Littlejohn, later Sir Henry, whose influence revolutionised health care, not only in Edinburgh but throughout the UK.[9]

The General Police and Improvement (Scotland) Act of 1862 helped to make the way clear for the appointment which was later called *Medical Officer of Health* (MOH). Dr Littlejohn's responsibility was to ascertain the existence of disease, particularly epidemic disease, to point out any local cause and to check its spread. Littlejohn's appointment in 1862 was a happy choice, warmly supported by the Royal College of Physicians of Edinburgh. His curriculum vitae includes not only the honour of being Edinburgh's first MOH but also Professor of Medical Jurisprudence of the University and, at the age of 71, he was appointed to the Regius Chair of Forensic Medicine. He had also served as President of the Royal College of Surgeons of Edinburgh 1875–76, was President of the British Institute of Public Health Care in 1891 and founder President of the Society of Medical Officers of Health of Scotland 1891–93. A brilliant and sought after speaker and lecturer he was known for his wit and sharp intellect at the University and as a formidable expert witness in the city courts. He was knighted in 1895.

Littlejohn's major achievements were, however, in the field of public health. It was largely due to his efforts locally [10] to implement compulsory smallpox vaccination that the Vaccination (Scotland) Act was passed in 1863, within 10 months of his appointment as MOH.

From the 1861 population census, Littlejohn derived the statistical information he needed to calculate the population density in the 19 'Sanitary Districts', into which he had divided the city. After meticulous research he produced his outstanding *Report on the Sanitary Condition of the City of Edinburgh* [11] of 1865 which is still regarded as a classic in public health literature. He showed that the more overcrowded the district, the higher its death rate compared with the death rate in the city as a whole. The districts he named – Abbey, Tron, Grassmarket, Canongate and St Giles – had mortality rates ranging from 28.8 to 37.1 per 1,000 compared with 25.9 per thousand for the city overall. These areas corresponded to the Royal Mile, High Street and the related neighbourhoods where over the centuries buildings had risen higher and higher creating a huge density of citizens per acre. The Abbey district, which was marginally less highly populated than the other four, was shown, however, to be the most deficient in sanitation. Littlejohn's *Report* also showed that in the 1848 cholera epidemic it was the overcrowded and unsanitary areas that fared worst.

Even as late as 1889 the public health Committee's *Report on the Sanitary Condition of Saint-Giles' Ward*[12] confirmed the direct association of overcrowding with mortality. Of the 4,454 houses inspected – excluding hotels and lodging houses – 375 were overcrowded and, of these, 28 were uninhabitable and 50 in serious disrepair. Overall 176 were condemned. Whereas the density of population in 1889 was 45 persons per acre in the city overall, there were 114.5 persons per acre in St Giles' Ward where the death rate was 22.11 per thousand compared with the city's overall death rate of 16.05 per thousand.

When Littlejohn was appointed MOH in 1862 he had only himself and two police assistants to supervise the health of the city.[13] The police sergeant inspected lodging houses and the constable checked new admissions to the fever wards in the Royal Infirmary every day and then arranged the disinfection of the homes of these patients. The sergeant and constable were also responsible for inspecting bake houses, dairies, meat markets and workshops and for the speedy transfer of patients into hospital during outbreaks of fever.

Years later the MOH and the Chief Constable cooperated with two Committees of the Town Council, one for Lighting and Cleaning and the other for Streets and Buildings. Both Committees came under the Council's Public Health Committee, which was inaugurated in 1872, as a result of the Public Health (Scotland) Act of 1867. Littlejohn also did much on his own initiative to improve the sanitary conditions of the city, without always bothering the Public Health Committee.[14]

Littlejohn's *Sanitary Report* of 1865 also described the condition of the city's workshops, byres, cowsheds, drains, trade in diseased meat and offal and the state of the cemeteries. He recommended paving and draining the closes and wynds, improving and repairing dwellings and introducing water and gas, cleaning of common stairs, reducing the number of people in apartments, lowering the height of buildings and pulling down those in a dangerous condition. Littlejohn hoped to have the most insanitary and overcrowded closes opened up to light and air with new streets. One of these was to run from the middle of Niddry Street in the west to the middle of St John Street in the east, so cutting a swathe through an area of narrow wynds and overcrowded tenements.[15] In addition the 'ticketing' of houses was introduced in Edinburgh as it had been in Glasgow.[16] A tin ticket, affixed to houses of three or fewer apartments or of a capacity of less than 2,000 cubic feet, showed the capacity of the rooms and the maximum number of people allowed to sleep there. Although difficult to enforce and so subject to abuse, this system did help to control overcrowding.

In his *Sanitary Report*, Littlejohn recorded the mortality figures for different districts as these were the only health statistics then available. They were of little use in the active management of an outbreak of infection as the records applied only to deaths and not to those alive but infected. Besides, the information came too late to be of practical value in the course of an epidemic. In 1877, a system of notification of infectious disease by the householder had been introduced in Greenock but was obviously subject to misdiagnosis by lay people. Littlejohn felt that the medical practitioner, rather than the householder, was the right person to notify infections[17] and that this should be done all year round and not simply in response to an epidemic as had been recommended by the Cholera Board of Health in the early 1830s. His idea was badly received by the profession and by both Royal Colleges in Edinburgh on the grounds that confidential patient–doctor relationships would be compromised.

Littlejohn persevered, however, and in November 1879 the Bill he had pioneered was passed by both Houses of Parliament. The Bill insisted that every medical practitioner practising in the Burgh should report within 24 hours every patient with smallpox, cholera, typhus, typhoid, diphtheria, scarlet fever, scarlatina, or measles occurring in his practice, stating the patient's address. Two shillings and six pence would be paid for each intimation. A penalty not exceeding 40 shillings was to be imposed for failure to comply with the Act.

Littlejohn pointed out that, during 1875, 'zymotic diseases' killed 873 people in the city yet only 12 doctors sent in intimations referring to a total of 18 cases.[18] After the Act was passed in 1879 much more realistic figures became available and the assistance to Littlejohn's team through notification must have been immense.[19] He even had the foresight to give every practitioner printed slips and stamped envelopes addressed to the local authority so as to facilitate rapid notification with the minimum of bother. He also insisted that the notification regulations applied to wealthy as well as to poor patients. Indeed one of the ways he had persuaded those initially against the Act that it was a good idea was to explain that disease was spreading from the poor communities in the Old Town into the more well-to-do areas of the New Town and that infectious diseases respected neither wealth nor status.

The eight diseases that were to be compulsorily notified under the *Edinburgh Municipal and Police Act* 1879 were smallpox, cholera, scarlet fever, scarlatina, typhoid fever, typhus fever, diphtheria and measles. In 1902, the Infectious Disease (Notification) Act 1889 came into force

	A. Form of Intimation.
	'EDINBURGH MUNICIPAL AND POLICE ACT 1879.'
No. .	No. .
Case of	To *Medical Officer of Health*, *Police Chambers*.
at No. .	There is a case of at 18 .
Reported 18 .	No immediate attention required. *Signature*

Infectious disease intimation form for the notification of smallpox, cholera, scarlet fever, scarlatina, typhoid fever, typhus fever, diphtheria and measles by medical practitioners. The 'No' preceding 'immediate attention required' could be deleted if appropriate. (From H. D. Littlejohn's *On the Compulsory Intimation of Infectious Diseases*. By courtesy of Edinburgh City Libraries)

under which measles was no longer to be notified but two streptococcal illnesses (besides scarlet fever) were to be included, namely erysipelas and puerperal fever. This interrupted the smooth accumulation of statistics but, nonetheless, important information regarding infections became available.[20]

There was an uphill struggle to have tuberculosis legally recognised. In 1888 Littlejohn warned of the danger of drinking infected milk. He was unsuccessful in getting tuberculosis included in the Contagious Diseases (Animals) Acts but did in fact get Edinburgh Town Council to enforce the 1885 Dairies, Cowsheds and Milk-Shops Order. Dr R. W. Philip, later Sir Robert and Professor of Tuberculosis, pressed strongly for the compulsory notification of tuberculosis in 1890 but Littlejohn was not so sure. Littlejohn had already correlated the high mortality from pulmonary tuberculosis with overcrowded Edinburgh districts. He therefore recommended the Town Council rather to improve sanitation and more regularly cleanse streets, closes and stairs. He particularly wished to discourage the habit of spitting, even the 'ordinary expectoration in our streets and public conveyances'.[21] Because tuberculosis was so rife, albeit not always infectious in every person, Littlejohn initially doubted whether compulsory notification would really reflect the incidence of the disease without the backing of a sputum sample showing tubercle bacilli. In 1900 the Town Council's Report 'On the Prevention of Consumption' made the way easy for sputum samples to be analysed (at the Corporation's expense) at the Laboratory of the Royal College of Physicians of Edinburgh and from 1901 at the Usher Institute of Public Health.[22] Eventually Littlejohn instituted the voluntary notification of pulmonary tuberculosis in 1903 and this became compulsory in 1907.

Much more could be told of Sir Henry Duncan Littlejohn and his success in pursuading Edinburgh, sometimes reluctantly, to espouse his sanitary reforms. Suffice to say his achievements could not be better summed up than in the following public health statistics quoted by both Dr Tait and Professor Crew in their eulogies of Sir Henry Littlejohn on the centenary of his appointment as the first Medical Officer of Health of Edinburgh.[23]

Year	Population	Birth rate	Death rate	Infant mortality rate	Phthisis death rate	Zymotic death date	Population per acre
1863	170,441 (from 1861 Census)	36.24	25.88	145	2.54	6.23	49.0
1908	350,761	21.39	13.37	114	1.12	0.69	30.7

PART TWO

Early Hospital Provision for
Edinburgh's Fever Patients

CHAPTER FIVE

The Royal Infirmary

Excluding the leper houses, like those at Liberton and Greenside, there was initially little in-patient provision for fever victims except during epidemics when hastily built huts in the city outskirts were used to isolate them. During these outbreaks the services of religious houses of charity like those of St Catherine of Sienna (now Sciennes) and the Chapel of St Roque (now in the Astley Ainslie Hospital) would be overstretched but there is reason to think they also provided for fever patients during the quieter, inter-epidemic periods. Bailie Pollard[1] records that in the reign of Mary Queen of Scots the city had at least eight houses for the relief of the infirm, all supported by charity. After the sixteenth century they had either closed, due to failing support, or else they became homes for the aged and decrepit rather than hospitals.

Sir George Drummond, six times Lord Provost of Edinburgh in the eighteenth century, was largely responsible for developing hospital accommodation. From its beginning in 1729 the six-bedded charitable Infirmary of Edinburgh provided some fever accommodation. Dr Logan Turner[2] mentions that in its first year 35 patients were treated in the 'Little House', as it came to be called, 37 in its second year and, by 1733, the number had risen to 49. Among the communicable diseases diagnosed were ague and consumption, and some cross-infection seems inevitable in so small a building. There was no geographical limit to the catchment area, patients being admitted from as far away as Caithness, Peterhead and the Island of Mull, and this must also have increased the risk of introducing and disseminating infection from all over Scotland.

Although a physician and a surgeon were both to attend the 'Little House' each afternoon, the only living-in staff were the Mistress or Housekeeper and one female servant. As Dr Logan Turner pointed out, the term 'nurse' had not yet come into use.[3] The patients were cared for on wooden bedsteads with a straw mattress and were covered with cotton sheets and a quilt. By the generosity of the Countess of Stair, blankets were later provided. Candle light was the only form of artificial illumination.[4]

According to Dr Logan Turner,[5] the exact location of the 'Little House' was unclear. He suggested it probably stood at the head of

Robertson's Close near its upper or south end and probably on its west side. Today, Robertson's Close remains a narrow passageway running northwards and steeply downwards from Infirmary Street to the Cowgate. Old houses are still present on its western side. It may seem a quaint, picturesque but insalubrious place for an infirmary, yet in the eighteenth century many of the Old Town gentry lived nearby.

Dr Andrew Fraser,[6] is quite clear that the 'Little House', was not in Robertson's Close but sandwiched between two other buildings, namely Scott's Laboratory to the west and the Partners' Laboratory to the east. Together with the house of the Professor of Divinity, they occupied the north side of the College Garden and fronted on to Infirmary Street, formerly Jamaica Street. Today a plaque on the north side of James Thin's bookshop records the site and, in the 1720s and 1730s, the Infirmary's patients were allowed to use College Garden as an 'airing ground'.

A Royal Charter from George II was granted in 1736, for the new Royal Infirmary of Edinburgh, under the guidance of the far-seeing Lord Provost Drummond. After a massive public subscription, the foundation stone was laid in 1738, although patients were not admitted until about 1741. By the 1750s the Infirmary accommodated 228 patients. It was designed by William Adam, father of the famous Robert Adam, architect of much of the Old College. The site chosen faced Infirmary Street to the north west with Drummond Street to the rear. Houses that later lined the east side of South Bridge, including the present Thin's bookshop, lay to the west of the Royal Infirmary building.

The elegant Royal Infirmary building of 1738 is described in the *Gazetteer of Scotland* of 1843[7] as consisting:

> of a body and two projecting wings, all four stories high, substantially built, and abundantly perforated with windows ... The central part of the body projects from the main line, and is elegant in its architecture ... The access to the different floors is by a large stair case in the centre of the building, so spacious as to admit the transit of sedan chairs, and by two smaller stair cases, one at each end. The floors are distributed into wards, fitted up with ranges of beds capable of accommodating 228 patients, – the smaller rooms for the nurses and the medical attendants, – a manager's room, a waiting-room for students and a consulting-room for the physicians or surgeons. Two of the wards, devoted to patients whose cases are considered most curious and constructive, are set apart for clinical lectures ... Within the attic, is a spacious theatre for surgical operations, capable of accommodating 200 students.[8] The house has separate wards for male and female patients, and a ward which is used as a Lock hospital;[9] but, even in ordinary

periods, it is utterly incompetent for the service of Edinburgh, and during the prevalence of an epidemic, affords a very fractional part of requisite accommodation.

The *Gazetteer of Scotland* pays tribute to Lord Provost Drummond whose enthusiasm and encouragement for the pioneers and contributors to the first Royal Infirmary was acknowledged by a bust of him set up by the Infirmary's Directors in the hall of the building.[10]

The Royal Infirmary of 1738 faced north west onto Infirmary Street. Both this site and the ground adjacent to it are also important in the story of the City Hospital, because that was where fever patients were long cared for by the Royal Infirmary Managers and their staff. The Royal Infirmary left there in 1879 for its third and present site in Lauriston Place. Except for the William Adam Infirmary itself, demolished in 1884, the remaining old buildings were taken over by the Town Council and used purely for the management of fever patients. The site extended north to the Cowgate, south to Drummond Street and east as far as the Pleasance where it was bounded by the old Flodden Wall. It included both the old High School and old Surgeons' Hall as well as the buildings surrounding Surgeons' Square.

Even with its eventual complement of 228 beds, the Royal Infirmary of 1738 could not provide enough accommodation for fever patients during epidemics. This problem became particularly acute in the early 1800s when the population was growing fast. Accommodation in the city was overcrowded with the families of poor Scottish and Irish labourers crammed into the insanitary Old Town, only recently vacated by the wealthy who had been slow to move away into the New Town.

The country was impoverished during and after the Napoleonic Wars whilst the recurrent bad harvests and crop failures led to hardship and malnutrition in the poorer classes.[11] Added to all this, and probably as a by-product of it, came several epidemics mostly of typhus and cholera. One clinical description of epidemic fever from 1818 included flea bites, rashes, eruptions, languor, lassitude, high fever, rapid pulse, headache and delirium.[12] Other characteristic features of fever patients were poverty, dejection, and a male preponderance among the Irish and the Highlanders engaged on public building works within the city. Employment opportunities attracted to Edinburgh 'labouring Irish who, without doubt, by their habits of filth and debauchery, have tended much to spread the disease, if not to introduce its present form into the city'.[13] Besides, the wives of the Irish labourers went begging in country districts where even the Society for the Suppression of Begging, the Magistrates and other public spirited persons found it difficult to stop them.[14] Doubtless the unfortunate Irish and their families, driven from their own country by famine and rapacious English landlords, became the scapegoats.

As there was no fever hospital as such in Edinburgh in the early nineteenth century, the Royal Infirmary frequently had to manage infectious disease patients. Normally two wards were available. Surprisingly Dr Logan Turner comments that even in epidemics there was no evidence of cross-infection from the fever wards to staff or other patients in the hospital.[15] As will be seen later, this did not apply to the Queensberry House Hospital where members of staff certainly did become infected. In the severe typhus epidemic of 1817–20 even the three extra wards provided by the Royal Infirmary could not cope with the outbreak. Additional accommodation for fever patients was becoming imperative.

CHAPTER SIX

Queensberry House Fever Hospital, 1818–35

Although not recorded at that time, the overflow of typhus patients in the 1817–20 epidemic may have been isolated in temporary wooden accommodation just as plague victims had been isolated on the Burgh Muir in the seventeenth century. The Lord Provost and 'a number of influential citizens',[1] however, persuaded the Government to let them use the unoccupied Queensberry House Barracks on the south side of the Canongate, close to Holyrood House. It was opened as a fever hospital on 23 February 1818.

Queensberry House was built between 1681 and 1686 by Charles Maitland, Lord Hatton, later the Duke of Lauderdale. It soon, however, became the home of the Dukes of Queensberry. Both Robert Chambers in the nineteenth century[2] and more recently Margaret Hume and Sydney Boyd[3] have documented the exploits of the colourful and sometimes eccentric Dukes and Duchesses of Queensberry who lived in Queensberry House for over a century.

In 1778 the Earl of March inherited the Queensberry title but, as the Duke of Queensberry, also known as 'Old Q', he seldom lived in Queensberry House. He eventually stripped the house of all its valuable ornaments in October 1801 and sold it. With its 85 rooms, 70 foot long gallery and garden, the upset of £900 was surprisingly low. It was snapped up for £1,170 by William Aitchison, a distiller from Wallyford,[4] who rented the house to Sir James Montgomery of Stanhope MP who later became Lord Chief Baron of the Scottish Court of the Exchequer. When he died in 1803 William Aitchison made a large profit by selling Queensberry House for £3,150 to His Majesty's Barrack Master General.[5]

The former great lodging of the nobility was remodelled in 1808 as a barracks and raised in height by one storey. Two guard rooms were placed on either side of the entrance on South Back of the Canongate (Holyrood Road). The one on the east side, the officers' guard room, still stands but the one on the west, the soldiers' guard room, has been demolished. A hospital was also erected in 1809, the Sir Andrew Murray Wing. It does not seem initially to have been used as such but rather as a dormitory capable of sleeping 520 soldiers.

The main building had full height, advanced wings enclosing the

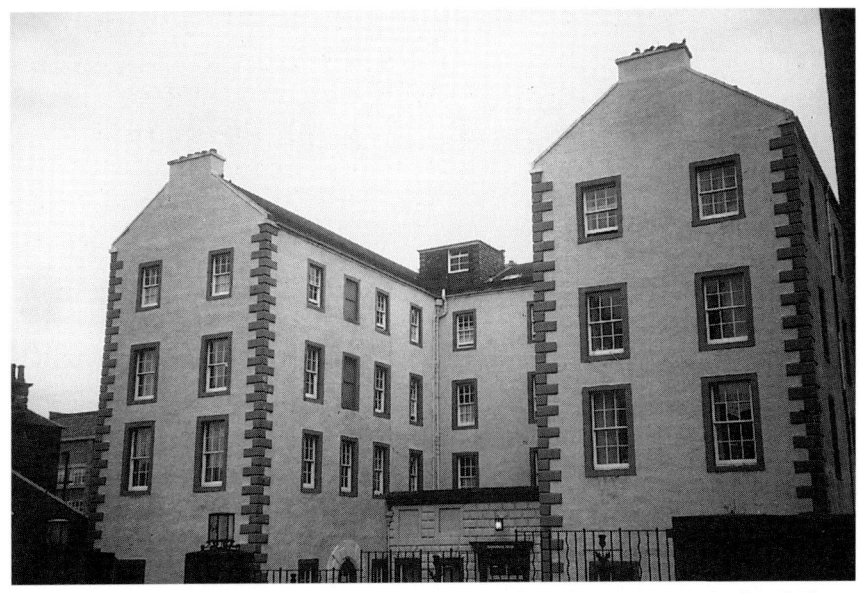

Queensberry House, built 1681–86, became a fever hospital, mainly for cholera and typhus patients between 1818 and 1835. (Photo: J. A. Gray)

entrance to the north on the Canongate. There were lower, square pavilions at the angles of the south front. The further storey added in 1808 when it became a barracks must have replaced the French roof, with storm windows in the style of Versailles,[6] so, by the time it was used as a barracks and later a fever hospital, it cannot much have resembled the original. Yet it still stands there, and was until 1996 a home for the elderly. The adjacent public well on the Canongate is dated 1817 and would have made a reasonably accessible water supply before piped water became available.

Dr Benjamin Welsh, MD, a Member of the Royal Medical Society, later a general practitioner in Haddington, was made the first Medical Superintendent of Queensberry House Fever Hospital.[7] His salary was £40 per annum. Visiting Physicians were Dr James Hamilton Snr, and Dr Thomas Spens, both physicians-in-ordinary to the Infirmary. Two physician-clerks were appointed as residents, namely Messrs Stephenson and Christison. Christison later became Sir Robert Christison, Professor of Materia Medica and Jurisprudence, and an eminent toxicologist. He graduated MD in 1819, but before this, whilst a physician-clerk in Queensberry House, he suffered twice from relapsing fever.[8]

Dr Logan Turner[9] describes the exchange of the old wooden bedsteads of Queensberry House Barracks for iron bedsteads and bedding which were transferred from Greenlaw Barracks (now Glencorse Barracks). Although he states that there was room for 60–80 patients when Queensberry House Fever Hospital was opened, Dr Welsh's detailed account [10] describes initially only 60 available beds. There may, however, have been more added later, possibly in the Murray Wing.

The following account is taken from Dr Welsh's *A Practical Treatise on the Efficacy of Bloodletting in the Epidemics of Fever in Edinburgh. Illustrated by Numerous Cases and Tables Extracted from the Journals of the Queensberry House Fever Hospital, Edinburgh*, which he wrote in 1819.[11] The *Treatise* describes in fascinating detail the accommodation and daily running of the fever hospital. Dr Welsh was an enthusiastic venesector. In his uncontrolled study of bleeding 872 patients with fever, he claimed 833 cured and that only about one in 22 died! He listed 23 indications for blood letting and insisted that copious venesection for epidemic fever lessened mortality, cut short the epidemic and, even when it did not save life, it protracted it in both the young and the old.

Dr Welsh's *Treatise* describes the former Queensberry House Barracks as having easy access from the High Street and the south back of the Canongate where there was a good airing ground. Presumably this was used by convalescent patients and was also where washed linen was dried. The ground floor of the building was below the street level in the front but open at the rear. On that floor were the kitchen, storerooms, apartments for the matron, the clerks, and the porter, together with waiting rooms for the physicians.

Accommodation for patients was on the four upper floors which were connected by an ample staircase. On each floor there were three wards measuring 18 ft × 18 ft, 21 ft × 18 ft and 30 ft × 15 ft with a ceiling height of between 9 and 12 ft. Each floor also had a good day room for the nurse and a bed closet for those employed at night. There were 15 beds on each floor, six in each of the two largest wards and three in the small. Each ward had a fireplace and windows to provide good ventilation. The stores for clean and foul bedding and for the patients' own clothing were separated from the sick rooms. Each patient had an iron bedstead, palliasse and bolster with a hair or woollen mattress and pillow, one pair of sheets, two blankets and a coverlet. A small table was placed between beds for drinking cups, 'spit-boxes' and medicines. There was much emphasis on cleanliness, washing of sheets and blankets and ventilating the palliasses, bolsters and mattresses in an airy part of the building or else fumigating them. The straw in the palliasses was frequently changed.[12]

Three nurses were allocated to each floor (15 beds) and there was always one night nurse available. The standard of nursing appears to have been high for its time. Dr Welsh commented that:

> everyone who has any experience in hospitals of this kind, will be aware of how much the order and regularity of the house, and comfort, nay, often even the lives of the patients, depend upon the attention and sobriety of the nurses; and I am happy to state, that, in general, we have had reason to be highly satisfied with the accuracy, cleanliness, and good conduct of the persons acting in that capacity in this hospital.[13]

The patients' diet consisted of milk, porridge, panada (bread boiled to a pulp and flavoured with white wine, sugar and sometimes nutmeg), milk-sops, beer, bread and milk, or beer, a basin of tea, arrowroot or weak beef tea. For those with actual fever, graduated first and second diets were prescribed.

Patients were conveyed in chairs 'belonging to the Royal Infirmary'[14] and admissions were to report by 1 p.m. to be seen by the physicians, this being their visiting hour. It was apparently up to the physicians to decide on admissions and accommodation and also to secure a 'recommendation from some respectable persons, binding themselves to remove the patient from the hospital when desired, or, in case of death, to be at the expense of the funeral'.[15] Help for those genuinely in need came from the Visitors of the Society for the Destitute Sick. About 9 out of 10 patients admitted came with such a recommendation.

On admission to the ward, patients were immediately undressed and their faces, chests, arms, feet and legs, or if need be their whole body, were washed by the nurses with tepid water and soap.[16] If they had not brought a shirt or shift and night cap with them, these were supplied and they were then put to bed. A list was made of all the articles of clothing that they had brought in with them, to which was added their name, date of admission and ward number. Their clothes were then conveyed to the ground floor, linens put in cold water until taken out for washing later and their clothes were either washed or fumigated. Ward clothes were changed as often as the nurses felt it appropriate. Patients got their own clothes back when they were eventually allowed out of bed, but not their own linen until they were finally discharged.

The patients were put to bed after admission, unless their symptoms were very urgent when they were attended to at once. Most lay in bed until the evening to recover from any faintness or fatigue resulting from their transfer to hospital 'so as to enable us to judge more accurately of the nature of their symptoms'.[17]

They were then clerked between 6 and 9 p.m. The next day, between

11 a.m. and 1 p.m., reports were taken noting the effect of any prescription given the preceding evening, how the patient had passed the night and what their present symptoms were. All this information was read to the visiting physicians between 1 and 2 p.m.:

> when they enquire as to the accuracy of the reports, make any additions they may judge proper, and give the necessary prescriptions.[18]

There was a daily report on each patient in the house throughout the course of the illness. Dr Welsh comments that:

> Besides regular daily visits of the physicians, all the patients are seen twice a-day, morning and evening, by myself and the resident medical officers.[19]

Changes in symptoms or alterations of treatment were recorded in a book for inspection by the visiting physicians. Dr Welsh was also in the habit of visiting the wards:

> at uncertain hours, to see that they are in proper order, are well ventilated, and the nurses attending to their duty.[20]

Bleeding, arteriotomy, cupping and the application of leeches were usually performed in the evening.

Visiting was strictly limited initially 'only to admit the nearest relations when the patients seemed likely to die'.[21] Later the regulations appear to have been relaxed in favour of occasional visits by friends provided permission was obtained beforehand. Even then, visitors were allowed to remain in the ward for only a very short time. Dr Welsh commented that infection had been caught during improper visits to the house. He also felt it should be illegal for items of food to be spirited in to the detriment of patients. He was surprised by the:

> ingenuity that some visitors, particularly females, display in concealing the articles they are conveying into the house.[22]

These rules of the house were drawn up by Dr Hope, one of the Managers, and Dr Spens, one of the Physicians, in the Royal Infirmary.

Despite all these precautions, cross-infection did occur. Dr Welsh commented that in the year following the opening of Queensberry House Hospital:

> my friends Messrs Stephenson and Christison, the Matron, two apothecaries in succession, the shop boy, washerwoman and thirty-eight nurses have been infected: four of the nurses have died.[23]

There were also examples of repeated episodes of infection of staff. Four doctors, the shop boy and nine nurses had two attacks and three of the nurses in all had three attacks.[24] Infection was also acquired by 'several students whom curiosity led too near the person of the patients ...'.[25]

Dr Logan Turner[26] records that between 1 March 1818 and 28 February 1819, 1,676 patients were admitted to Queensberry House of whom 1,605 recovered and only 71 died, making a relatively low mortality of just over 4.2 per cent. The difficulty for the Infirmary was that the cost of maintaining both the Infirmary and its annex (Queensberry House) was £8,376 which was very much more than any previous annual outlay.[27] Nonetheless Queensberry House continued to be used until the autumn of 1823, when the Government had hoped to sell the building. The Managers, however, decided in 1825 to lease Queensberry House for a further 10 years at a rent of £80 per annum.[28] This proved to be a wise decision because the second typhus epidemic of the century, between 1826 and 1829, was much more severe. Queensberry House was again opened and somehow 140–150 beds were maintained and continuously occupied to supplement those used for fever patients in the Royal Infirmary itself.

Dr Logan Turner describes the consternation in Edinburgh at the outbreak of Asiatic cholera which came to the city in 1831.[29] This prompted the setting up of the Cholera Board of Health.[30] By the end of June 1832, 600 people had died of cholera in Edinburgh. The Managers of the Royal Infirmary tried to prevent cholera patients being admitted to their own hospital, having them transferred both to Queensberry House and 'a house situated at Fountain Bridge'.[31] It is unlikely the latter was the same poorhouse 'in a field westward of Lothian Road' as is mentioned in the *Gazetteer of Scotland* of 1843;[32] this more likely refers to St Cuthbert's Charity Workhouse built in 1759 further north, partly on the site which eventually became the Caledonian Hotel.[33] It is therefore unclear where the house at Fountainbridge actually was but it may have been one of several that were from time to time taken over for fever patients during epidemics.

Queensberry House was used in 1832 'as an Hospital for persons complaining of cholera'.[34] Cholera suspects could also be detained there if the doctors so advised. On 31 January 1832, for example, Archibald Scott, Procurator Fiscal, petitioned 'the Honourable the Sheriff of Edinburghshire' to keep nine cholera contacts in Queensberry House for five days of isolation.[35]

During this cholera outbreak, Dr Logan Turner quotes a minute of the Town Council of 4 January 1832, stating:

> the College of Surgeons at the earnest solicitation of the Board of Health granted to that body the use of the old building and, conditionally, that of another house of which they are proprietors for the important purpose of

providing accommodation for cholera patients, if such accommodation should be required.[36]

The old Surgeons' Hall was opened temporarily as the Drummond Street Cholera Hospital which accommodated the patients treated with intravenous fluids by Dr Thomas Latta.[37] It was used again in 1848 to cope with a further epidemic of Asiatic cholera. The Managers of the Royal Infirmary had by this time purchased the old Surgeons' Hall to be used as the capital's fever hospital on the understanding that the Royal Infirmary, whilst supplying beds, bedding and nurses, should not be liable for any other expense incurred in looking after cholera victims.

During the third epidemic of typhus in 1837, two years after the lease on Queensberry House expired, the Infirmary provided nine wards (approximately 140 beds) for fever patients. Dr Logan Turner[38] explains that this had become possible following the transfer in 1832 of surgical patients to the old High School building which had been purchased in 1829. The Fever Board of the city took over a house in the same grounds and the Lock Hospital of 30 beds (previously used for treating sexually transmitted disease) as accommodation for patients with typhus. The Fever Board provided the running costs. Between 1 October 1837 and 30 September 1838, 2,244 patients were treated and between 30 September 1838 and 13 December 1838 a further 527 patients were treated.[39]

During the next two epidemics of typhus fever, 1842–43 and 1846–48 the accommodation and funding resources of the Royal Infirmary were stretched even further. Besides the buildings already mentioned, temporary accommodation was set up near the Infirmary, in tents that had been borrowed from the Ordinance Store at Edinburgh Castle and from the Archers' Hall. Even the Infirmary Chapel was temporarily requisitioned to accommodate fever patients. Altogether, 17,542 patients with infectious fever were under the care of the Royal Infirmary between 1841 and 1848.[40] The New Surgical Hospital, as distinct from the use made by surgical patients of the old High School building, was yet to be constructed. When it came, it was a long Renaissance style block designed by David Bryce (1848–53) and had additions made to the rear (north side) by Rowand Anderson and Balfour Paul in 1906–07. It was later to provide much needed fever accommodation after the Royal Infirmary moved to Lauriston Place in 1879. It now houses the University's Department of Geography.

CHAPTER SEVEN

The First City Fever Hospital: The Canongate Poorhouse

A 'Report by the Town Clerk and Medical Officer of Health as to the Present and Prospective Arrangements for Treatment of Infectious Diseases in the City', dated 5 November 1884, summarises some of the problems concerning the accommodation and management of fever patients in the second half of the nineteenth century.[1]

In 1860 some relief came both to the Royal Infirmary, which had always found difficulty in accommodating children with infectious diseases, and to the local authorities which were together responsible for their management. The children's hospital, newly established at Meadowside House overlooking North Meadow Walk on the present Royal Infirmary site, took over the care of children with infectious diseases, so lightening the burden of fever patient accommodation for a while. In 1876 one third of the children in Meadowside House had infectious diseases including typhus, scarlet fever, typhoid and measles. In 1885, however, the Royal Hospital for Sick Children, following the lead of the Managers of the Royal Infirmary, refused to admit fever patients and so the old problems of accommodation recurred.[2]

The Report of 1884 also mentions that, as the popularity and reputation of the Edinburgh Medical School increased, so also did the demand for medical and surgical beds in the Royal Infirmary. This pressure on hospital accommodation rose dramatically in 1866 when a further outbreak of cholera forced the Managers of the Royal Infirmary to tell the Town Council that they could no longer admit patients with cholera. The Town Council, feeling obliged to make provision for the cholera epidemic, took temporary possession of the 'City Poor House Hospital' in Forrest Road where cholera victims were treated at the expense of £2,423 14s.[3]

The *Gazetteer of Scotland* describes the building as follows:

> the city Poor's house, built in 1743 is situated within the angle formed by Bristo-street and Teviot-row, considerably back from the roadway, so as to look down on an open area. The edifice is of four stories very spacious

The First City Fever Hospital

but of plain and dingy appearance. In its vicinity are a bedlam and a children's hospital.[4]

This building, however, may later have become the Ragged School shown as a large L-shaped block in the triangle formed by Forrest Road, Teviot Row and Bristo Place (not Bristo Street).[5] The even larger Charity Workhouse, west of Forrest Road between Greyfriars' Churchyard and Lauriston Place, is also shown on Johnston's Plan of Edinburgh and Leith, 1851.[6] This is more likely to have been the temporary fever hospital. Its remaining north wing, much altered, is the harled building still seen on the north side of Forrest Hill, the cul-de-sac leading off Forrest Road.

Dr Henry Littlejohn, the MOH, then urged the Town Council to obtain a permanent infectious diseases hospital, rather than continue with the make-do-and-mend system which had previously failed.[7] The Town Council therefore bought for £1,600 the Canongate Poorhouse,[8] at the foot of a wynd behind the Canongate Tolbooth,[9] and had it converted into a fever hospital. When this opened on 19 December 1870 it became known as the first City Fever Hospital,[10] although this ignores the previous considerable contribution of Queensberry House Fever Hospital from 1818 to 1835.

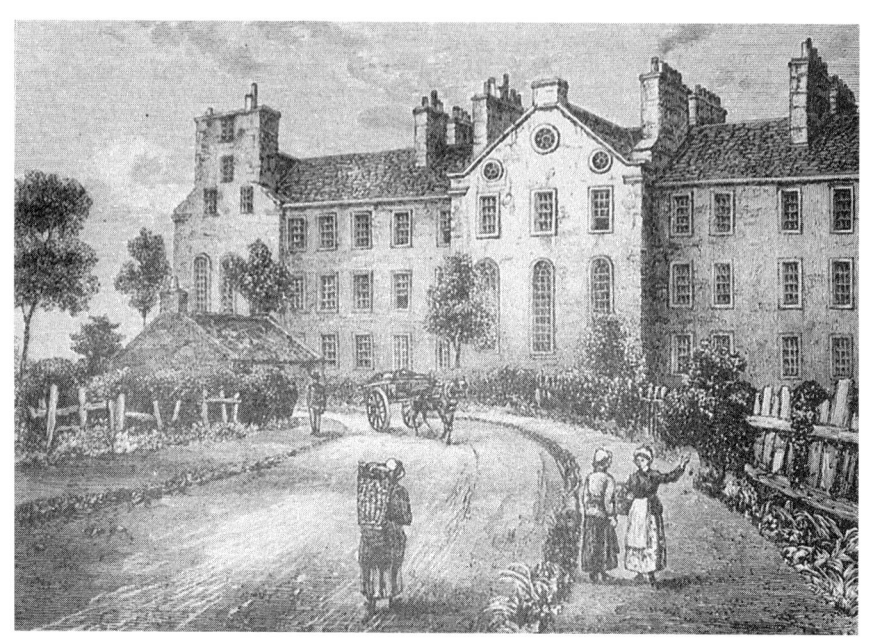

The Charity Workhouse, west of Forrest Road. This or the City Poorhouse was used for cholera patients in the 1866 epidemic. (From James Grant's *Old and New Edinburgh*, Vol. II, p. 324)

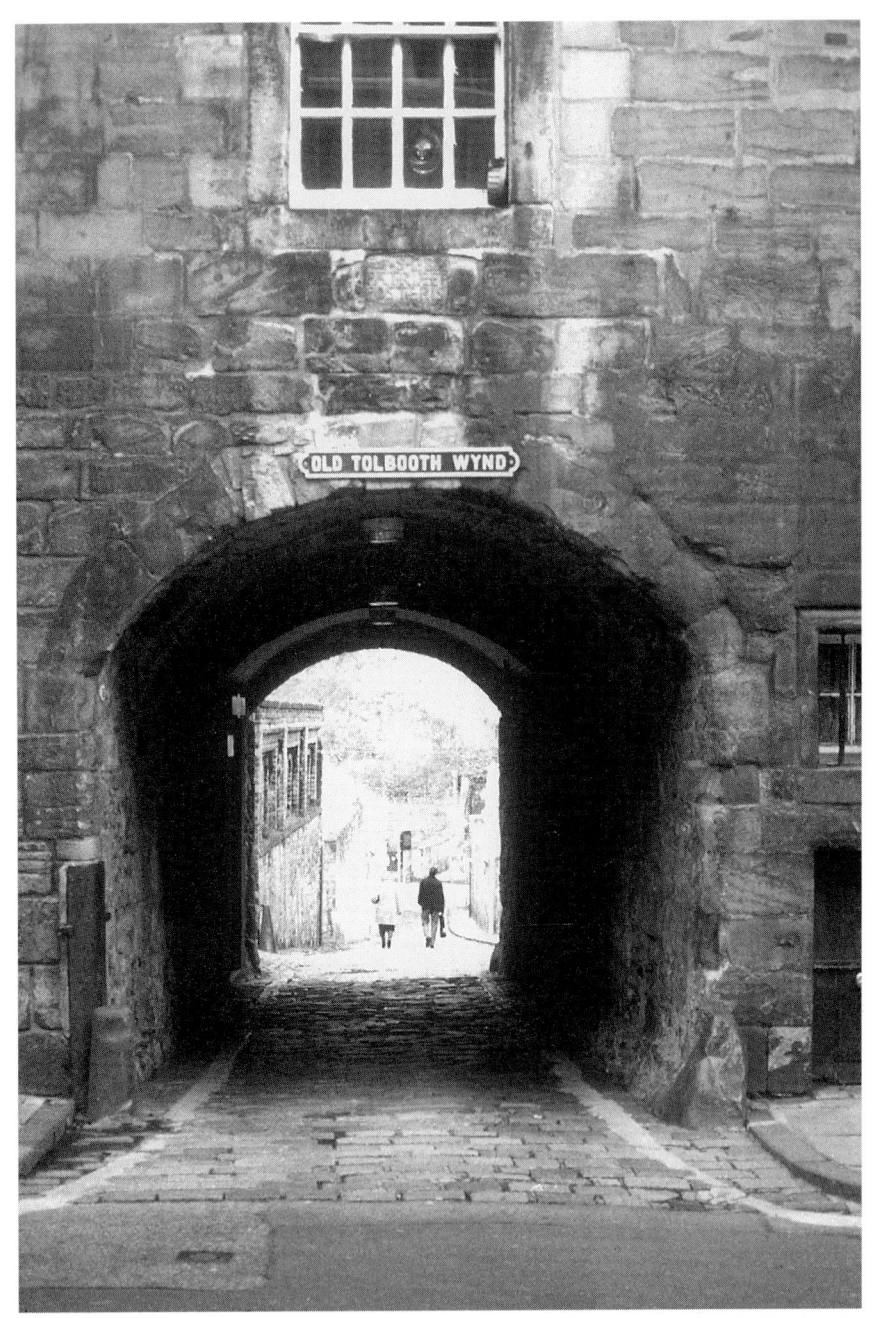

Old Tolbooth Wynd looking north to Calton Road (formerly North Back of Canongate). On the right (east) at the foot of the wynd stood the Canongate Charity Workhouse or Poorhouse that became the first City Fever Hospital in 1870. (Photo: J. A. Gray)

From 1870 onwards the Canongate Poorhouse was much used for cholera and smallpox patients. The print of a view sketched in 1822 looking south east from Calton Hill unfortunately shows no more detail of the Canongate Poorhouse than a long, pitched roof, parallel to Tolbooth Wynd, with a plain chimney breast at either gable end.[11] Situated between the Canongate Church burying ground and North Back of Canongate (now Calton Road), its front lay along the east side of the narrow Tolbooth Wynd near its junction with North Back of Canongate. Johnston's Plan of Edinburgh and Leith, 1851 refers to it as the Canongate Charity Workhouse. It had been established in 1761 by subscription but by the 1840s it had fallen into disrepair and was described as unfit for the debilitated and aged.[12]

By 1868 a new poorhouse was opened at Craigleith and later became the Western General Hospital. In 1873 this poorhouse, which was under St Cuthbert's Parish Board's supervision, amalgamated with the Canongate Poorhouse.[13] This became known as the St Cuthbert's and Canongate Combination, but by that time, the buildings, although not the outdoor poor relief responsibilities of the Canongate Parish, had come under the aegis of the Town Council.

Even with the additional beds in the Canongate Poorhouse from December 1870, the Town Council had insufficient hospital accommodation to cope with outbreaks of infectious diseases. In 1871 when it was suspected that a smallpox epidemic in England would soon reach Edinburgh, the Royal Infirmary Managers told the Town Council that they would not admit cases of smallpox. Since the Public Health (Scotland) Act of 1867, the Town Council was obliged to provide accommodation for smallpox patients but had great difficulty in finding suitable premises. Its proposed additional accommodation in King's Stables Road proved inadequate. The Royal Infirmary Managers then permitted the Town Council to look after smallpox patients on a temporary basis in George Watson's Hospital, which they had recently bought at the Lauriston Place site for £75,000.[14] During the epidemic of 1870–71, therefore, the Town Council had to pay £6,035 11s 1d for the use of George Watson's Hospital and £2,912 7s 6d for City Fever Hospital at the Canongate, in order to accommodate smallpox patients.[15]

Both the MOH and the Public Health Committee felt it was imperative for smallpox patients to be admitted quickly. During a further outbreak in 1877, therefore, the Committee's Convener wrote to all the doctors in Edinburgh and Leith urging them to speed up smallpox admissions to the Canongate Poorhouse Hospital. His printed circular,[16] which follows entire, was accompanied by a Report from the MOH regarding the proper notification of infectious diseases.

Public Health Office
Police Chambers
EDINBURGH
21 February 1877

Sir,

I am directed by the Public Health Committee of the Town Council in view of an outbreak of Small-pox in the City, to intimate to you that the Hospital at the foot of Tolbooth Wynd, Canongate, is now open for the reception of persons affected with that disease. On intimation being made to this Office, or at any of the Police Stations, the Hospital Conveyance will be sent at any hour, with attendants, and every assistance given in the removal of Patients; also with fumigation of houses, the disinfection, and, where necessary, the destruction of any infected articles of clothing or bedding.

In the event of death in a private house, the Authorities will aid in removing the body to a special mortuary, and thence to the place of interment, at any time arranged by the friends. The fumigation of the house, removal of infected articles, etc., will also be attended to as soon as the body is removed.

I am also instructed to draw your attention to the enclosed Report by the Medical Officer of Health, on the importance of early intimation of infectious diseases being given to this Office. In the only case of Small-pox which has as yet appeared in Edinburgh, a delay of two days unfortunately occurred, in consequence of the intimation which was given by the Medical Attendants, having been posted late on a Saturday, and only delivered here on the Monday morning.

I am Sir, your obedient servant,

JAMES GOWANS
Convener of Public Health Committee

NB. A copy of the above Circular and Report referred to, sent of date to all the Medical Practitioners in Edinburgh and Leith.

The first City Fever Hospital at the Canongate Poorhouse continued to be used for smallpox outbreaks well into the 1890s.[17] By this time, however, the second City Hospital east of the old Royal Infirmary site had become well established. Even then, accommodation for fever patients remained precarious until Colinton Mains Fever Hospital was opened in 1903.

CHAPTER EIGHT

Who Should Care For Fever Patients? The Second City Fever Hospital at Infirmary Street

It is interesting to compare the pressure on accommodation in Leith Hospital during epidemics in the late nineteenth century with similar difficulties being experienced in Edinburgh. Dr Boyd's account[1] draws many parallels. The directors of Leith Hospital were in conflict with Leith Town Council. As in Edinburgh, various buildings were used as temporary hospitals during epidemics but not until the opening in 1896 of East Pilton Fever Hospital (later the Northern General Hospital) was Leith Hospital totally relieved of the responsibility of caring for fever patients.

Similarly in Edinburgh from the 1870s till 1885 there was a prolonged controversy between the Managers of the Royal Infirmary and the Town Council regarding accommodation for fever patients both during and between epidemics.[2] An Act passed on 20 June 1870 committed the Royal Infirmary to buy George Watson's Hospital with money from the subscriptions already received and to move the Royal Infirmary from its site facing Infirmary Street to Lauriston Place. The Town Council was quick to point out that the Infirmary had been incorporated for the free relief and cure of patients from all quarters and that a fever hospital had also been part of the plan. In addition to the ordinary medical and surgical wards, there was to be a pavilion devoted to the treatment of fevers, possibly including scarlatina, which was then regarded as slightly different from the other infectious diseases.[3]

The Act of 1870, amongst other things, provided for the construction of a sewer to connect the new Royal Infirmary with a public sewer running westwards near the east end of Lonsdale Terrace.[4] After many meetings between the Managers of the Royal Infirmary and representatives of the Town Council regarding both fever accommodation and the drainage of the new building, the Managers refused to provide more than 50 fever beds in the new building although requested by the Town Council to provide more. Eventually at a joint conference held on 28 January 1875

Sir Robert Christison [for the Royal Infirmary] made a statement reference to the capabilities of the New Infirmary, the result being, that accommodation within the Hospital could not be provided for more than fifty patients, but the accommodation for a number not exceeding twenty-four additional, would be obtained by the appropriation of three iron buildings adjacent to the Fever Hospital, which are to be erected by the Infirmary Managers for the treatment of other infectious diseases, in so far as these buildings may be at the time available. The members of the Town Council present expressed their unanimous assent to this proposal.[5]

All seemed well but unfortunately the architect then found difficulty in using the natural line of drainage towards Lonsdale Terrace. In the Session of 1875 the Managers inserted into a second Bill a provision to relinquish the sewer previously authorised and instead to run a new sewer eastwards connecting the new Royal Infirmary's drainage with the main public sewer at St Leonards. Unfortunately, this new line of drainage was also connected with drainage from George Square, Buccleuch Place and part of the Grange. The inhabitants of these areas under which the sewer was proposed to pass protested against the danger of infection to which they felt they were exposed. As rate payers they appealed by petition and sent a deputation to the Town Council to protect their interests.[6] The Town Council's response by opposing the Bill in Parliament could have interfered disastrously with the building of the new Royal Infirmary. Despite learned debates between the Town Council and the Managers as to possible ways in which the sewage outflow might be deodorised and the drains properly ventilated, no one came up with a satisfactory answer. Eventually the matter was settled. The Town Council's petition against the Bill was withdrawn from March 1875 subject to the proviso:

> that no sewage from a fever ward shall be allowed to pass into the sewer by this Act authorised, without the consent of the Magistrates and Council of the City of Edinburgh, and subject to such regulations as may be made by them from time to time.[7]

It was hoped that this would end the controversy but this was not to be. On 13 March 1875 the Town Clerk wrote to the Clerk of the Royal Infirmary that the Lord Provost's Committee still wished 74 fever beds to be provided by the Royal Infirmary.[8] This amounted to a trade off for the withdrawal of opposition by the Town Council to the Managers' plans to connect their new drainage to the St Leonards sewer.

In late March 1875, the Managers of the Royal Infirmary replied[9] explaining that they had instructed their architect to abandon the erection of a new fever hospital at Lauriston Place. In its place they would retain the eastern portion of the old Infirmary ground. This contained the present fever hospital (the City Infectious Hospital) with three wards for 35 patients, the previous fever hospital (the Infirmary Fever House), then a nurses' home and formerly the original Surgeons' Hall, which they claimed could accommodate 50 patients, a kitchen attached to that building, a laundry and a three-storey house also used at that time for a nurses' home. The Managers were also prepared to treat up to 74 patients with infectious diseases not in the proposed new Royal Infirmary but in the old Infirmary grounds and to give the Town Council, as the local authority for the treatment of fever patients, every facility to manage any in excess of the number of 74 in the buildings at the old Infirmary site.[10]

This proposal from the Managers was unanimously accepted by the Town Council. There was little doubt that the Managers had wished to have a small fever hospital of, say 50 beds, at Lauriston Place, so as to provide clinical teaching in infectious diseases for medical students. The Town Council also felt the Royal Infirmary had an unwritten obligation to provide some fever accommodation. Besides it was surely expected by those who had contributed to the Royal Infirmary's appeal for funds that the Infirmary should not neglect infectious diseases and that their services to fever patients should continue as they had in the past. The Managers and the Town Council then agreed that the Infirmary should treat cases of typhoid fever, scarlet fever and erysipelas. The Town Council, however, should be responsible for patients with typhus, measles and smallpox in the 70 beds available in the former Canongate Poorhouse.[11]

In 1881 the Town Council purchased from the Infirmary the Surgical Hospitals for £16,000 and the Medical Hospital for £8,500, both at the west of the old Infirmary site. £5,000 had already been paid to refit the Surgical Hospitals with 200 beds with special arrangements for the isolation of smallpox patients, and with separate nursing and cooking establishments. Special provision was also made for managing measles and typhus. This left other diseases such as typhoid, scarlet fever and erysipelas to be treated in the eastern group of the old Infirmary buildings (to be called the Infirmary Fever House) still belonging to the Managers which were then only separated by the distance of a few feet from the former Medical and Infectious Hospitals, now called the City Infectious Hospital.[12]

In November 1884, there took place a 'Friendly Conference', unlike the previous meetings which had frequently been contentious.[13] The Subcommittee of the Public Health Committee of the Town Council met a Subcommittee of the Managers of the Royal Infirmary about the time the City Infectious Hospital, now largely based on the old Infirmary site, was about to be occupied.

Two proposals were put forward. The first recommended that the Managers continue to treat typhoid, scarlet fever and erysipelas in their own Infirmary Fever House whilst the adjoining City Infectious Hospital should accommodate patients with typhus, measles and smallpox. The Town Council was to pay the Managers for every patient treated at the City Infectious Hospital and to cover the cost of furnishing and maintaining it as a suitable hospital. The building itself and its furnishings would remain the property of the Town Council. Unfortunately the Managers rejected this proposal and recommended a second proposal instead: that the Managers were to transfer 74 beds from the new Royal Infirmary to the new City Infectious Hospital and to dispose of their existing fever hospital at Lauriston because they felt that the 74 beds for infectious diseases there would necessarily interfere with the suitable treatment of other diseases; the Town Council should not insist on the treatment of smallpox in the City Hospital but that, along with cholera, smallpox should be treated by the Town Council in some separate building (suggesting a continuing use of the Canongate Poorhouse Hospital); with that accommodation provided, it would allow the Managers to treat satisfactorily all cases of infectious disease except for smallpox and cholera; the Town Council should pay the Managers a sum such as might be subsequently agreed on for all cases treated in the new City Infectious Hospital over the number of 74.

The old arguments were trotted out by the Managers that the Public Health (Scotland) Act had made it the responsibility of the Town Council as the local authority to look after infectious disease patients and that it was always better for a single body to have overall control of infectious outbreaks in the city. This would include the speedy transfer of patients to hospital, the disinfecting and fumigation of homes and the enforcement by the police of these recommendations.[14] The Managers did not feel that any of that was their responsibility.

For their part the Town Council stressed the huge public contributions which had been given to the new Royal Infirmary being built at Lauriston Place and the fact that fever patients would be aggrieved at not being admitted to the new Royal Infirmary, having subscribed to its building. Besides, the Royal Infirmary motto 'Patet omnibus' suggested that the Royal Infirmary should admit all patients, including those with fever. The Town Councillors further argued that contributions to the Infirmary would fall off if the local authority took over the total responsibility for fever patients. Moreover patients might be reluctant to go into a hospital under the charge of the Magistrates and Council but rather more willing to go into a fever hospital run by the Royal Infirmary.[15]

The Managers' Committee quoted extensively from experience in

Glasgow where infectious disease was managed totally by the municipal authorities. Even fever patients from outside Glasgow could, on the payment of £8 each, be managed in the Belvidere Hospital.[16] The Managers of the Royal Infirmary of Edinburgh also commented that under the provisions of the Public Health Act of 1867 their conveyances should not be used for the transfer of infectious disease patients without appropriate permission. Indeed, the transport of fever patients should be entirely the responsibility of the Town Council.

The Managers said nothing had changed since April 1882 when they had proposed that the Infirmary should continue to treat infectious diseases but be relieved of the expense. They felt that there was no benefit in entering into new negotiations with the Town Council albeit giving them time to make appropriate arrangements by a certain date (1 July 1885) to take over all fever cases at the old Infirmary site (City Infectious Hospital). They would put the existing Infirmary Fever House at the Town Council's disposal for a price to be agreed.[17] In fact the income and expenditure records of the Royal Infirmary show that in the year 1880–81 the building fund for the new Royal Infirmary had been boosted by the sum of £24,336 18s 6d, being the price of the old Infirmary site buildings sold to the Town Council, which was then applied to the reduction of the debt on the new Infirmary buildings.[18]

At a special meeting of the Managers of the Royal Infirmary – with *ex officio* Town Council representatives – on 27 February 1885, the second, alternative, proposal of the November 1884 'Friendly Conference' was again debated.[19] Lord Shand, seconded by Mr Edmund Baxter on behalf of the Managers of the Royal Infirmary, moved the approval of the recommendations. The Lord Provost, seconded by Bailie Turnbull, however, moved that the Report (amounting to the second proposal of the Conference of 27 February 1885) be not approved. Various Managers spoke in support of Lord Shand's motion and a division was taken. All the Managers present, with the exception of the Lord Provost and Bailie Turnbull, voted to approve the Report which was then adopted. The Clerk of the Managers was then directed to communicate the Report and its resolution to the Town Council with special reference to the item that the new Royal Infirmary should no longer admit infectious disease patients.[20]

At last it was the responsibility of the Town Council alone to look after all fever patients. The old Infirmary Buildings at Infirmary Street were set up as a 260 bedded fever hospital and opened with good isolation facilities for patients with typhus and smallpox in addition to reception accommodation for family contacts. The buildings included the old Surgical Hospital and old Surgeons' Hall, which became part of the second City Fever Hospital. Although the old High School (old Surgical Hospital) was disposed of and pulled down,[21] the first City Hospital (the former Canongate Poorhouse) remained available for smallpox cases during the 1890s.[22]

The minutes of the Royal Infirmary of 22 June 1885 record that the Managers unanimously agreed that, if the Magistrates and Town Council took over the treatment of all cases of infectious disease by 1 July 1885, they would offer to them for the sum of £4,000 the fever hospital with all its fittings,

> it being understood and agreed all cases of infectious disease and including Erysipelas occurring, in the Infirmary, will hereafter be taken in the City Hospital in the same way as cases occurring in any other part of the City.[23]

On 1 July 1885 an offer was therefore made by the Town Council for the Fever House grounds and buildings for the sum of £4,000. The offer was accepted by the Managers, with the proviso agreed above. A further minute of 27 July 1885[24] records that Councillor Baxter reported that the whole management of the Fever House had been taken over by the city authorities. It was only in the third week of September 1885, however, that the Treasurer of the Royal Infirmary could report that during the previous week he had signed the conveyance of the Infirmary Fever House in favour of the City of Edinburgh and had received the sum of £4,000 (less £56; one half of the expense of conveyancing) which he had applied to the reduction of debt on buildings.[25]

The second City Fever Hospital was established at last and a Medical Superintendent, Consulting Physician, Matron and staff appointed. The Consulting Physician was responsible for the clinical teaching of medical students and the Medical Officer of Health started a school for nurses with certificates of proficiency and silver badges for those successful in fever nurse training.[26] Private patients could also be accommodated in the hospital for £2 10s a week per person.[27]

Dr Logan Turner's book[28] gives a plan of the old Infirmary site after the new Surgical Hospital was built in 1853 and it shows the area available for development as the second City Hospital from 1885. Dr Littlejohn was upset when the Town Council started to sell off land adjacent to the hospital and preclude its expansion.[29] The School Board, for instance, secured part of the area near where the old Infirmary had been and built South Bridge Primary School upon it in 1885. Immediately to the east of this the City Architect built the Corporation Baths between 1885 and 1887. Later still between 1905 and 1906 the red sandstone St Patrick's Roman Catholic School was built near the former east wing of the old Infirmary where a scarlet fever airing ground had been. By

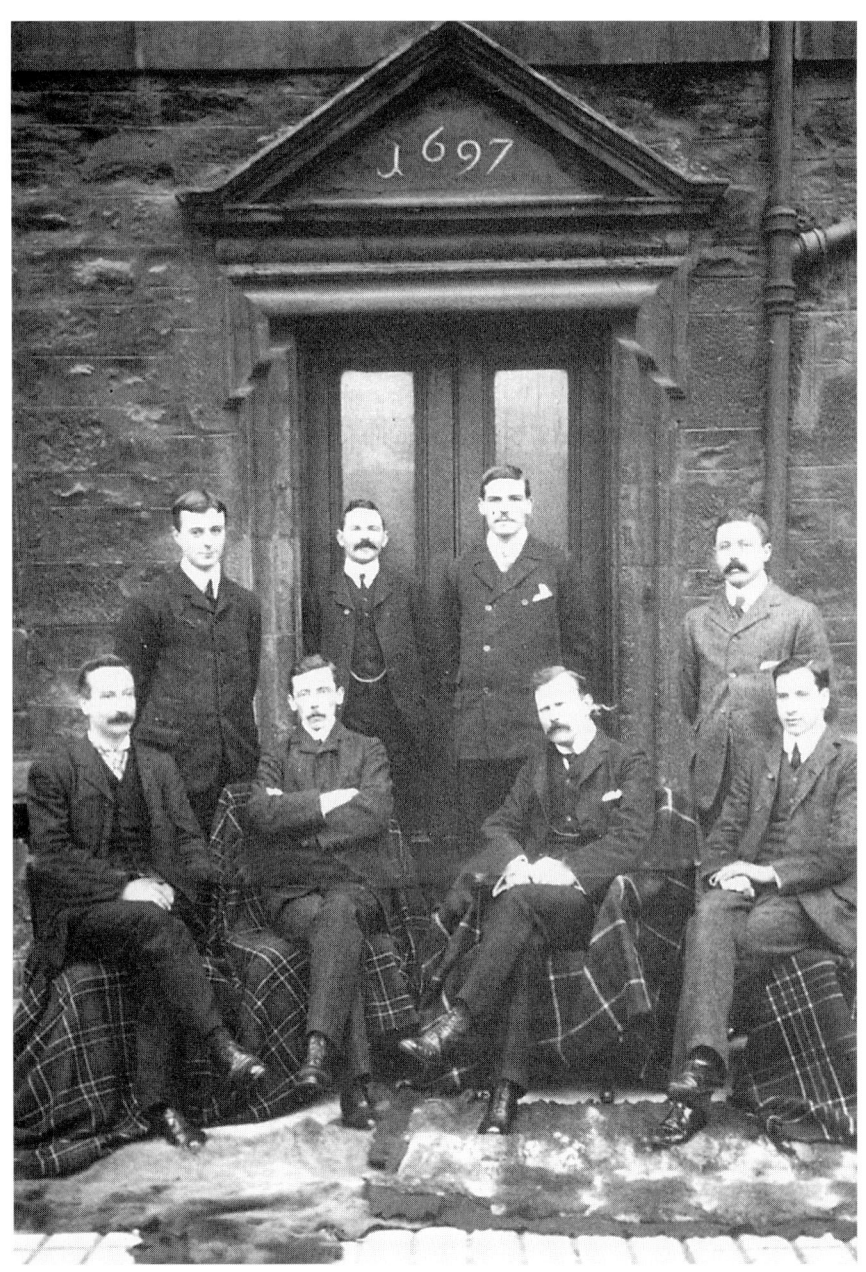

Second City Fever Hospital medical staff (ca. 1897–1903) outside old Surgeons' Hall. Standing left to right: Drs. E. C. Pritchard, D. Macrae Aitken, D. C. L. Fitzwilliam, J. G. McBride. Sitting left to right: Drs R Raeburn, J. H. Meikle, C. B. Ker, (Medical Superintendent), R. Dodds Brown. (Photo: A. Swan Watson, Bruntsfield, Edinburgh)

this time, however, the third City Hospital at Colinton Mains had been completed.

Despite the space available, the ability of the second City Hospital to cope with epidemics remained stretched. Even with the use of small fever hospitals like those at Portobello and Slateford, the contribution made by the 30 convalescent fever beds at Campie House in Musselburgh and the intermittent use of the Canongate Hospital, accommodation remained inadequate during outbreaks of infection. In the smallpox epidemic of 1894–95, temporary wooden huts were hastily erected in the Queen's (Holyrood) Park. Some alternative solution became imperative. In the meantime Sir Henry Littlejohn (knighted in 1895) and the City Fathers were planning a major expansion of the second City Hospital on the old Infirmary site as the next chapter will show.

CHAPTER NINE

The Reorganisation and Expansion of the Old Infirmary Site

The early Public Health measures introduced by Sir Henry Littlejohn to prevent and control infectious diseases were implemented by Dr William Chambers, Lord Provost from 1865 to 1869, in his Improvement Scheme. Despite this and, in 1893, a further Improvement Scheme brought in by a medical doctor, Lord Provost Sir J. A. Russell, major epidemics continued into the late nineteenth century.

Although the population was increasing, conditions for the poor had improved in terms of housing, sanitation and water supply. Bailie James Pollard, Convener of the Public Health Committee, explained how Public Health measures were having an impact.[1] In 1864 just before Littlejohn's *Report on the Sanitary Condition of the City of Edinburgh* was published, Pollard wrote that there were only 9,746 inhabited houses for a population of 161,000 (more than 16 persons per household). In 1898, by contrast, there were 60,000 inhabited houses for a population of 298,000 (fewer than 5 persons per household). Despite the increased population, the city's total annual mortality in 1898 was only a very little over that of 1864. Pollard therefore calculated that, had the 1864 slum conditions prevailed in the city until 1898, there would have been an additional annual loss of 3,200. Some progress was obviously taking place.

By 1885 Edinburgh had around 260 beds for infectious disease patients at the old Infirmary site and, from 1870 onwards, the refitted Canongate Poorhouse Hospital could accommodate about 70 smallpox or cholera patients. In the mid-1890s, even without patients, that is in a non-epidemic year, the Canongate Hospital cost £300 annually to maintain: £200 for the wages of the gatekeeper and the other servants, and £100 in repairs, furnishings and insurance.[2]

From 1889 to 1910, the 30 convalescent fever beds at Campie House were in constant use. This large house in spacious grounds was situated south of Market Street in Musselburgh. After 1910 it became a school[3] and was later demolished to make way for sheltered housing. In the 1890s, convalescent, and relatively non-infectious, patients were conveyed to Campie House by train. The Town Council's Public Health

Committee Minutes are peppered with repeated requests by the MOH, Dr Littlejohn, for the sum of £10 to cover the cost of rail fares for these patients.[4] The draft Provisional Estimates (1894–95)[5] show that the likely annual cost of maintaining Campie House would be £875, of which the Lady Superintendent's salary was £80. Before it was reopened for patients after a refit in 1891, the Lord Provost and Mrs Boyd, the Lady Superintendent, were planning a celebratory garden party in the grounds of Campie House.[6] The recovering convalescents of Campie House played golf free of charge on Musselburgh Links with the permission of Musselburgh Town Council[7] so their well-being was also being supported locally. But not even the extra accommodation in the Canongate, Portobello and Slateford Hospitals and in Campie House could obviate the building of temporary accommodation to cope with epidemics.

Dr Tait[8] describes 'Houses of Reception' that were used both for convalescent patients and for the family contacts of those infected. The local authorities commandeered private accommodation during emergencies. For instance in 1873, following a further threat of cholera, a Mrs Jones who owned lodging houses in Cowgatehead, Blackfriars Street and the Grassmarket gave permission to the Corporation to make use of these premises, although on that occasion they were eventually not required.

A formal Reception House was designated on the old Infirmary site when the second City Hospital opened there in 1885.[9] By 1905 the reception building, situated at High School Yards, could accommodate 20 persons. As late as the 1920s, long after the third City Hospital was opened, it was used for children with scabies. The building may originally have been George Heriot's Hospital School at the north east end of High School Yards at the corner of the Pleasance and the Cowgate.[10] In the 1893 Extension Plan it takes up an area labelled 'House Servants and Quarantine'. This building, later the Salvation Army's Men's Social Service Centre, was built in 1840 in the seventeenth-century style. Its arcaded ground floor which was originally a covered playground,[11] could have been adapted as an airing ground for quarantine patients. The estimated annual cost of maintaining this 'Temporary Quarantine or Reception House in Cowgate' was £200, of which £100 was for wages of ward assistants and others, and £100 for repairs and furnishings.[12]

Much consideration was given to the welfare of the Matron, head nurses, both day and night under-nurses, as well as the ward assistants, kitchen and laundry servants on the old Infirmary site. In his Report of January 1891[13] the City Superintendent of Works, Robert Morham, planned to provide bed and dayroom accommodation for the nursing staff much further away from their wards than previously. In the north east cluster of buildings he proposed to site more nurses' bedrooms, single bedded for the head nurses and 2–3 bedded for under-nurses. A parlour for the head nurses and the bedroom and sitting room for the Matron were to be preserved. A large room in the east block was to be reassigned for a nurses' dining room with a covered way connecting the east and west blocks. The former nurses' dining room was then to become the ward assistants' and servants' dining hall. They too were to have a room furnished for their use – perhaps a common room – on the ground floor of the lecture theatre block. Mr Morham's plans, therefore, suggest that changes were being implemented to improve the comfort and well-being of staff.

Information about accommodation for the fever patients on the old Infirmary site is contained in a Report by Sir Henry Littlejohn and Robert Morham, entitled 'City Hospital Extension', dated 9 December 1893.[14] As early as 30 May 1892, the Public Health Committee had submitted to the Fever Hospital Subcommittee a remit to consider 'the suitability of the City Hospital for the satisfactory treatment of Typhus Fever and other Infectious Diseases'.[15] Jointly with the Lord Provost's Committee, they were to debate reconstruction and rebuilding of the City Hospital. The Minutes of a Public Health Committee meeting of 28 February 1893,[16] record that the MOH spoke to the Committee about the enlargement and reorganisation of the City Hospital and suggested that plans and estimates be submitted. Councillors Pollard and Mitchell Thomson with the MOH and the City Superintendent of Works were to report back.

The remit of the Fever Hospital Committee in 1893 empowered them:

> to report on – (1) The capacity of the present site and property adjoining to be acquired under the Police Act of 1893; and (2) the rental of properties over the Pleasance now proposed to be acquired for the required Hospital accommodation, the probable cost of the buildings they would recommend should be erected on this additional area, and submit a plan showing how they would propose to adapt the additional area.[17]

This was a bold and potentially expensive enterprise especially if the expansion east of the Pleasance was to be incorporated. It certainly showed that the city authorities were dissatisfied with the continuing necessity to build temporary fever accommodation each time an epidemic came along. They were determined to think big this time.

In 1893 both the Fever Hospital Committee and Public Health Committee must have echoed some of the deliberations that took place between 1864 and 1869 regarding the future of the Royal Infirmary itself and the adjacent complex of buildings. In the 1860s the structure of William Adam's Infirmary was failing and there were complaints too about the old and new Surgical Hospitals. Some advocated moving the Royal Infirmary to a new site at George Watson's Hospital between Lauriston Place and the Meadows; others recommended that a new medical hospital be built on the Royal Infirmary site to replace the old, after removing some of the buildings on the east of South Bridge opposite the Old College so as to increase the amount of light and the circulation of air. If the old site was to be retained, the complex around High School Yards should be bought, and thought given to expanding east of the Pleasance connecting a new site on St John's Hill with the old site via one or two iron bridges. This 'Battle of the Sites' was described by Dr Logan Turner[18] and even earlier by William Cowan.[19]

The Royal Infirmary moved to Lauriston in 1879, and the old Adam building was pulled down in 1884. Ten years later, however, the Public Health Committee and Fever Hospital Committee were determined, initially at least, to redevelop the old Infirmary site for the new City Hospital. Although the dream of Lauriston had long been realised by the Royal Infirmary Managers, the Town Council in the early 1890s had not even begun to dream of Colinton Mains.

So keen were the members of the Public Health Committee to get their plans right that, in their meeting on 11 April 1893, they discussed sending a deputation to visit Berlin and other continental cities to obtain information on hospital accommodation 'in the matter of the proposed additions and alterations to the City Fever Hospital'.[20] They argued whether the deputation should consist of the Medical Officer of Health, City Superintendent of Works and the Burgh Engineer or only a single representative and, if so, whom. It was decided eventually to send the Convener of the Committee and the City Superintendent to visit Berlin. Apparently not even this plan materialised. Later, however, before the decision had been made to construct an entirely new fever hospital (at Colinton Mains), Bailie James Pollard, the Convener of the Public Health Committee, was dispatched alone in September 1894 on a European fact-finding mission. He attended the International Congress on Public Health in Budapest and then visited a number of fever infirmaries on the continent. Mr Morham, the City Architect, joined Bailie Pollard later in his trip and together they inspected 'the best of the German and Danish hospitals'.[21]

The plans to upgrade the City Fever Hospital included better accommodation for the staff, the house servants and the quarantine patients. Patients in each disease category had to be segregated both in their accommodation and airing grounds and be, ideally, as far away as possible from staff living quarters. The main diseases were 'scarlet fever, measles, typhoid, typhus, erysipelas, hooping [sic] cough and diphtheria'.[22] Interestingly 'cerebrospinal meningitis' is not mentioned despite its prevalence at that time. The daily average number of patients treated in the hospital rose from 96 in 1888 to 219 in 1892.[23] Scarlet fever gave rise to the largest numbers of patients on any one day followed by typhoid fever with less than half that number.[24] The Canongate Hospital was taking smallpox cases, seven being the most on any one day in 1892 but, by 2 June 1893, 19 cases were under treatment there.[25] Many more were to come in the epidemic of 1894–95.

Today antibiotics dramatically shorten the course of most bacterial infections and, it is hoped, cure many within days. By contrast in 1893, the Consulting Physician, Dr Claud Muirhead pointed out that the length of admission for scarlet fever patients was 'on the average, eight weeks or thereby'.[26] Part of this time would have been spent convalescing in hospital. In the pre-antibiotic era this would reduce the risk of convalescent patients transmitting residual infection after being discharged home.

In 1893 there were 182 beds for scarlet fever patients. An additional 24 beds were to be provided by building an extra storey on top of the old Surgical Hospital, so increasing the number of scarlet fever beds to 206. Convalescing patients were to be separated from those at an early stage of the illness in an attempt to prevent reinfection in hospital. Measles patients were to be accommodated in the wards at the east end of the site formerly used for erysipelas and whooping cough. By adding another storey there, 70 cases of measles could be housed. Typhoid was to be managed in 30 beds in the former nurses' home. Typhus, erysipelas and whooping cough would be relocated in newly built blocks with 70 beds north of the High School Yards. Ten beds for diphtheria in a new block would complete the whole complement of 386 beds.[27]

In the alternative plan of 1893–94,[28] three wards now earmarked for typhoid, diphtheria and typhus were to be oriented on a north–south axis. The idea was to allow each ward to receive the maximum sunshine without overshadowing its neighbour, a plan Robert Morham adhered to when he designed the third City Hospital at Colinton Mains.

Accommodation for epidemics and for quarantine patients would be in the basements of the new blocks, especially those running north and south. Owing to the very steep fall of the land towards the Cowgate at the north end of these buildings, there was a lot of extra space underneath which would require extensive underpinning. As it happened, the former George Heriot's Hospital School was appropriately adapted as the Temporary Reception and Quarantine House.

In the original but not in the alternative plan, diphtheria patients

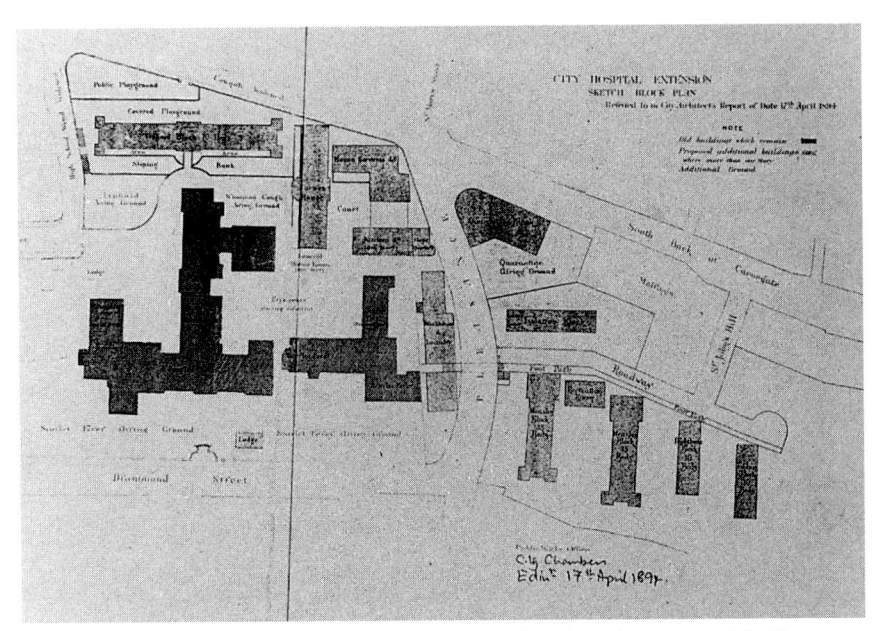

City Hospital Extension Plan, 17 April 1894, showing the proposed bridge over the Pleasance and an isolation block and wards for measles (2), diphtheria and typhus fever oriented on a north-south axis on St John's Hill. (Public Works Office. By courtesy of Edinburgh City Libraries)

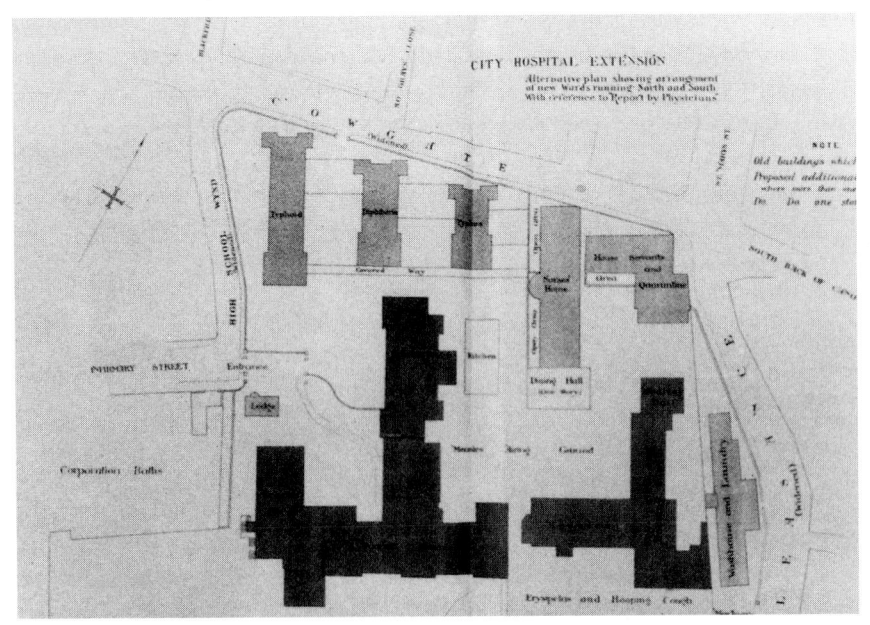

City Hospital Extension (Alternative) Plan, 10 May 1894, showing wards for typhoid, diphtheria and typhus fever to the east of High School Wynd. No extension east of the Pleasance. (Public Works Office. By courtesy of Edinburgh City Libraries)

would occupy a small 10 bedded ward squeezed into the north west corner between the Cowgate and High School Wynd. The proposed new accommodation would accommodate 386 patients as follows:[29]

Scarlet Fever	206 beds
Measles	70
Typhoid	30
Diphtheria	10
Hooping [sic] Cough, Erysipelas, Typhus, Quarantine & Emergency beds	70
	386

The airing grounds for scarlet fever, typhoid and measles were close to the relevant wards. The largest was for scarlet fever. It lay to the south west of the present Drummond Street frontage and its eastern part was for typhoid patients. In May 1893 the Public Health Committee recommended measures to prevent contact between patients and the public and also between patients with one infection and those with another. One recommendation was to construct a railing across the Drummond Street airing ground to ensure that scarlet fever and typhoid convalescents did not mix. The airing ground for measles patients, the former Surgeons' Square, was sufficiently enclosed to prevent its patients mingling with others.

The Consulting Physician, Dr Claud Muirhead, his Assistant and other medical staff were to be accommodated in the north easterly buildings, then partly occupied by nurses. The Lady Superintendent of Nurses would move from the main block to a suite with sitting room, office and bedroom in the new nurses' home. The new home would house 70 nurses and comprise:

> three flats above the general level of the Hospital Grounds and lower storey in the under buildings towards the north end so far as the levels permit; each flat consisting of a series of rooms for the Nurses, arranged on each side of a central corridor running from end to end of the building, with a staircase midway in length, and a large room opposite it on each flat, to be used as a recreation room and having at the south end a dining hall 50 feet by 30 feet.[30]

Sick rooms, linen stores, bathrooms and lavatories were to be provided at both ends of the central corridor. If separate coal fires were to heat the rooms, rather than 'steam coils', as in the Royal Infirmary nurses' home at Lauriston, a lift was to be installed, presumably to facilitate the delivery of coal. Wherever possible, staircases and corridors were to be of fire-proof construction.

The house servants were to be accommodated in the extreme north east of the site in the corner made by the Pleasance and the Cowgate, where Heriot's Hospital School had previously stood.[31] This 'Messrs. Rankine's Property', was still to be acquired. The quarantine patients would be lodged in the lower flat of this building, suggesting that here at least there was not quite so much staff–patient segregation as had at first been envisaged.

The porter's lodge, with a visitors' waiting room, would be in Infirmary Street. The outer gates were to be kept closed to prevent unwanted people entering. In June 1893, glass panels were authorised for the Infirmary Street entrance and a commissionaire was appointed at the main entrance of the hospital for a short trial period.[32]

If it was decided not to extend the hospital east of the Pleasance, the kitchen in the south west corner would remain where it was, adjacent to the scarlet fever block. If the development east of the Pleasance was to be pursued, however, the kitchen would be moved to a more central site.[33]

In both plans the wash-house and laundry occupy the buildings on the east side of the original site, just within the Flodden Wall. Should it be decided to have 'steam coil' heating in the nurses' home and hospital blocks, the boiler would be situated in the laundry area. Alternatively, Bailie Macpherson of the Public Health Committee[34] asked what would be a reasonable sum to be charged 'with respect of the motive power supplied by the Boiler at the Corporation Baths to the City Hospital Hydro Extractor and Disinfector', so it may be supposed that the new hospital might have ultimately been linked with the heating system in Robert Morham's Infirmary Street Baths, which were built between 1885 and 1887. Finally the mortuary at the south east of the original site might later be connected to the hospital blocks by a discrete subway.[35]

If the hospital buildings were to be extended eastwards across the Pleasance, various problems were envisaged besides the resiting of the hospital kitchen. First, the cost of purchasing the existing property and a further 3.25 acres of ground would be £24,284. Secondly, a communicating bridge would be needed over the Pleasance posing an engineering problem in that the ground to the east was much lower than on the original site. This bridge, with the new buildings, and the removal of the kitchen to a central position, would alone cost an additional £6,000.[36]

The Fever Hospital Subcommittee had met in October 1893 and January 1894 and asked the opinion of Dr Littlejohn, Dr Claud Muirhead, Consulting Physician, and Dr A. F. Wood, Medical Superintendent, to respond to their questions about the new plans.[37] Dr Littlejohn agreed with the overall design. Dr Muirhead suggested some alterations on the siting of different categories of patients. Dr Littlejohn and Dr Wood both felt there would be no overcrowding. Dr Muirhead would have preferred more ground space and greater cubic capacity for children but agreed that this depended on the ventilation of the wards. Questioned about the advisability or otherwise of moving elsewhere, Dr Littlejohn said 'In my opinion no better site than the present one can be got in the City or County'.[38] He also felt that emergency accommodation could be made available on the present site, but Drs Muirhead and Wood were less sure.

There seems little doubt that the Town Council intended to upgrade the old Royal Infirmary site into a modern infectious diseases hospital of about 400 beds. Dr Littlejohn himself gave the plans his blessing, saying than they would:

> afford suitable provision, in my opinion (As the Medical Adviser of the Corporation), for the next ten to fifteen years.[39]

Dr Claud Muirhead added that provision should also be made:

> for the erection of a well appointed Bacteriology Laboratory, in the neighbourhood of the Mortuary, or other convenient place.[40]

A memorandum to this effect had been submitted to the Public Health Committee in March 1893 by the Edinburgh Medico-Chirurgical Society in connection with the 'Cholera Hospital', as the building on Drummond Street was still sometimes known.

The intention to stay on the old Infirmary site was also supported by the Joint Subcommittee of the Lord Provost's and Public Health Committees. In February 1893 they decided as follows:

> The Sub Committee examined Mr Morham's plan of suggested additions to the City Hospital. The Sub-Committee are strongly of the opinion that the present site of the City Fever Hospital is the best one, and that with the acquisition of the properties at present scheduled there will be a sufficient area for a sufficiently equipped Hospital for a very long period of years.[41]

Two major objections were made by Dr Muirhead[42] regarding the alternative possibility of erecting 'on a large open isolated plain' an infectious diseases hospital 'built according to the most recent theories of hospital accommodation, and worthy of the great Edinburgh School of Medicine'. He said firstly that, as no site was available within a two mile radius of the city centre, the long journey to hospital would increase mortality, especially among very ill typhoid patients. Secondly he anticipated that the clinical teaching of infectious diseases for medical students would suffer if the fever hospital moved far out of town.

It seemed certain that the old Royal Infirmary site was where the developments would take place. In addition to the railings to separate the public from patients and patients with different infections from each other, many other upgradings continued to be made. In 1892, the use of the Drummond Street entrance by fever patients brought a complaint from a Mr W. H. Anderson, perhaps worried about the spread of infection if more than one entrance was kept open. The Public Health Committee therefore recommended in September 1893 that the Drummond Street Gate be covered with sheet iron.[43] The Infirmary Street gates remain a fine example of the work of William Adam with a concave entrance area and fluted gate piers surmounted by 'wonderfully elaborate urns carved with grotesque heads and foliaged swags'.[44] They were moved from the Infirmary Street entrance to their present Drummond Street site about 1906–07.[45]

Other upgrading procedures recommended on the old Infirmary site included the provision of urinals in the water closets, improved bathing and disinfecting areas for scarlet fever patients[46] and better drainage at the front door on Drummond Street.[47] In September 1894 a recommendation was made to renew wash-house tubs and certain baths at the City

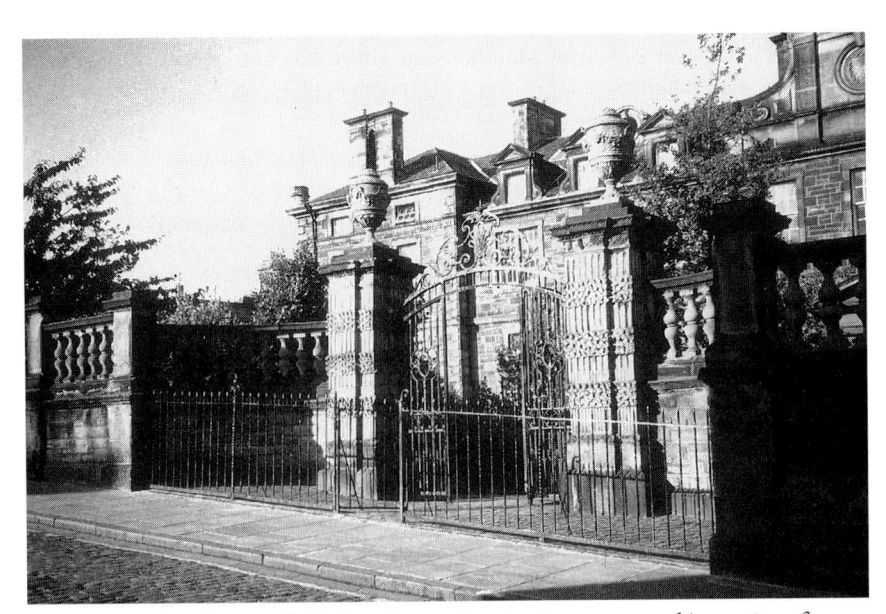

The Royal Infirmary of Edinburgh gates (1738–48) were moved in 1906–07 from Infirmary Street to Drummond Street. Behind is the new Surgical Hospital (David Bryce, 1848–53), now the University Department of Geography. (Photo: J. A. Gray)

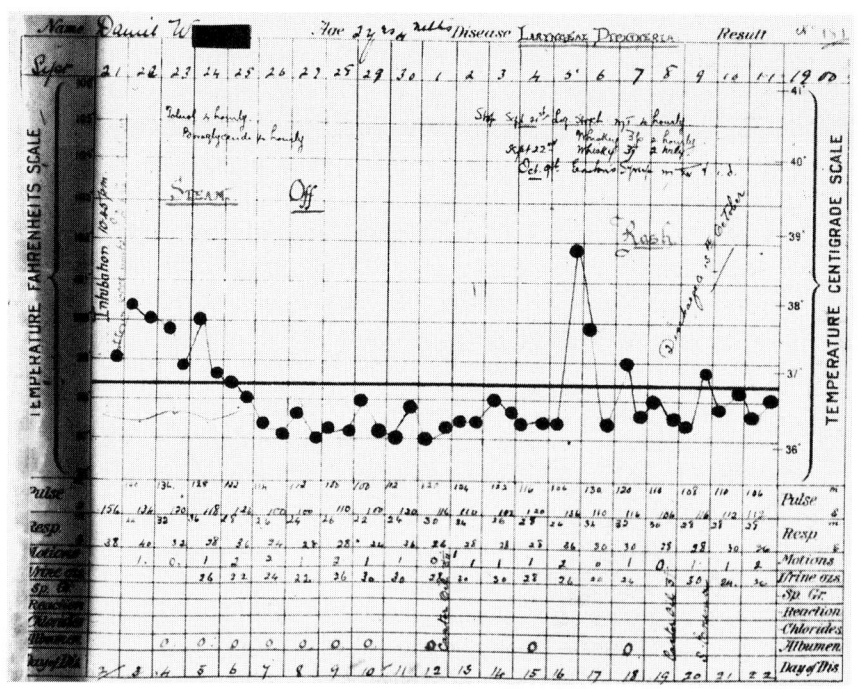

Temperature and progress chart of a boy aged 2 yr 4 mths with laryngeal diphtheria, Sept-Oct. 1900 at the second City Hospital. He was treated by immediate intubation and steam and received diphtheritic anti-toxin which caused a fever on day 16 of admission and a rash two days later. Note the use of strychnine, whisky and castor oil. (By courtesy of Lothian Health Services Archive, University of Edinburgh Library, LHB 23)

Hospital.[48] and, in November, provision for a galvanised iron lining for the railings at the west of the Drummond Street enclosure was to be costed.[49]

Owners of property adjoining the hospital, such as A. Grey & Son, enquired whether their premises would be required for the extension of the City Hospital.[50] They were told that the property was likely to be needed by Whitsunday 1894. As late as 23 February 1895, Messrs Rankine offered to sell their property at the north east corner of the site which the MOH felt might be suitable as accommodation for nurses. On 28 May 1895 a supply of 'motive power' from the Corporation Baths in Infirmary Street to the City Hospital was considered again.[51] Plans were also made the same day to convert a disused passage adjoining the hospital kitchen into a cold meat larder. Some of these improvements could be regarded as purely for maintenance but others not. All the pointers were that the old Infirmary site would continue to be the infectious diseases centre for Edinburgh.

The draft Provisional Estimates, 1894–95[52] showed that the overall annual running costs of the City Hospital amounted to £10,900. The Medical Superintendent received a salary of £300, the Visiting Physician £150, the Chaplain £100 and the Resident Medical Assistant and Registrar £50. Dr Jamieson, Visiting Physician to the City Hospital, had a salary increase to £200 recommended on 24 November 1891[53] though this may never have been implemented. The Lady Superintendent, Housekeeper, nurses, ward assistants, laundresses, cook, kitchen-maids, cleaners, gatekeeper, porter, etc. were on weekly pay amounting to a total of £2,300 per annum. In September 1896 the Public Health Committee recommended that the Lady Superintendent's salary should go up from £100 to £135,[54] but at the same time the Lady Superintendent at Campie House had her salary fixed at £60 per annum.[55] Certainly the Town Council appreciated the work done by the nursing staff even if their remuneration remained meagre. They proposed an 'At Home' in the City Chambers on 23 January 1896 at 1s 6d per head so that they could meet them.[56] This may have been in response to the extra work imposed on the nurses in the previous outbreaks of infection. On 16 October 1895 the Public Health Committee recommended an honorarium of £50 for the Resident Physician and £30 for the Lady Superintendent 'in recognition of their services in connection with the smallpox epidemic'.[57]

In addition to his many other duties as MOH, Dr Littlejohn seems to have been responsible for many aspects of daily living and working at the City Hospital. His Rules for the Hospital[58] insisted that the day and night staff were drilled by the Fire Master. This was just as well for a small fire did break out in the Quarantine Building on the Cowgate on 8 September 1894.

The Public Health Committee also asked the MOH to enquire into any grievances by patients as, for example, when a Mr Waterston complained about the treatment his wife and children received in the City Hospital.[59] One sad event on 2 January 1894, in which the MOH was again involved, related to the accidental death by poisoning of Helen Swan, one of the servants in the Hospital. It is unclear what happened to her but Dr Littlejohn recommended a solatium of £100 to her mother and £25 towards legal expenses without admitting any legal liability.[60] The Sub Committee appointed to report on the death disagreed with Dr Littlejohn, however, stating that the Night Superintendent could not be absolved from blame.[61] The eventual outcome remains obscure.

One final example of the duties of the MOH in connection with the City Hospital related to smallpox contracted by the driver of a carriage taking an infected patient to hospital. In contrast to the inevitable lengthy litigation process that would happen nowadays, Dr Littlejohn simply instructed a weekly payment of 10s to be made to support the driver's family.[62] There being no further entries in the Minutes about his illness, it must be supposed the driver survived.

This case of the carriage driver pointed to the reason why, despite all the plans to upgrade and expand the City Hospital at the old Infirmary site, this did not actually happen. In 1894 Edinburgh was in the grip of a smallpox epidemic. The acute shortage of accommodation for fever patients once again became very serious and was a catalyst for the volte-face. The old Infirmary site would not be developed after all. A new green-field site would be sought for a grand, purpose-built, third Edinburgh City Fever Hospital.

CHAPTER TEN

The Smallpox Outbreak 1892–95 and a Change of Plans

In the late summer of 1894, it had looked as if the old Infirmary site, probably including the extension east of the Pleasance, would be developed as Edinburgh's 400 bedded fever hospital. Yet there were already signs pointing to the inadequacy of this plan. Even if the new complex had been ready with 400 beds in 1894, there would still have been a major shortfall of proper accommodation.

A glance at the Notifications of Infectious Diseases, compiled by the MOH gives the explanation.[1] Figures for typhoid, diphtheria and particularly scarlet fever had risen steadily in the preceding three years. Although typhus fever was numerically not a problem in 1894, over 70 cases were to be reported in 1898. In the typical pre-immunisation pattern, measles notifications fluctuated biennially with just over 1,000 reported in 1894 but as many as 7,000 reported the next year. The problem was that on top of the scarlet fever notifications, which nearly reached 3,000 in 1895, there was an unexpected outbreak of smallpox despite Sir Henry Littlejohn's efforts to improve vaccination uptake in the city. There had been no smallpox notifications for the three years, 1889–91, then a trickle of eight began in 1892, followed by a stream of 51 in 1893 and finally a flood of 537 cases in 1894. The outbreak only came to an end in 1895 after a further 109 cases had been notified.[2]

Leith, whose port may have been the source of this smallpox outbreak, was having similar problems. During the epidemic of 1893–94, 384 patients from Leith were admitted to hospital with smallpox. Fifty died including seven children.[3] The East Pilton Fever Hospital was not due to open till 1896 and so a wooden hospital was built on Leith Links and maximum use made of various other temporary premises in Leith.[4]

In Edinburgh too, the local authorities were under great pressure during and after the smallpox outbreak to provide adequate accommodation. The Canongate Hospital was again in use. Dr Littlejohn was concerned about its furnishings and requested the Public Health Committee to have a further flat there placed at the disposal of the Medical Officer.[5] In May 1894 the City Superintendent of Works requested telephone links between the Public Health Office through the Canongate Police Station to the Canongate Hospital and also from there to the City Hospital[6] presumably to improve communication and maximise the use of the beds available in the city. The Public Health Committee agreed to receive cases of smallpox from the Royal Infirmary even 'at anytime after 8 o'clock evening'.[7] Additional mattresses were ordered from the Royal Blind Asylum to cope with the outbreak.[8] There were pleas for more accommodation and the MOH was to report directly to the Lord Provost on the progress of the outbreak.[9]

Dr Littlejohn was doing everything he could. He even encouraged free vaccination of 'poor people' between 15 June and 31 August 1894 and reimbursed 1s 6d to the dispensaries for each one carried out.[10] This offer was later extended to 15 September as the outbreak continued.

The Public Health Committee[11] authorised the use of a former Masonic Lodge in High School Yards for scarlet fever patients in the emergency. It was the continuing load of scarlet fever patients that made the superimposed smallpox outbreak so difficult to cope with. Dr Littlejohn was also to explore a site near Easter Road, which might be used as a temporary cholera hospital in the event of a cholera epidemic becoming an additional problem.[12] He introduced in August 1894 temporary notification of both 'British cholera and choleric diarrhoea'[13] for two months so there must have been a lot of gastrointestinal infection adding to his many problems. Meanwhile permission was given by the Public Health Committee[14] to use the temporary accommodation already erected in the Queen's Park if an outbreak of cholera should occur. The Minute of 11 September 1894[15] suggests that the temporary smallpox accommodation was already being used for cholera patients and was the subject of a letter (probably of complaint) from Her Majesty's Office of Works.

On 25 September 1894, Dr Littlejohn reported to the Public Health Committee on hospital accommodation for cholera.[16] After the same meeting, the proposed site for a temporary hospital for infectious diseases off Easter Road was reported on by the City Superintendent of Works. In June 1895 the MOH got the Public Health Committee to make an offer for about two acres of a field off Easter Road at a rent of £10 per acre for two years.[17] By November 1895 the Public Health Committee had received a letter from the secretary of the Local Government Board approving the proposed temporary hospital at Quarryholes off Easter Road.[18] In September 1896 the Dean of Guild Court of Leith granted permission to the Town Council of Edinburgh to erect, north east of the Eastern Cemeteries on what would now be Quarryhole Park, a temporary hospital to be used 'for the treatment of cholera cases only'.[19] This was to consist of three wooden pavilions, one covered with a roof

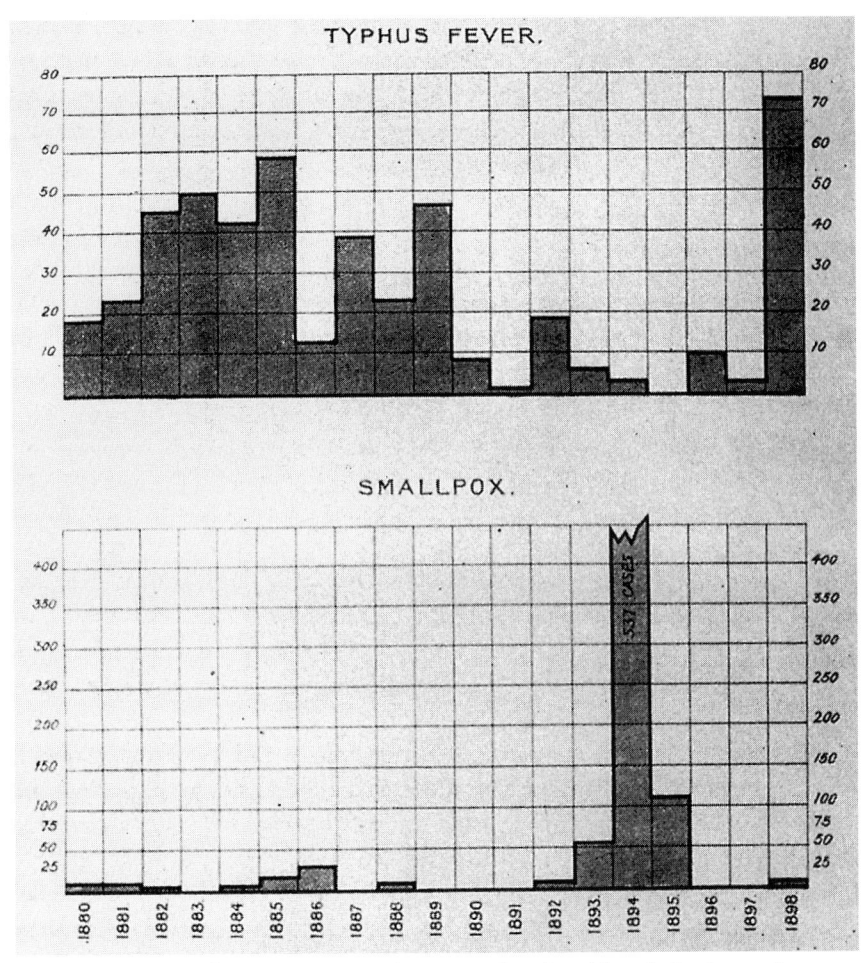

Typhus and smallpox, 1880–96. Histograms showing (above) the last major outbreak of typhus fever in 1898 and (below) the smallpox outbreak of 1892–95. The smallpox outbreak peaked in 1894 with 537 cases and demonstrated that the second City Hospital had too few beds to cope with epidemics. This ultimately led to the decision to build a new, larger hospital elsewhere. (Annual Report of the MOH, 1898. By courtesy of Edinburgh City Libraries)

of felt, the other two with corrugated iron roofs, a small gate lodge at the entrance and an incinerator with a chimney 50 feet high, not of 30 feet as originally designed. The incinerator, moreover, was to be enclosed in corrugated iron and have a covered way extending between it and the pavilions. The whole area was to be surrounded on the north west, north east and south east sides with 'a fence of close boarding' presumably to prevent cholera patients getting out or the uninfected populace getting in by the back door.[20]

It is unclear whether this hospital was ever constructed or used. Events were moving fast elsewhere and, as it happened, the cholera problem diminished. Nonetheless the Public Health Committee must have viewed the matter urgently as they were considering building estimates for the Quarryholes Hospital at their meeting on 1 September 1896,[21] seven days before the Act & Warrant was minuted by the Town Council. For the builder work, John Lownie (of whom more later) tendered £1,989 for day work or £2,100 for working day and night and for the plumber work, Barton & Son tendered respectively £240 and £260.[22] The Public Health Committee must have been anxious to have the hospital built and in use very quickly or they would not have invited these more expensive tenders for working round the clock.

The MOH, now Sir Henry Littlejohn, reported an outbreak of measles at Portobello and told the Public Health Committee that he proposed opening a hospital there.[23] This presumably did function then for a further Minute of that Committee on 4 May 1897 actually comments on the furnishings for that temporary hospital with 40–60 beds.[24] It was situated at Duddingston Yards immediately north of the Niddrie Burn and west of what became Duddingston Park. Every effort was therefore being made in the later 1890s to find additional accommodation even though by that stage the smallpox epidemic was over.

In the meantime the Public Health Committee and the Town Council must have been smarting under the barrage of criticism regarding the way the smallpox outbreak of 1892–95 had been handled. Mention has already been made of the Canongate (Poorhouse) Hospital and the Houses of Reception and Quarantine that were pressed into use to cope with the epidemic. Most controversial was the decision to build temporary wooden accommodation not only within the grounds of the City Hospital itself, but also in the Queen's Park. In June 1894 the Public Health Committee heard a report by the City Superintendent of Works about the erection of a temporary ward for smallpox patients in the playground between High School Yards and the Cowgate. So urgently was this accommodation required that the Committee did 'approve and grant authority' regarding the furnishings and 'especially to have cots supplied without estimates'.[25]

Only the next month the Public Health Committee was to hear letters of complaint from a Mr Daniel Donworth of Lutton Place and from the Secretary of the Irish National League of Great Britain (W. E. Gladstone Branch) regarding the erection of the temporary smallpox hospital in the Cowgate.[26] The ratepayers of St Giles' Ward also petitioned for its removal.[27] In the meeting of 24 October 1894, the Public Health Committee heard that the timber wards had been shifted from the

Cowgate side of the City Hospital area southwards to the Drummond Street side.[28] In the interim it seems that the Canongate Hospital was not to receive new cases of smallpox[29] and it was later ordered to be thoroughly cleansed.[30]

The temporary accommodation in the Queen's Park also came in for much criticism. Perhaps with the Canongate Hospital being less used, or more difficult for staff to terminally disinfect after use, and with the ongoing controversy over the wooden buildings on the City Hospital site itself, it was felt necessary to build in the Queen's Park. On 19 June 1894 during the height of the smallpox epidemic, the Public Health Committee authorised:

> if the Office of Works grants sanctions, provision for treatment of the whole cases occurring in the City in the Park and remit to Convener powers to instruct City Superintendent to take immediate steps for the erection of the temporary buildings.[31]

A 'letter from HW Primrose, HM Office of Works, London as to the temporary Hospital in Holyrood Park' was remitted to the Fever Hospital Subcommittee by the Public Health Committee and representation was made by the City Superintendent of Works about the temporary hospitals in the Cowgate and in the Park.[32] He was 'to report as to what may be got for the wood ...'[33] suggesting that, if not burnt, the timber of any buildings not used might be recycled when the epidemic was over.

In the meantime the Town Council expressed confidence in the way the Public Health Committee had handled the smallpox outbreak so far. This was despite a letter being:

> presented from the Chairman of a Public Meeting of Citizens held in the Literary Institute intimating that a deputation would wait upon the Town Council to present a resolution passed at the meeting, and a protest in reference to the proposed Smallpox Hospital in the Queen's Park.[34]

On 27 November 1894 the Public Health Committee not only approved of the Convener's action in opening the hospital in the Park in the emergency and of the expenses incurred, but also authorised the erection of further wards.[35] This brought about another complaint this time from the 'agents of the Lessee of Pasture in Queen's Park ...'.[36]

There were problems too with the builders of the temporary accommodation in the Park. The Public Health Committee learnt on 11 December 1894 that 'works specified at Hospital did not fall under Mr Lownie's jobbing contract.'[37] It will be recalled that John Lownie, Builder of Gilmore Park, was to tender for the temporary hospital at Quarryholes

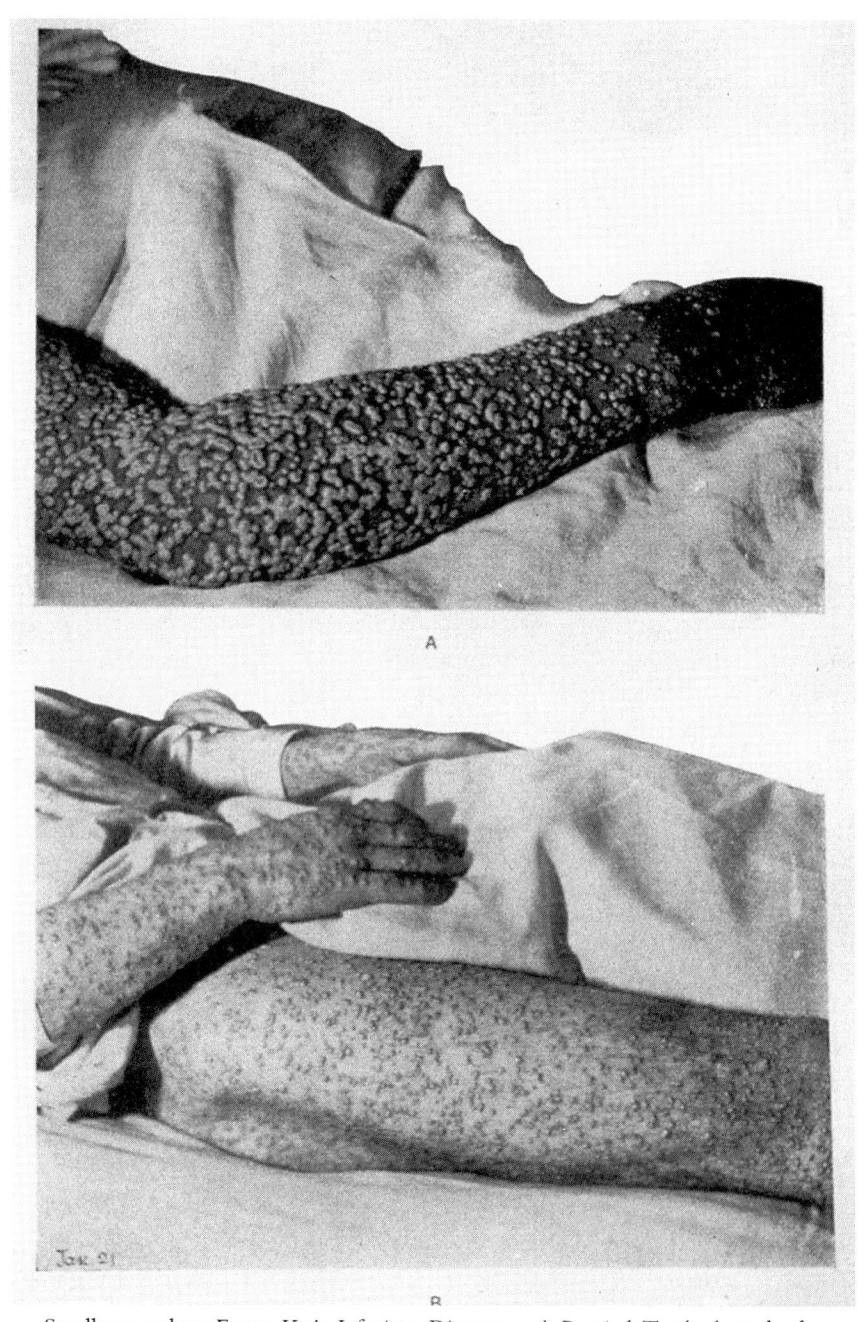

Smallpox rashes, From *Ker's Infectious Diseases – A Practical Textbook*, 3rd edn., C. B. Ker, Revised by Claude Rundle, 1929, p. 160. (By permission of Oxford University Press)

in 1896 and later still, but more significantly, he tendered for most of the mason work at Colinton Mains Hospital. Mr Lownie now complained that some of the work was being given to another contractor.

This could have meant a lucky escape for Mr Lownie's builders for, in January 1895,[38] the Public Health Committee declined to provide an allowance 'in respect of workmen engaged at St. Leonard's Smallpox Hospital having contracted that disease'. Two heating engineers belonging to Messrs D. Lowe & Sons as well as workmen for Colin Macandrew, Builder, and Ness & Barton & Sons were similarly affected. It is not recorded whether they contracted smallpox on the site or as part of the city epidemic nor is it recorded whether they survived. Colin Macandrew, Barton & Sons, Plumbers, and Lowe & Sons, Heating Engineers, had their tenders accepted in November 1895 for the re-erection, at Colinton Mains, of that part of the Queen's Park temporary smallpox hospital that had not been used and was not to be burnt down. It must therefore be supposed that the workmen all survived or, alternatively, that their firms were gluttons for punishment.[39]

As the smallpox epidemic subsided in 1895 an assessment had to be made of the permanent and temporary accommodation available for fever patients. The Canongate Hospital was to be reopened, this time prompting a letter of complaint from the Secretary of the Canongate Ward Advanced Liberal Committee,[40] whilst consideration was being given simultaneously to closing the temporary hospital in the Queen's Park. Indeed a letter from the Secretary of HM Office of Works was received by the Public Health Committee in May 1895 intimating that the First Commissions thought it desirable that the Queen's Park Hospital be removed as soon as possible.[41] The Town Clerk replied that, as the epidemic was subsiding, the buildings would be removed 'at a very early date'. In August 1895, as nothing had happened, a Mr A. H. Morham wrote to the Public Health Committee asking for the Queen's Park Hospital to be removed immediately. Again the Town Clerk was instructed to say it would be 'at earliest possible moment'.[42] In October 1895, with pressure on accommodation still present, now more from scarlet fever patients than those with smallpox, the MOH persuaded the Public Health Committee to use the Canongate Hospital again, this time for scarlet fever.[43] They decided definitely to remove the unused wooden buildings from the Queen's Park and in November 1895 to re-erect them at Colinton Mains Farm.[44] The remainder were to be burnt.

Some timber accommodation, however, still remained at the old Infirmary site in 1895. That autumn the Public Health Committee discussed the heating of the wooden wards in Drummond Street[45] and the painting of their exterior.[46] It is likely that these wards were being kept serviceable in case of another epidemic. No one was taking the chance of being caught out again.

Yet the view was being expressed during the smallpox outbreak that even an upgraded City Hospital on the old Infirmary site might not cope. Besides there was obvious dissatisfaction with the need to use temporary accommodation so often. A change of plan was formulated. Those who had previously been so enthusiastic about expanding the City Hospital at the old Infirmary site, including Sir Henry Littlejohn himself, now embraced the concept of building a brand new fever hospital on a green-field site. The next chapter will explore how this came about.

PART THREE

The Planning, Building and Opening of the Third City Fever Hospital, 1894–1903

CHAPTER ELEVEN

Choosing a Site for the Third City Fever Hospital

Bailie Pollard, Convener of the Public Health Committee, wrote that between 1885 and 1893 the general public had become increasingly confident in the City Hospital. Paternalistically he declared that:

> Prominent Citizens in whose homes fever in one form or another has broken out did not hesitate to use the hospital, and thus a wholesome example was given to all classes of people.[1]

The old Infirmary site was well situated within the city yet close to the Queen's Park and it had excellent drainage. Despite its old fashioned buildings and its proximity to an 'inferior class of property', the hospital had never caused infection to its neighbours, 'the poorest in the city'.[2]

Yet the Town Council also noted, with dismay, that the annual cost of running the hospital had quadrupled between 1885 and 1893.[3] Moreover the Council and its hard working Public Health Committee were constantly criticised because of the unpopular, wooden wards that had to be built in response to epidemics both within the hospital grounds and in the Queen's Park.[4]

No sooner had Robert Morham's plans to expand and modernise the old Infirmary site received general approval than an alternative scheme was being considered, namely to build a new hospital on a green-field site. Even with the proposed 400 beds at the old Infirmary site, the use of the Canongate Hospital, the measles hospital in Portobello, Campie House in Musselburgh and the proposed cholera hospital at Quarryholes, the despised temporary wards would still be necessary during future epidemics. The whole fever hospital service was scattered, disjointed, and inefficient. Bailie Pollard, therefore, wrote on 14 May 1894 to the Royal College of Physicians of Edinburgh asking for advice 'On the subject of the site, that is whether we should extend the present site or build a new hospital in the suburbs'.[5] They felt the two important considerations were 'the proper treatment and cure of the patients entrusted to us and ... the usefulness of the Hospital to the Edinburgh Medical School'. At an Extraordinary Meeting of the College on 28 May

1894 only one of the Fellows, Dr Claud Muirhead, also Consulting Physician to the City Hospital, was in favour of keeping and expanding on the existing site; others felt a new hospital in the suburbs would be advantageous. It was then decided to form a committee with Dr David J. Brakenridge as convener to report back as soon as possible.[6]

The 'Report by the Committee of the College on the New City Hospital Site' was presented to the College on 7 August 1894.[7] It objected to the proposed extension of the existing City Hospital site for several reasons: the much lower level of the ground to be acquired east of the Pleasance, the inadequate size of the proposed site (8 acres) and its awkward shape which would not allow a proper arrangement of buildings. The connecting bridge over the Pleasance 'in the opinion of the committee would be highly objectionable'. Finally, the proximity of large buildings connected with breweries both north and south of the site was considered most undesirable.

As the East Pilton Hospital proposed for Leith's fever patients might also eventually serve the population of north Edinburgh, a site on the south side of the City seemed most appropriate for the new hospital. The Report therefore suggested firstly a 17 acre site in the south Grange including the Craigmount Cricket Field (later the ground of the Carlton Cricket Club) together with the large house 'South Park', and the whole of Grange Terrace. Their second choice was a 30-acre site, now Craigmillar Park Golf Club, on the east slope of Blackford Hill and south of the road leading from the Harrison Arch to the Blackford Hill Observatories. The Committee preferred the first site as it was closer to the Medical School, and for the same reason, rejected the alternative sites in Morningside and on Corstorphine Hill.

The Report opposed the suggestion that, if a new green-field site was selected, typhoid fever patients should still be managed at the existing City Hospital. Dr Claud Muirhead again expressed his grave concern about typhoid victims being transported to a hospital so far away but his recommendation to keep some wards available at Drummond Street for enteric fever was overruled.[8] Dr Muirhead was little consoled to hear that the journey time for patients was steadily decreasing as ambulance transport was improving.

Why did the Town Council not choose south Grange or Blackford Hill? It may have been because of Lord Provost, Sir Andrew McDonald. At the meeting of the Town Council on 21 May 1895 he moved:

> that it be remitted to the Lord Provost's Committee to consider and report as to the expediency of the acquisition by the Corporation of one of the Poorhouses for a City Hospital.[9]

Choosing a Site for the Hospital

One of those considered was the Craiglockhart Poorhouse, later known as Greenlea Old People's Home and now The Steils. It had opened in 1870 to replace the old Charity Workhouse at Bristo Port.[10] Whilst the Lord Provost's Committee were investigating this possibility, they quickly appreciated the potential of the farm land immediately south of Craiglockhart Poorhouse for their new hospital, in preference to developing the Poorhouse itself.

From then on events moved fast. Less than a month after the Lord Provost's Committee took on the task of finding a site, the Magistrates and Council suspended the standing orders at their meeting on 18 June 1895 to adopt a motion by the Lord Provost. This read:

> that it be remitted to the Public Health Committee to consider the suitability of the Grounds adjoining the Craiglockhart Poorhouse, and belonging to the City Parish Council, as a site for a new City Hospital, with powers to employ experts, and if so advised, to negotiate with the Parish Council and complete a provisional agreement for the acquisition of a sufficient portion of the property, at a price to be fixed by arbiters mutually chosen.[11]

In September 1895 the Public Health Committee presented the Town Council with their findings on the advisability of purchasing Colinton Mains Farm, backed up by reports from the MOH, Sir Henry Littlejohn, the City Superintendent of Works, Robert Morham and Burgh Engineer, John Cooper.[12] The whole estate of 131½ acres largely comprised the farm of Colinton Mains, then on lease to Messrs John Lockhart, senior and junior, 4 acres feued to a Mr Beatson and 1½ acres feued to the Water Trust. Both the smaller feus lay to the west of the site proposed for the actual hospital buildings but there was a clause in Mr Beatson's agreement that no buildings except separate dwelling houses or villas were to be erected within 100 yards of his property.

If the Town Council became proprietors of the whole estate they would receive an income of £606 0s 0d per annum from the lease of the farm and the feu duties on the other two properties less £57 12s 9d, being the average public parochial and local burdens and property tax, leaving a net income of £548 7s 3d. Although there was a 19-year lease on the farm itself, the proprietors could at any time take off and resume possession of land for any purpose, including building, at an abatement of rent of £4 6s 0d per acre per annum plus a further £4 6s 0d per acre to compensate the tenant for land profits – a total £8 12s 0d per acre. On resumption the proprietors would have to pay compensation for the 'value of any growing crop injured by them or unexhausted manure'.[13]

The MOH[14] favoured putting the new hospital on the fields immediately to the south of the Craiglockhart Poorhouse because of their elevated situation and excellent drainage. Water supply was no problem. He countered the argument that the proposed site lay outside the city boundary by emphasising that no suitable site was available within the boundary. Besides the distance was never more 3½ miles as the crow flies from the furthest patient catchment areas such as London Road and Leith Walk. Unlike Dr Claud Muirhead, he did not expect any risk to patients being conveyed these long distances. He felt that the size of the site would permit ample airing grounds, separation of different classes of infectious patients and satisfactory temporary accommodation in times of epidemics.

Mr Morham, City Superintendent of Works, in his Report[15] also favoured building on the 30 acres in the north east of the farm. This would be sunny and sheltered to some extent by the Wester and Easter Craiglockhart Hills to the north and the Braid and Blackford Hills to the east. The site was between 350 and 400 feet above sea level. Although at the time covered with crops, he considered that the subsoil consisting of sand and clay would not hinder proper building.

Mr Morham also commented on access, favouring a new roadway (later Greenbank Drive) to connect the new hospital with Comiston Road, rather than using the old Poorhouse Road, most of which lay immediately to the south of and parallel to the Craiglockhart Burn. He considered the Poorhouse Road too narrow and too close to domestic property to be suitable for conveying infectious patients and yet much of the Greenbank Drive eventually lay only a few yards south of the Poorhouse Road. To the west he proposed widening Greenbank Farm Road and establishing it as a right of way. The slope of ground on the hospital site was sufficiently gentle to the south as not to require much underpinning of buildings. The drainage, water and gas supplies would not cause any problems. Overall he was delighted with the prospect, regarding:

> an elevated site on a gentle slope and on dry soil, where the free circulation of the air about the hospital buildings was not interfered with, and where an abundant and wholesome water supply with reasonable facilities for drainage were available, as having distinct advantages over sites differently circumstanced.

Finally Mr Cooper, Burgh Engineer, reported on the outfall drainage of the proposed site.[16] This seemed relatively simple bearing in mind the elevated situation of the site and the two natural drainage channels: the Craiglockhart Burn to the north and, to the south, the Braid Burn which carried nearly all the drainage off the agricultural land. There was currently a proposal to extend the city boundary southwards and the

Burgh Engineer pointed out that, as soon as one house was erected within that area, it became the responsibility of the city authorities to provide outlet drainage. Feuing could not be granted without this and to provide an outfall drain to receive the sewage of a wide suburban district as proposed would mean connecting the area of Colinton Mains Farm to Cameron Bank on Dalkeith Road, a distance of 5,350 yards and at a cost of £12,000. Mr Cooper felt such an expense was out of the question.

The farm stood at 358 feet above sea level and the site selected for the hospital at 368 feet – a difference of 10 feet which Mr Cooper could exploit by running a private drainpipe of fire clay, 10–12 inches in diameter, solidly encased in concrete, 1,100 yards eastward to join the public sewer on Comiston Road. This would cost £1,000, or £1,200 if much rock cutting was required. An automatic flush tank at the top of the system would make the hospital drain self-cleansing. Mr Cooper had felt that joining the City Hospital drainage to the Craiglockhart Poorhouse drain would raise objections by the parish authorities. Besides, the drain, which ran along Craiglockhart Burn Valley, was too close to dwelling homes anyway and was not in good condition.

Bailie Pollard reminded the Town Council that if it offered before 31 October 1895, the whole estate could be obtained for £20,500 together with Mr Beetson's and the Water Trust's feus.[17] The alternative was to purchase only the 30 acres actually needed for the hospital buildings at a price not exceeding £20 per acre, or a capital sum of £15,000. The Town Council's Minutes of their meeting of 17 September 1895 record:

> After full consideration, the Committee, on the motion of the Convener, seconded by Councillor Mitchell Thomson, unanimously resolved to recommend the Magistrates and Council to purchase the whole subjects, in terms of the option, at the price of £20,500, with entry at Martinmas first. Signed James Pollard, B., C.[18]

The Town Council Records go on 'The Magistrates and Council approved the foregoing Report, and resolved as therein recommended'.[19]

It had only been just over a year before that the Council had approved the upgrading and extension of the City Fever Hospital at the old Royal Infirmary site with all the constraints which that cramped, uneven and awkwardly shaped area would have imposed on any new developments. There was after all a silver lining to the smallpox outbreak cloud of 1894. The Town Council now had the opportunity to plan an ambitious, modern hospital for infectious diseases at Colinton Mains Farm. The three men most involved in this project are described next.

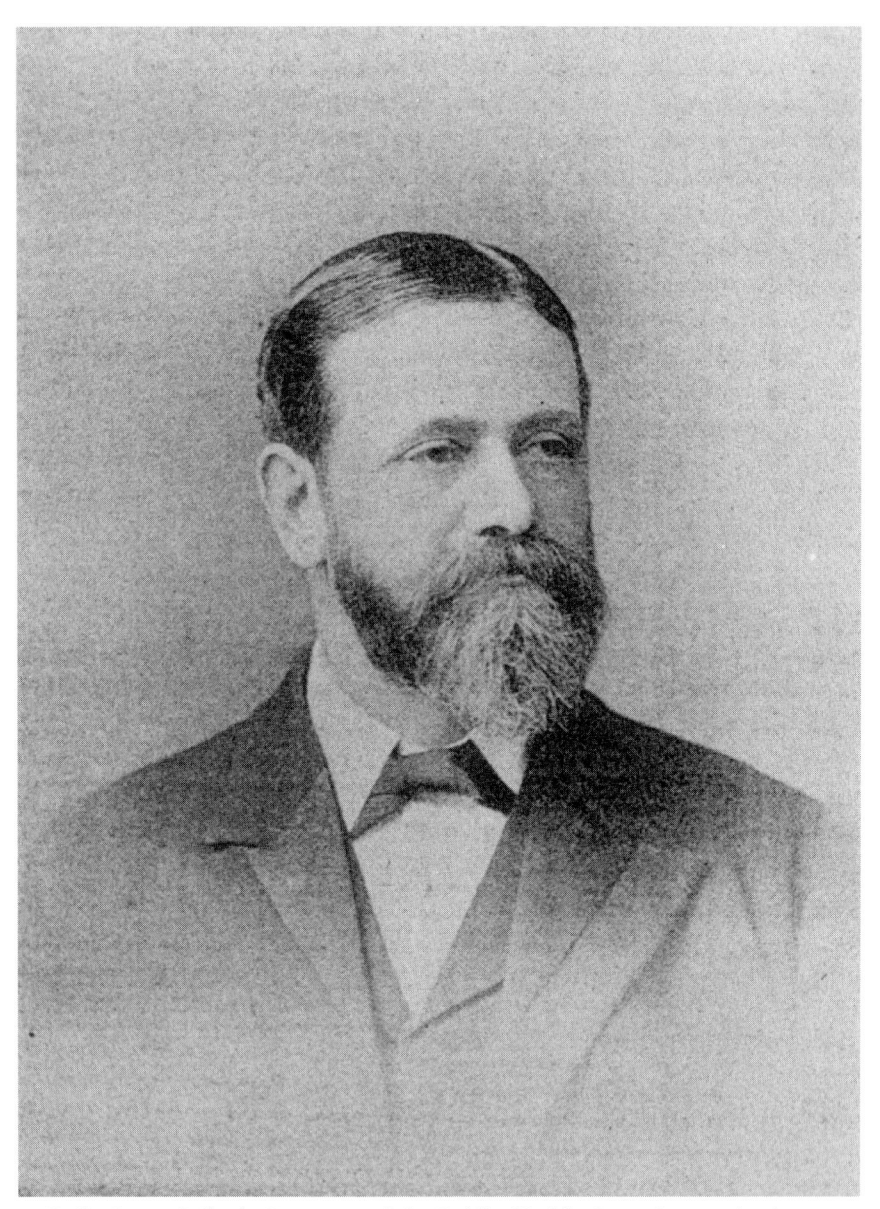

Bailie James Pollard, Convener of the Public Health Committee and prime figure in the planning of the third City Hospital. From *Men of the Period – Scotland: the Records of a Great Country*, p. 80, London, ca. 1895. (By kind permission of the Trustees of the National Library of Scotland, NLS:Biog. D.5.I. M)

CHAPTER TWELVE

The Bailie, the Architect and the Builder

Once the decision had been taken to build the new hospital at Colinton Mains, the MOH gave the project every encouragement. Besides Sir Henry, three other men had important roles to play in the construction of the hospital. They were Bailie James Pollard, Convener of the Public Health Committee, Robert Morham, City Architect and Superintendent of Works, and John Lownie, the Edinburgh Public Works Contractor. Dr Claude B. Ker, successor to Dr A. F. Wood as the Superintendent of the City Hospital, was also much consulted.

Two biographical sketches outline the career of Bailie James Pollard.[1] He was born in Dublin in 1845 but spent almost all his life in Edinburgh. His boyhood was a struggle as his parents died when he was young and his own health was poor. He attended Heriot Watt College but was otherwise largely self-educated. By the age of 17 he entered the firm of John Scott Moncrieff and Thomson, chartered accountants (CAs), with whom he stayed for 12 years. Both James and later his brother, William, served their indentures with the firm. James qualified CA in 1873 and, after three years in accountancy practice, he took in his brother to form the successful firm, James and William Pollard, CA.

In 1883, whilst keeping the business going, James entered public life joining the Edinburgh Town Council as member for the Calton ward. He was so popular with his constituents that, when he retired from the Council six years later, they persuaded him to re-enter local politics. He became Convener of the Public Health Committee in 1891 and a Bailie in 1894 and was influential in the planning of Colinton Mains Hospital. In 1888 he was a member of the Commission for Peace for the County and City of Edinburgh and wrote a treatise on the Municipality of Berlin for he regarded Berlin's internal government as an ideal model. In the 1880s he was a keen debater and often attended the Parliamentary Debating Society which met in Queen Street Hall. In politics he was a liberal. He was a member and elder of the Free Church of Scotland and member of that church's General Assembly. As the Secretary of the Edinburgh Chamber of Commerce and Manufacturers he played an important part in both local and national affairs. He encouraged the Town Council to buy the Edinburgh and Leith Gas Light Companies which resulted in an improvement to the public supply and a reduction in the price of gas. Somehow or other he also managed to be a Fellow of the Royal Statistical Society of London and the British Economic Association and served on the Council of the Geographical Society of Scotland. He was made a Governor of George Heriot's Hospital in 1883 and served again from 1892 until his death in 1901.[2]

As convener of the Public Health Committee, Bailie Pollard contributed immensely to the benefit of Edinburgh. He persuaded the Town Council to buy Campie House, Musselburgh, whose 40 beds were used between 1889 and 1910 for convalescent fever patients,[3] so relieving some of the pressure on infectious diseases beds in Edinburgh. Like Sir Henry Littlejohn, Bailie Pollard had originally favoured the redevelopment of the old Infirmary site for the new City Fever Hospital. In the mid-1890s, however, persuaded that an entirely new site was to be preferred, he worked tirelessly to achieve this and encouraged the Town Council to purchase Colinton Mains Farm.

In 1894 Bailie Pollard toured continental fever hospitals with the City Architect, Robert Morham, and so became well informed on the latest designs. It is a tribute to the joint work of James Pollard and Robert Morham that the final building was so successful. In May 1897 Bailie Pollard must have enjoyed watching Lady Provost McDonald 'breaking ground' to inaugurate the building programme at Colinton Mains. Sadly, however, Bailie Pollard died on 26 September 1901, so he saw neither the Royal Opening in 1903 nor the completion of the work to which he had devoted so much time and energy. Overall his contribution to the city's health and welfare was immense.

Robert Morham is rightly given credit for his enlightened plans for the new City Hospital at Colinton Mains and he also deserves recognition for battling with considerable difficulties during the six long years it took for those plans to materialise. His biographical sketch appears appropriately beside that of Bailie Pollard in C. J. Smith's *Historic South Edinburgh*.[4] Miss P. A. Morham, his granddaughter, has also kindly supplied information.[5] The City Architect's grandfather, Robert Morham (1778–1868), was a butcher in Edinburgh. His first wife, Jane Edmonstone, died in 1819. Their eldest child was another Robert (1812–89) who became Deputy City Clerk. He married Janet Aird in 1836. Of their six children, the second eldest was yet another Robert Morham (1839–1912) who became the City Architect.

This third Robert Morham was born in Edinburgh and attended successively Newington Academy, the High School of Edinburgh, the Watt Institution and School of Art, and the Board of Manufacturers' Art School. The Architectural Institute of Scotland awarded him their silver

Mr Robert Morham, City Architect and Superintendent of Works, who designed the third City Hospital. (Photo. by Hyman Davis, Edinburgh. By courtesy of Miss P. A. Morham)

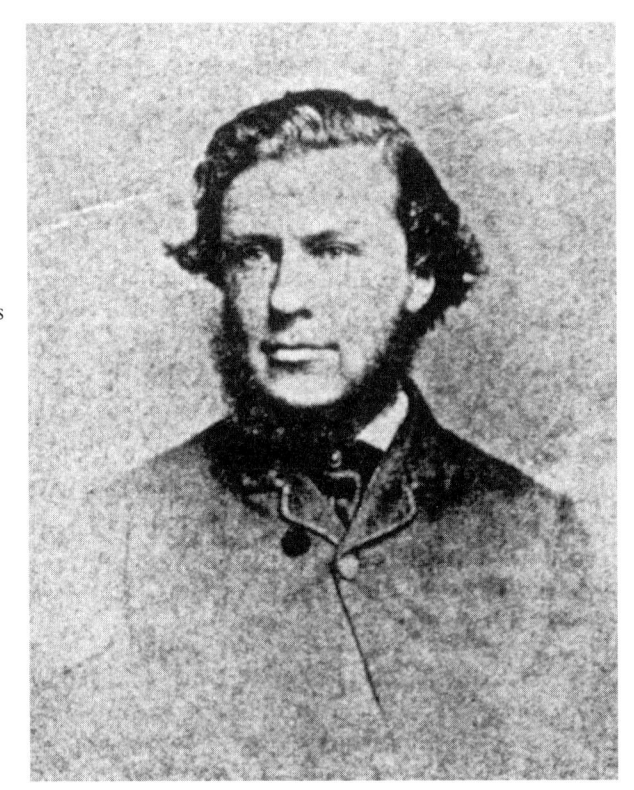

medal for the best perspective drawings of an architectural subject during the 1857–58 session. He was first apprenticed to architect David Rhind for five years and then to David Bryce for three years. David Bryce was the architect of the new Surgical Hospital which opened in Drummond Street in 1853 and, between 1872 and 1879 with his nephew John, he designed the Royal Infirmary at Lauriston Place. After his apprenticeships Robert Morham worked in London for W. E. Nesfield and returned to Edinburgh in 1866 to be assistant and then partner to David Cousin, City Architect and Superintendent of Works. When Mr Cousin retired in 1873, Robert Morham succeeded him as the City Architect.

Although still entitled to conduct private architectural practice, Morham, worked exclusively for the Corporation. As the City Architect he was responsible for the first Waverley Market and various other city markets, four swimming baths, including those at Infirmary Street, five police stations, several public wash-houses, the Fire Station at Lauriston Place, a bridge over the Water of Leith and Marchmont St Giles Church on Kilgraston Road. He made additions to several other public buildings and designed the layout of four public parks.

His greatest achievement, however, was to design Colinton Mains

Fever Hospital and to see the whole enterprise completed between 1897 and 1903. He had joined Bailie Pollard in September 1894 and they both inspected modern Scandinavian and European fever hospitals, when they were seeking inspiration for improvements to the second City Hospital at the old Infirmary site.

Ideas obtained during this trip were incorporated into his plans for redeveloping the second City Hospital site where several of the new pavilions were to be oriented on a north–south axis so as to obtain the maximum of sunshine. At Colinton Mains he employed the same principle for all the pavilions whose south-facing balconies remain efficient sun-traps. Following the lines of continental fever hospitals also, the interconnecting roofed corridors at Colinton Mains were left open-sided to encourage the maximum circulation of air. The whole was to be finished in lovely red Dumfriesshire sandstone in the same style as the Central Fire Station at Lauriston Place. This gave a warmth and intimacy to the structure which might otherwise have followed the typically austere architectural style of contemporary civic and public buildings.

Robert Morham's Building Specification[6] for Colinton Mains Hospital is extraordinarily meticulous. He could certainly envisage the whole plan but his insistence on having every detail so exactly right may have irritated others, notably John Lownie, the builder. Although the builder later accused Mr Morham of altering the Building Specification, making delays in the works schedule inevitable, there were also faults on Mr Lownie's side in failing to have materials readily available for the workmen to use. The differences that sadly arose between the two men are detailed later. Mr Morham was presented to the King at the Royal Opening of the hospital on 13 May 1903 but it is doubtful if Mr Lownie was even invited.

Mr Morham was also a family man. In 1873 he married Anne Isabella Cunningham, a surgeon's daughter, and they had five sons and a daughter. Latterly they lived in No. 13 Lauder Road, where Robert Morham, the Architect, died in June 1912 having had the satisfaction of seeing his great work, the Edinburgh City Fever Hospital, operating successfully for the first nine years of its existence.

A biographical sketch of John Lownie, the building contractor for most of the work at Colinton Mains, appears in *Men of the Period*[7] which was probably published about 1895 well before the completion of the hospital. The Honourable Judge Ralph Lownie has kindly supplied details about his family.[8] He is a grandson of John Lownie who built the hospital and the only one of his generation to work for the family firm before it was wound up on the death of his uncle in 1946. As a boy in 1932, Judge Lownie found himself as a patient in the hospital his

Mr John Lownie, Builder of Gilmore Park, who was awarded the major building contracts for the third City Hospital. From *Men of the Period – Scotland: the Records of a Great Country*, p. 86, London, ca. 1895. (By kind permission of the Trustees of the National Library of Scotland, NLS:Biog. D.5.I.M)

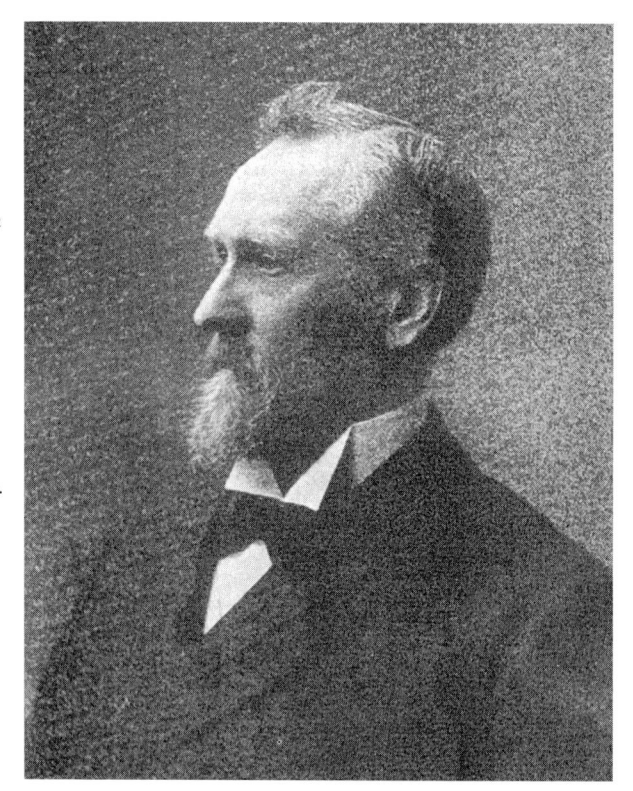

grandfather built. He can still recall being incarcerated for weeks in one of the scarlet fever pavilions, the only solace being the lovely view southwards to the T-wood above Swanston village on the slopes of Caerketton Hill.

John Lownie was born in 1841, educated in Perthshire, and then apprenticed as a house builder and carpenter. In the 1870s he moved to Edinburgh and set up on his own in Wrights' Houses at Bruntsfield. By 1886 he had become successful and moved to Gilmore Park close to the North British Rubber Works where he had a three storey brick house, extensive sheds and yards, saw mills and steam operated engines 'all of the newest type'.[9] He became Edinburgh Public Works Contractor[10] and 'one of the foremost builders in this part of this country'.[11]

Before constructing Colinton Mains Hospital, John Lownie's major undertaking had been the masonry and joinery work of Craighouse Asylum for the Commissioners of the Edinburgh Lunatic Asylum. This opened in 1894 and cost £150,000.[12] The architect was Sydney Mitchell but the inspiration for the designs came from Dr Clouston, later Sir Thomas Clouston, after whom a clinic is still named in the Royal Edinburgh Hospital. Dr Clouston had visited modern mental institutions in the USA and Europe to get up-to-date ideas much in the same way that Bailie Pollard and Robert Morham were to visit European and Scandanivan fever hospitals in 1894 when they were planning the redevelopment of the second City Hospital.

Other works by John Lownie include Dalry and Roseburn Schools, nurses' homes for both the Royal Infirmary (Red Home of 1892) and the Royal Hospital for Sick Children, and additions to many public works. He constructed private homes and terraces, including Admiral Terrace where he and his family lived in the 1880s.[13] By the 1890s he rarely had a staff of less than 200 and frequently nearer 400.[14]

In the early 1900s, the family firm moved to offices in a tenement block they had built in Harrison Road with extensive yards along West Bryson Road. John Lownie was later assisted in the business by three of his five sons. He died in July 1920.[15]

It was unfortunate that two such eminent men as Robert Morham and John Lownie should have had so many differences of opinion during the building of Colinton Mains Hospital. The confrontation between the Town Council and the Contractor is described in Chapter 14.

CHAPTER THIRTEEN

Planning the Hospital

Following the Town Council's decision to accept the Public Health Committee's recommendation of September 1895 to purchase the whole estate of Colinton Mains Farm, the MOH, now *Sir* Henry Littlejohn, and the Architect, Mr Robert Morham, submitted a Report on 7 December 1895 on the general character of the buildings for the proposed hospital which they named 'Colinton Hospital'.[1] For each disease they favoured a distinct pavilion. The pavilions were to be well separated from each other, mostly two-storey, the lower floors being at least 4 feet above the asphalted ground underneath. There was to be no internal communication between the upper and lower wards which should be no bigger than to accommodate a number of patients easily managed by the nursing staff. The actual bed numbers in each ward were not given at this early stage. The administrative and other offices were to be separate from the wards but connected to them by open-sided, covered passages.

Largely on the ground of cost, brick buildings were preferred:

> but in view of the antipathy to brick in this country, except for the most utilitarian structures, a stone exterior would probably be, on the whole, more satisfactory.[2]

Whether brick or stone was to be used for the exterior, the internal walls were to be of brick and separated from the main walls by a 2–3 inch gap 'to aid in maintaining equality of temperature within'. In addition to the cavity walls, the ward windows were to have secondary glazing, both surely innovations in the 1890s. Fire resistant, airproof floors were to be installed throughout. To make cleaning easier, all internal surfaces were to be of non-absorbent material, re-entrant angles hollowed, salient ones rounded and in general all unnecessary projections and recesses avoided. In addition to the general heating by hot water pipes, there should also be fire places or stoves. Ventilation must be 'on the most approved principles'.

An elegant water tower was to be provided in case of any temporary interference with the water supply, to improve the water pressure on the relatively elevated site, and for use in case of a fire. Although it is

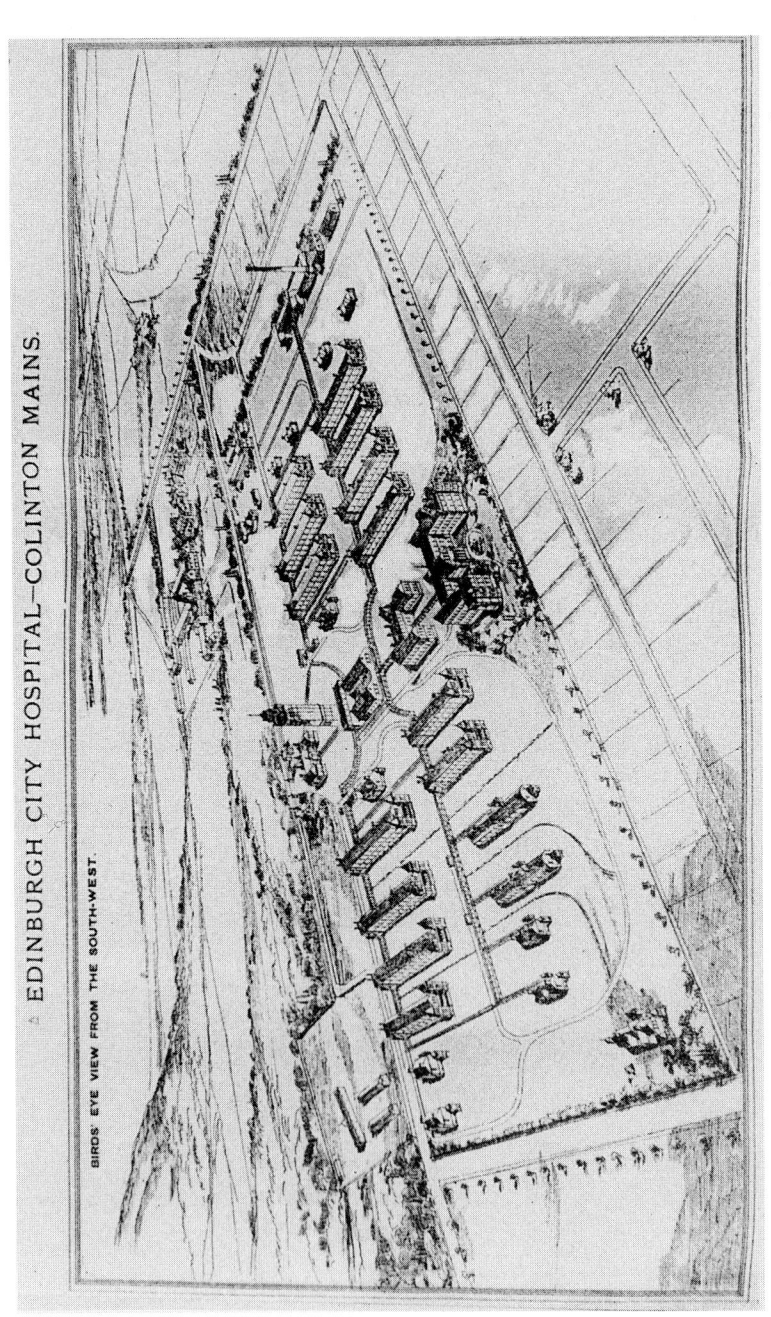

EDINBURGH CITY HOSPITAL–COLINTON MAINS.
BIRDS' EYE VIEW FROM THE SOUTH-WEST.

Bird's-eye view of Edinburgh City Hospital from the south west. The temporary smallpox hospital is at the extreme north west. Centrally is the projected water tower. Ward 22 (typhus) is in the south west corner. In the far distance is Craiglockhart Poorhouse. From Description and Sketch Plan, Public Works Office, 5 October 1896. (By courtesy of Edinburgh City Libraries) shown on the plans and drawings situated centrally in the courtyard between the general offices and the general store, it was never built. Perhaps anticipating the hugely improved water supply from the Talla Reservoir, incidentally not completed till 1905, a 100,000 gallon cistern was constructed on higher ground north west of the hospital, instead of building the water tower.[3]

Bailie Pollard had visited Budapest in September 1894 to attend the International Congress on Public Health. *En route* he visited 20 fever hospitals with bed complements from 200 up to 900. His report was not published until June 1896 and then in the form of a memorandum 'On Fever Hospitals on the Continent, with Reference to the New City Hospital about to be Erected at Colinton Mains, Edinburgh'.[4] He visited hospitals in Zurich and Innsbruck which had just been completed and he anticipated that they would incorporate some of the best designs. The isolation hospital in Basel was empty so he could not see it in working order. He was surprised to find Berne with no fever hospital at all.

Bailie Pollard congratulated the Hungarians in Budapest on making great progress in sanitary provision and noted that their new isolation hospital had a whole section for the care of patients with rabies. Vienna disappointed him although there were some signs that the Austrians would soon make progress in managing infectious diseases. Similarly Prague had the potential, but not the inclination, to change from an insanitary, badly housed city to one with excellent facilities. It was, content to spend:

> in numberless fetes and celebrations money which might be infinitely more usefully employed in clearing away its foul habitations and in developing its almost boundless natural possibilities for the promotion of public health.

Prague had obviously lacked the equivalent of Sir Henry Littlejohn.

In Berlin, Bailie Pollard's spirits rose when he visited Moabit Hospital with 900 fever beds, Friederichshain Hospital built in 1874, the Urban Hospital of 1890, the Koch Institute and experimental hospital for tuberculosis and lupus near the Charite Hospital and, finally, the Emperor and Empress Frederick Fever Hospital for Children. In all of these he was impressed by the close association of clinical and laboratory disciplines stemming from the pioneering work of Professor Koch[5] whom he met there. In Hamburg Bailie Pollard noted the thoroughness of the public health services' methodical supervision of water, milk and food and the number of disinfecting stations throughout the city. In the 2,000 bedded Eppendorf Hospital, 3,000 cholera patients had been managed efficiently during an epidemic in 1892.

In Copenhagen at the Blegdam Hospital 'situated on an open plain' and constructed mainly with single-storey pavilions, he found superb facilities for fever accommodation using materials such as steel, glass and stone and very strict isolation procedures. He wrote that 'in the general hospitals antiseptic treatment may be almost said to run wild'.

Bailie Pollard was accompanied for part of his trip by Mr Morham. They noted that these continental fever hospitals never had a mortality lower than 10–12 per cent compared with a mortality of only 6 per cent in Edinburgh. Pollard attributed this discrepancy in part to the 'weaker vitality' of continental children versus those in Scotland. He also commented that whilst it was admirable for a fever hospital to be run on the German model with efficiency, smoothness and precision, the chief quality of nursing staff 'ought to be tenderness and sympathy in the care of their patients'. Despite the skill and regulation in German hospitals, their nurses 'cannot yet be said to have learned to fully exercise what may be called the humanities of their profession'. Pollard felt this difference must have an 'influence upon the less favourable results obtained in Germany compared with those in Scottish hospitals'.[6]

Pollard concluded from his visits to continental hospitals that sunlight and fresh air were of paramount importance in the siting and construction of the new hospital at Colinton Mains. After all Professor Koch had exclaimed to him at his Institute in Berlin 'Sunlight is the great germicide'. It seemed that Colinton Mains was perfect in this respect. Although one-storey blocks would be ideal, two-storey blocks would be much cheaper and, with the open airy situation at Colinton, probably as efficient and acceptable. Sound construction in stone or brick, preferably the former, was advised for the Scottish climate but Pollard 'would sacrifice nothing to outward appearance at the cost of practical usefulness'.[7]

Clearing of the farm ground, especially where heavily manured, rendering basements impervious and having the first floor several feet above ground were important considerations. Floors, walls, ceilings and furnishings should be simple, with an emphasis on easy cleaning and with maximum access to sunlight. To this end sunrooms should be incorporated in the wards on the lines of continental hospitals. In the diphtheria and croup pavilions, small operating theatres should be available for tracheotomy to be performed. Good individual sleeping accommodation and recreation facilities for nurses and domestic staff were important considerations. Drainage and heating of the hospital demanded attention, and electricity rather than gas was preferred for lighting.

A bacteriology laboratory and pathology museum were to be incorporated within the new hospital to investigate the cause of fevers and for the instruction of medical students. Insufficient research and teaching had taken place in the previous City Hospitals and this deficit was to be made good along the lines of German hospitals.

On 3 December 1896, the Fever Hospital Committee approved the provisional plans drawn up by Mr Morham:

> On the understanding that the construction of the covered ways, the provision of a private installation of electric light, and the building of two of the scarlet fever pavilions, be not proceeded with at present.[8]

Councillors Brown and Waterston had urged Mr Morham to report on the number of beds the hospital should accommodate. On 8 December 1896 the same councillors put forward a motion to the Public Health Committee that provision be made for 400 beds only. This caused some controversy so on 17 December the Town Council, whilst approving the plans in general, remitted back to the Public Health Committee the task of obtaining estimates for a hospital containing 600, 500 and 400 beds respectively.[9]

Mr Morham reported that for 600 beds the cost would be £225,700 (£376 per bed); for 500 beds, which would mean omitting the two larger and two smaller scarlet fever pavilions, the cost would be £204,678 (£409 per bed); for 400 beds, which would mean omitting a further scarlet fever pavilion, the cost would be £176,989 (£437 per bed).

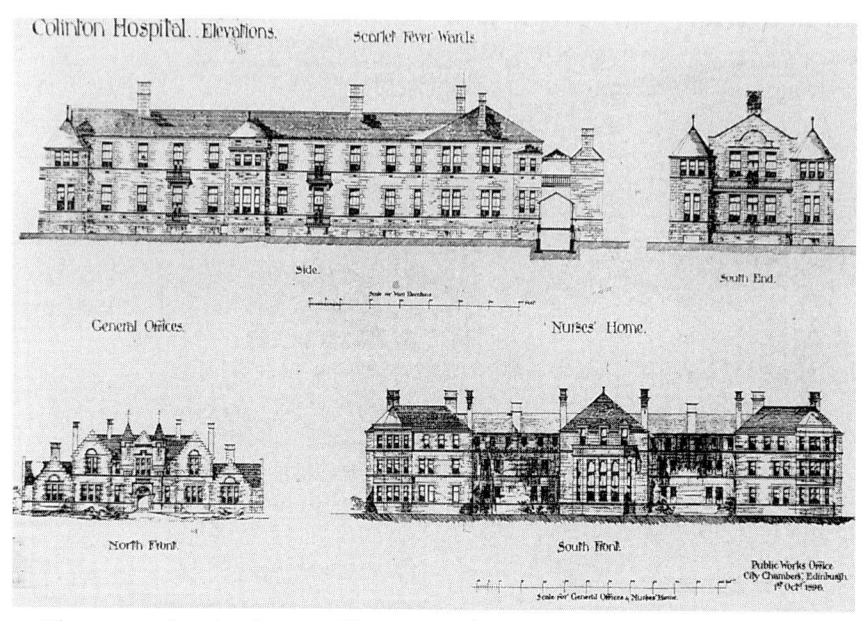

Elevations of scarlet fever pavilions, general offices and the nurses' home. A cross-section of a covered way is shown with subway beneath. Compare the appearances here with the finished buildings in subsequent illustrations.
From Description and Sketch Plan, Public Works Office, October 1896.
(By courtesy of Edinburgh City Libraries)

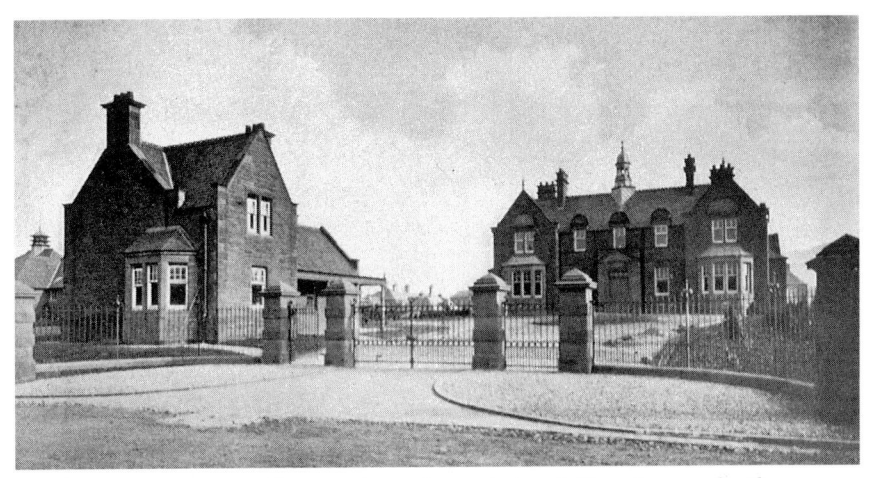

The main entrance with porter's gatehouse lodge (left) and general offices (right) 1903. From *Edinburgh City Hospital, Colinton Mains,* Presentation copy, 1903. (Photo: J. C. McKechnie, Castle Street, Edinburgh)

Mr Morham then realised that, the more beds there were, the more accommodation would be needed for nursing staff and the more ward furnishings. He therefore hurriedly submitted revised estimates on 16 February 1897[10] as follows:

600 beds	£233,700
500 beds	£212,678
400 beds	£181,989

Sir Henry Littlejohn now argued for 600 beds. He pointed out that the second City Hospital sometimes had as many as 459 beds filled and could accommodate only 50 per cent of the cases of infectious diseases referred. He therefore supported the Public Health Committee's recommendation of 600 beds saying 'This amount will certainly tide us over for some years to come'.[11] He suggested the following allocation of beds:

	Scale of 600	Scale of 400
Scarlet Fever	320	200
Typhoid	80	60
Typhus	10	10
Diphtheria	30	20
Measles	80	50
Chicken Pox	20	10
Hooping [sic] Cough	20	20
Erysipelas	30	20
Probationary	10	10
Total	600	400

Planning the Hospital

Dr John Wyllie, now the Consulting Physician to the City Hospital, also favoured 600 beds so that the wards could be disinfected between epidemics and he declared:

> To be safe from cross infection a fever hospital ought to have a greater number of beds and of wards than would probably be required for occupation in ordinary time.[12]

Dr Claude B. Ker, the new Medical Superintendent of the City Hospital, also supported the 600 bedded hospital plan. After a complicated series of motions and amendments, the Magistrates and Councillors voted on 26 February 1897 to approve the Public Health Committee's recommendation for 600 beds, by a majority of 25 to 5, only Treasurer McCrae and four other councillors having favoured the 500 bedded option. The Public Health Committee were then remitted to obtain estimates in accordance with Mr Morham's plans.[13]

By 15 April 1897 the Public Works Office had produced a 14 page Building Specification for the New City Hospital at Colinton Mains.[14] The plans and relevant documents could be consulted at the Public Works Office, City Chambers and, on receipt of a three guinea deposit, were to be supplied to intending competitors for the tenders. The three guineas were refundable on receipt of bona fide tenders and return of the completed Schedules and Specifications. A Preliminary Contract would cover a main service road from Colinton Road to the further end of the site, an office for the Clerk of Works, a water pipe to the centre of the site and a barbed-wire fence enclosing the area.

As would be expected from the meticulous approach of Robert Morham, the Building Specification was extraordinarily detailed. Under the general provisions he made careful stipulations, some of which became points of contention and litigation later, as the building works progressed too slowly. Whilst emphasising that strict adherence to the specifications and a high quality of work were mandatory, Mr Morham was careful to give himself freedom to make alterations during the progress of the work without invalidating the contract. He would arrange subsequently to add or deduct pro rata from the agreed sums of payment to contractors. Yet he would specifically reject any claims for additional work which did not have his written permission.

It was vital that each contractor finished work on time to allow the next skilled worker to complete his schedule. If the masonry work was delayed, the wrights, plumbers, plasterers, slaters and smiths would all be held up by a domino effect. Another stipulation therefore stated that, within two years of the completion of the temporary access roadway, each group of buildings must be ready for painting, fitting and furnishing under a penalty of £3 for each day's delay. If any difference of opinion arose between the contracting parties the question was to be referred to Mr Morham, Architect, whom failing Mr Walter W. Robertson, Surveyor of Her Majesty's Board of Works. The decision of either should be final and binding upon both parties.

Individual specifications were laid down for the work of each trade. In the builders' work, foundations were to be of best Craigleith or Hailes stone with walls of best rubble from Hailes Quarry dressed with stone from quarries at Corncockle near Lockerbie, or Corsehill near Annan, both in Dumfriesshire. Failing a supply of stone from these, 'others approved by the Architect' would be accepted.[15]

According to one authority[16] the facing stone came from Closeburn Quarry in the Dumfries and Galloway Thornhill basin. Both Closeburn and possibly also Locharbriggs may have provided stone besides the Corsehill and Corncockle quarries to which Mr Morham referred in his Building Specification. The correspondence of March 1899 between Mr Morham and Mr A. L. Thomson, for J. Murray & Sons, Quarry Owners, Corsehill, makes it clear that at least some of the stone used for the hospital came from Corsehill.[17] The warm red sandstone from south west Scotland was popular at the turn of the century for buildings in Edinburgh

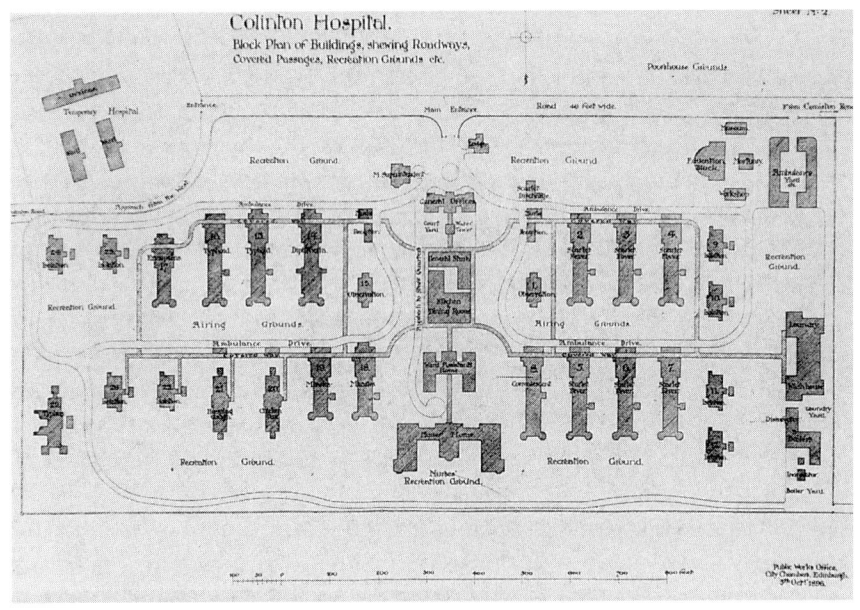

Block plan from Description and Sketch Plan, Public Works Office, 5 October 1896. The temporary smallpox hospital is shown at the north west and, centrally, between the general offices and stores, is the projected water tower that was never built. (By courtesy of Edinburgh City Libraries)

notably the King's Theatre, Caledonian Hotel, the Scottish National Portrait Gallery, Edinburgh College of Art and Mr Morham's own Central Fire Station in Lauriston Place. The stone was transported to Edinburgh by rail; J. Murray & Sons had notepaper headed with *Corsehill Quarries Siding, Solway Junction Branch, Caledonian Railway.*

Larger sizes of stone were to be used for the wards and smaller ones with more carefully split faces and flat cleavage for the general offices and the Medical Superintendent's house. The recommended 2½ inch gap between the outer stone and the inner brick walls was to be carefully preserved and the two walls bonded with galvanised wrought iron ties, two to every yard of surface. These were to be the only points of contact between them, and care was to be taken that no lime fell into the space between stone and brick. Precise specifications about the composition of mortar and cement were also laid down showing how well Mr Morham knew his job and how great a perfectionist he was. It would have been difficult for a tradesman to short-change him in respect of materials or quality of workmanship.

Similarly detailed requirements were specified for wrights' work. The timber was to be 'well seasoned, free from sapwood, shakes, large or loose knots, and all other defects'.[18] Carpentry was to be carried out in best St Petersburg redwood. All white wood was to be 'of the best from Russian or north German ports'.[19] Joiner work was to be in American yellow pine or selected pitch pine, carefully chosen and cut to show figure in the wall lining, cove and ceiling of the nurses' recreation room and other interior furnishings. Most of the floors were to be laid on thick, inodorous felt for deafening, with meticulous tongue and groove wooden joints bedded and set in bitumen. Ward floors were to be made of 1¼ inch thick, 4½ inch wide, teak planks with felt below, grooved and tongued and closely jointed and securely nailed to breeze concrete with steel wire nails of flat cross-section. Any defect in these floors due to lack of seasoning of the timber and found before the buildings were occupied was to be made good by the contractor. Most of the ward floors have since been covered with linoleum, so it is difficult to appreciate the original craftsmanship.

Details of doors, fittings, screens, and windows included, for example, the McLean's patent hinges and 12 inch long, strong, brass bar lifts for the windows in Matron's residence. Following the preliminary specification, all ward windows were to be double glazed. Plumbers and plasterers were also given meticulous instructions to use specific materials such as Keene's cement or Adament cement, best polished terrazzo paving with a red cement hollow at the walls. The slaters were to use best galvanised wrought iron nails weighing 12 lb per thousand to hang best, full-sized Ballachulish or Easdale slates double nailed every third row over a layer of thick, inodorous felt. The instructions for iron work were similarly exact.

The Town Council Minutes[20] recorded that the Local Government Board approved the plans of the new City Hospital and expressed their 'appreciation of the skill and care which have been applied to render the plans so thoroughly complete'. Certainly the whole Building Specification is a tribute to Mr Morham's dedication to detail. Tenders were invited for the first group of buildings comprising the general offices and staff quarters, and for the second group consisting of the scarlet fever pavilions. Offers could be made by one contractor for a group of buildings but would require their own and individual sub-contractors' tenders to be listed.

A separate tender for the construction of the service access from Colinton Road was awarded to John Lownie, for the sum of £1,078 10s 0d. The access road was to be built as quickly as possible and preferably within six weeks from the Building Specification of 15 April 1897. It was to consist of railway sleepers and cast iron rails, gated at the Colinton Road end, well maintained and made available for access by any of the contractors using the site until the hospital was completed.

In the meantime Mr Morham wrote to the Public Health Committee on 5 July 1897 that the cost of the whole building operation was now estimated at £237,716 rather than the previous quotation of £233,700 because the cost of building had risen.[21] Moreover he suggested a further increase of £6,000 if the Council's wish for fire proofing was to be carried out on the roofs of all 12 two-storey buildings at £500 per block.[22]

The estimates for buildings became available in late June 1897. Only one contractor, Mr John Lownie, had tendered for all departments (i.e. masonry, wrights' work, plastering, plumbing, slating and iron work) in both groups of buildings at a total cost of £96,477 6s 0d. The lowest tender for all departments and all groups came to £90,536, headed by Colin Macandrew, and with the same builder with other tradesmen tendering *separately* for the two groups the cost would be reduced to £89,616. The Public Health Committee, however, felt that with the additional expenditure now estimated at £104,087 to complete the hospital, rather than the general offices, staff quarters and scarlet fever pavilions only, it would be wise to get the whole hospital built by a single contractor or at least by a sole contractor for each building group. Tenders were then received from Colin Macandrew for £93,317 10s 0d and from Kinnear Moodie & Co. for £94,683 0s 0d for the whole

Planning the Hospital

work. After voting, the Committee decided to recommend the Town Council to accept Colin Macandrew's estimate.[23]

All therefore seemed set when Mr Macandrew unexpectedly wrote to the Public Health Committee withdrawing his offer for the mason work.[24] The Committee therefore voted on whether to accept Mr Lownie's tender at £18,470 for the mason work of the general offices and £37,747 for the masonry of the scarlet fever pavilions. This was then agreed and an amendment to offer him the whole of the building contract for £96,477 6s 6d was rejected. At their meeting on 31 August 1897 the Public Health Committee[25] had several tenders and variations of agreements from different contractors to consider. One of these was a letter from Messrs Thomson, Dickson & Shaw for Mr Lownie. The Committee agreed to depart from the condition of a cautioner in Mr Lownie's contract (money deposited on condition of satisfactory work). The Town Council's representative also provisionally agreed to omit a clause which had stated that, in the event of a general strike (rather than a local confrontation between the builder and his workers) or else in the event of exceptionally bad weather, the builder would not be fined £3 daily for each day's delay if the work was not completed by the appointed time.[26]

It became apparent very soon that the hospital would take much longer to build than had been expected. The delays, together with claims and counter claims about alterations and additions to specification, became the subject of a protracted lawsuit between the Town Council and Mr John Lownie.

CHAPTER FOURTEEN

Building the Hospital: The Town Council v. John Lownie

The Scotsman reporter[1] wrote that it was a dull, mild but dry afternoon in Edinburgh on Friday 14 May 1897. With due ceremonial, Lady McDonald, wife of Lord Provost Sir Andrew McDonald, inaugurated the building operations of the new City Hospital by cutting the first sod. The invitation card requested the presence of over 100 ladies and gentlemen at the 'breaking ground'. The Lords Provost of Edinburgh and Leith, the ex-Lord Provost of Edinburgh, the Magistrates, Councillors and their friends attended and notably Bailie James Pollard, Convener of the Public Health Committee, who had done so much to forward the project. The church and medical profession were well represented. Dr Claude B. Ker, appointed Medical Superintendent of the second City Hospital earlier that year, was also present. Others attending were University and Royal Infirmary medical staff, a publisher, a lawyer, and the Governor of Craiglockhart Poorhouse. Especially welcome were Miss Sandford, Lady Superintendent of the second City Hospital, and a contingent of her nurses.

Mr Morham, the City Architect, was also there to witness the start of his project. After the ceremony, in which he received fulsome praise in Bailie Pollard's speech, Mr Morham pointed out to everyone the full extent of the hospital site which was marked out by flags stuck in the ground. One notable absentee was Sir Henry Littlejohn, Medical Officer of Health, although both he and Mr Morham would attend the opening ceremony in 1903. Sadly by that time Bailie Pollard would be dead.

The proceedings began with a prayer offered by Dr Cameron Lees. Bailie Pollard next asked Mrs McDonald to break the ground with a spade handed to her by Mr Morham. This she did and 'in a purpose-like way, lifted and turned over a bit of turf (in front of the small stand which had been erected) amid cheers'.[2] When the official party had adjourned to an adjacent tent, the turf turned by the Lady Provost was 'pounced upon by the nurses and others and broken up into small pieces and carried off as souvenirs of the occasion'.[3]

Within the large tent, tea and light refreshments were provided by Mr Sawers of Hanover Street. The Lord Provost asked Bailie Pollard to make a statement which he did at length and with intermittent applause. He described the patterns of infectious disease going back to 1645 when plague victims were cared for on the Burgh Muir. More recently plans had been made to expand and extend the City Hospital (old Infirmary) site at which fever patients had been admirably looked after since 1885 when the Corporation took over their care from the Managers of the Royal Infirmary. The Town Council, willing pupils of the Public Health Committee, agreed six years previously to spend £20,000 on an extension to the old hospital. Yet their ideas had expanded to a new-build site costing £240,000, a figure which the Town Council were willing to face without blanching. He enumerated the reasons for the move, not least improved ambulance transport and the necessity to have 600 beds in the new hospital compared with 400 beds. Besides caring for the sick he hoped this new institution would be used to instruct nurses and medical men. The importance of a laboratory was therefore stressed, though Councillor Waterston, an anti-vivisectionist, interjected with 'That has not yet been decided, Bailie'.[4]

Lady McDonald was then presented with a photograph of herself and Sir Andrew in an inscribed silver gilt frame. A portentous speech was delivered next by Dr Turnbull Smith who praised the work of the Public Health Committee and Bailie Pollard. His 'text' was *Prosperity to the undertaking and to the city* and he eulogised on the government of the city by the Lord Provost and Council over the previous three years. This mutual back-slapping continued at length and won some further applause.

Finally the Lord Provost's reply alluded to the cost of the new building. There was no problem if the city could borrow 'three quarters of a million of money at 2½ per cent as it did a week previously and lend it at 7 per cent [Applause]! That was what he called business'![5] Although the new hospital was expensive, the Lord Provost said:

> the benefit the city would derive from having a well-equipped hospital for the treatment of infectious diseases could not be estimated in pounds, shillings and pence. [Hear, hear][6]

It would not cost the rate payer more than 1d or 1¼d. Bailie Pollard and the Town Council were then thanked for the handsome souvenir of the occasion presented to Lady McDonald, three cheers were given and further compliments exchanged. That ended the proceedings.

It was now up to Mr Morham to see the work through. Few at the ceremony of 'breaking ground' could have anticipated what an uphill task this would be. It was not until a full six years later that enough buildings were completed for the royal opening on 13 May 1903. Even then the finished parts of the hospital consisted only of the administrative and general offices, the Medical Superintendent's house, nurses' and servants' homes, boiler house and Pavilions 2–8 for scarlet fever. The exterior of other pavilions was barely complete.

The delays in building caused much irritation to Mr George Ballingall, Clerk of Works, all of whose 343 informative Weekly Reports on Works in Progress have been carefully preserved.[7] Even more frustration was felt by Mr Robert Morham, who bore the ultimate responsibility for ensuring the hospital was satisfactorily completed according to his detailed plans. His correspondence with the builder, Mr John Lownie, who was successful in tendering for Contracts 1 and 2, starts in a civil and friendly manner, but over the months Mr Morham's annoyance at the delays is plain to read. Copies of this correspondence and the Weekly Reports are retained in the Edinburgh City Archives together with documents concerning the subsequent protracted legal action which took place between the Town Council and Mr Lownie.

According to Mr Morham, things started badly at Colinton Mains and got steadily worse. To be fair, some delays were caused by bad weather but these were allowed for in the contractual agreement. For instance for the six days ending Saturday 24 February 1900, Mr Ballingall reported 'No building done because of frost and snow'[8] Some inside joiner work was done in the servants' home and in Pavilion 5 that week, but the 35 masons or brick layers would have lain idle or been paid off.

However, bad weather was an unusual reason for holding up the work. More commonly a want of essential materials delayed progress. In his first Weekly Report dated 7 August 1897, Mr Ballingall records that the service road from Colinton Road to the hospital site was marked off so that the contractor (Mr Lownie) 'can start operations on Monday'.[9] Imagine Mr Ballingall's frustration when he reported two weeks later 'Formation of service road now at a stand still owing to railway sleepers not being delivered', and two weeks later still 'Unsatisfactory progress on service road for want of sleepers'. In Weekly Report No. 8 on 25 September 1897, he records 'The progress of the service road is still unsatisfactory owing to the transplates not being ready'.[10] Only by 23 October 1897 was the service road complete to the front of the scarlet fever pavilions. A job that should have taken only six weeks had taken more than nine to complete.

The route taken by the Dumfriesshire quarried stone from the Caledonian Railway to the City Hospital site is unclear. Mr Ballingall's Reports record that access was from Colinton Road. His references to 'transplates and sleepers' and, in the Building Specification, Mr Morham's reference to 'cast iron rails', indicate a temporary railroad, but whether horses or locomotives were used remains conjectural. When the nearby Redford Barracks were under construction about 1913, there was a tramway from Slateford Station to the building site. This took the line of the present Allan Park Road, south-eastwards, then curling south-south-westwards along what is now Craiglockhart Road and the Royal Soldiers' Home to reach the barracks' site. A contemporary picture postcard shows wagons belonging to Messrs Colin Macandrew standing at the barracks during their building.[11] As Mr Macandrew eventually worked on the smaller Contract No 3 at the City Hospital, it is tempting to suggest that the City Hospital stone was delivered by a similar route despite contemporary maps not showing the metal bridge over the Union Canal nor even a proposed tramway before 1911–12.[12] However, it is apparent that Colin Macandrew had the tramway from Slateford built about 1909–11 expressly for the construction of the barracks.[13] Stone for the interior walls and foundations of the hospital was probably carted direct from the relatively nearby Hailes and Craigleith quarries. The consensus view of several experts consulted suggests that steam traction engines may have been used to carry the local and more distantly quarried stone to the hospital building site.

On 13 November 1897, the Clerk of Works wrote about Pavilions 1–3:

> The progress of the work at this date is very unsatisfactory principally owing to want of rubble. *Note:* The Contractor has today promised to send on a better supply of material.[14]

Yet, by the next week, there was still no rubble delivered. For two consecutive weeks in December, Mr Ballingall reported further lack of progress, this time because the contractor was employing too few builders. The Weekly Reports of 19 February and 5 March 1898 again record delays because of insufficient stone.

Two early letters between Mr Morham and Mr Lownie set the scene.[15]

11th December 1897

> Visiting premises this afternoon with Bailie Pollard and doctors, we were disappointed to see so much of the work lying back. There seems no good reason why the Ward buildings (except Convalescent) should not all have been as far forward as the north-east one, or getting as for it; whereas beyond the concrete foundations some of them have nothing done to them.
>
> Then for the Servants' and Nurses' Homes, except southern extremities of the latter the foundations plans have been out of hands for some considerable time, and the General Office plans have all been ready from the first. I

must ask you to take measures for operations on a much more general and progressive scale, and your best attention for seeing this will much oblige.

Yours etc. R Morham.

On 10 March 1898, Mr Morham wrote again to Mr Lownie:

I regret to learn from the Inspector of Works' reports that there appears to be a serious short-coming of material both in ruble [sic] and in cement for the concrete work. As there is plenty of work – too much – before us, it seems strange that there should be any short-coming in either of these materials. With regard to the latter – the cement – the Inspector's Statement is that in order to his testing it in good time it must be forward some time before it is actually required.

Your best attention to remedy these complaints will much oblige.

Yrs. etc. R. Morham.

Throughout June 1898, Mr Ballingall, Clerk of Works, recorded his frustration that so little mason work was being done through lack of red stone. Insufficient brick layers at work were also holding up the progress with fire-proof floorings. Shortage of stone tempted the masons 'to cut hewing work out of common rubble. This I have ordered to be stopped'.[16] On 22 August 1898, Mr Ballingall reported that other

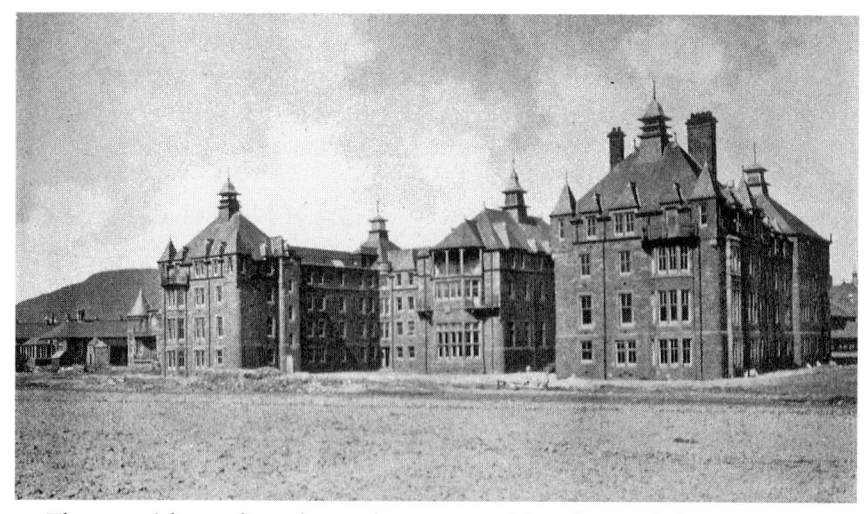

The nurses' home from the south east, 1903. Note the south-facing sun balcony above the many windowed recreation hall in the centre. From *Edinburgh City Hospital, Colinton Mains*, Presentation copy, 1903. (Photo: J. C. McKechnie, Castle Street, Edinburgh)

work had halted because the masons' work had not progressed. 'This ought not to have happened had Mr Lownie carried on the work in anything like a tradesmanlike manner'. Two days later he commented '. . . the way in which the building is carried on it is more like an old ruin than a new building, just a bit up here and there'. On 27 October, Mr Ballingall wrote:

> ... I am afraid things are getting rather serious with us now. Little or no material is coming in from any of the Quarries, in fact to keep things moving the men have to be changed from one section of the buildings to another to work up whatever can be got.[17]

In his defence Mr Lownie wrote to explain that his problems had been made worse by the unsettled and cold weather. He claimed to have his stone-cutting machines working 22 in every 24 hours and to be employing night as well as day workers.[18] Mr Morham, however, could not reconcile the quarrymasters' statements with those of Mr Lownie.[19] One quarrymaster was not told that the quantities were insufficient and Mr Lownie's casual ordering of 'a waggon or two of good rubble – if they have it'[20] did not convey any sense of urgency that the supply was so low as to be hindering the works. Mr Lownie reported temporary breakdowns at quarries in September 1898 but these hardly justified the long continued problem caused by his casual ordering of stone.

Mr Lownie was next accused of employing untrained workmen and Mr Morham ordered some defective brickwork to be taken down and properly rebuilt. On 10 May 1899 for instance, Mr Morham complained that a workman whom Mr Lownie claimed had 20 years' experience in concreting turned out to be a mere plasterer's labourer. He also appeared not to pay sub-contractors what they felt they were due.[21] In March 1900, sub-contractor Messrs M. Potter threatened to cease work 'on Saturday next if not paid £270 owed them by John Lownie'. Next a tiling firm went bankrupt causing further delays with Mr Lownie trying unsuccessfully to palm Mr Morham off with samples of different coloured and sized tiles from another firm. The special Shepwood partition bricks for the sanitary towers in the wards were not ordered although Mr Lownie claimed they had been. This led to even more delays according to Messrs Morham and Ballingall.

By 25 March 1902, Mr Morham's patience was running out. He wrote to Mr Lownie:

> I regret to learn that there is only *one* man working at the terrazzo in the General Offices, and none in the Servants' Home, and no word yet of the Shepwood bricks &c.

This is really most vexing, and I am at a loss to see how, at this rate of progress, your promise to the Committee can be made good. Do please see if something cannot be done to push matters on not simply *better but as they should*.[22]

On 29 March 1902, Mr Lownie received from Mr Morham the following:

The promise of extra men has been made good by the addition of one, while there is room for a dozen; and the tiling at the Nurses' Home which, when the Committee met you on the premises in January, they were assured was just about to proceed, remains as it was then; what can be the meaning of this? Please say, as I am being urgently enquired by the Committee as to these delays ...[23]

He wrote again to Mr Lownie on 1 April 1902:

2 terrazzo men on the job are going about idle today for want of material. I am sorely at a loss to know what to think of such methods of conducting work. In this matter there can be no question of Kilns going wrong.

Then the tile border for the General Offices – a very ordinary matter – ordered nearly a month ago there is not word of yet, and this is keeping back work at this part ...[24]

In November Mr Lownie lamely claimed one reason for the few tile layers at work was that 'some of the men had been drinking, and Messrs Field & Allan were obliged to pay them away'.

As early as November 1898 Mr Lownie had gone behind Mr Morham's back to the Public Health Committee claiming he was not being paid properly. Mr Morham strongly objected and said he would be paid when all the Measurer's reckonings were available. Mr Lownie replied that he could not wait that long.[25]

Thereafter protracted arguments began. Mr Lownie claimed that Mr Morham had made him do extra work not in the Building Specification which therefore required extra payment. Mr Morham countered with complaints about the delays for which he blamed Mr Lownie alone. He could not now possibly meet the deadline for completing the works as agreed in the contracts of October 1897.

It will be recalled that Mr Walter W. Robertson, Surveyor in Scotland to Her Majesty's Board of Works, was to act as arbiter in any dispute between the Town Council and the contractor which could not easily be settled by Mr Morham in the first instance.[26] The second arbiter was to be an Edinburgh surveyor, Mr William Ormiston. On 25 May 1898 the Town Council and Mr Morham, both already dissatisfied with the rate of progress of the buildings, wrote to Mr Robertson to ask if he

Building the Hospital

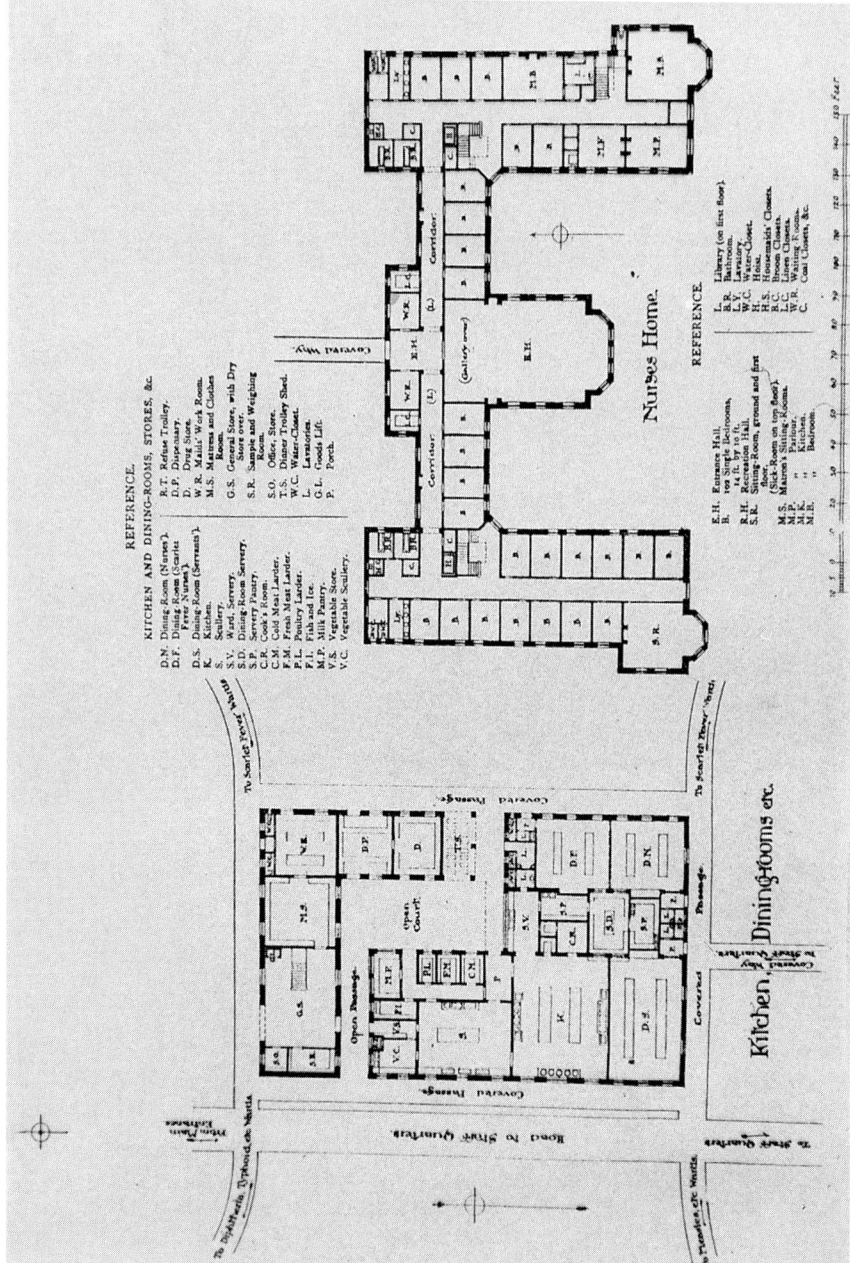

(a) Plans of kitchens and dining rooms (left). Note the segregation of scarlet fever nurses (DF) from other nurses (DN) in south east corner of the dining rooms. (b) Plan of the nurses' home (right) with its large, central recreation hall (RH) and, at the south east corner, Matron's apartments, (MS, MP, MK, MB). The nurses' sitting room is at the south west corner. From Description and Sketch Plan, Public Works Office, 5 October 1896. (By courtesy of Edinburgh City Libraries) accepted the office of arbiter but he declined. On 1 June 1898, therefore, the Town Clerk wrote to Mr Ormiston who did accept the offer. Mr Ormiston disposed of the questions which had then been raised as to the progress of the buildings in June, July and September 1898 but at no time recommended the work be taken out of Mr Lownie's hands.[27]

In his Report of 17 June 1898 Mr Ormiston stated that 'At the present rate of progress the Building will not be ready to receive painting etc. within the time specified'.[28] He quoted the difficulties the contractor had in procuring builders despite wide advertising and pointed out that the 103 builders on site at that time represented $\frac{1}{7}$ or $\frac{1}{8}$ of the total number present in Edinburgh. Secondly, owing to an engineers' strike from the end of October 1897 to 25 January 1898, he was unable to get machinery forward to start on the engineering and boiler work. Lastly, two additional stone-sawing machines and one moulding machine had not been properly utilised 'owing to labour troubles'.

Mr Ormiston wrote that he had:

> impressed on the Contractor the necessity of pressing on at every possible point and of using every means for expediting the work. I would consider it would be most unwise for the Corporation in the meantime to interfere in the manner provided for in the contract as such a proceeding would only lead to much greater delay, increasing cost and general dissatisfaction.[29]

The Town Council perhaps felt Mr Ormiston was not being forceful enough on the contractor. He should have insisted that, despite past delays, future agreed deadlines for completion must be met. Mr Lownie doubtless felt relieved.

The next turn of events concerned the suitability of Mr Ormiston to act as Arbiter.[30] He was elected Dean of Guild in November 1898, a post which he held by annual re-election till November 1902. This was considered by the Town Council – but contradicted by Mr Lownie – to debar him completely as arbiter since the Dean of Guild was *ex officio* a member of the Town Council. Moreover, since Mr Ormiston as Dean of Guild had given some advice to the Council early in the building programme, the Council argued this too debarred him from being able to act impartially.

The legal battle continued. The Town Council was prepared to have Mr W. W. Robertson, the original arbiter, reinstated and he was now prepared to accept. Mr Lownie, however, objected to this and in the interim the whole of the buildings and materials in Contracts 1 and 2 were remeasured at considerable cost. Ultimately, but not until early 1904, Mr James Walker, Surveyor, 122 George Street, Edinburgh was approved as a suitable arbiter by both sides.

Building the Hospital

№ 31

Weekly Report on Works in Progress in
New City Hospital, Colinton Mains
The Property of The City of Edinburgh
For the week ending 5th March 1898

NUMBER OF MEN EMPLOYED.		STATE OF THE WEATHER.	
Excavators,	18		
Masons ~~and~~ Bricklayers, *Hewers*	77	Monday,	Good
~~Wrights~~, *Apprentices*	11	Tuesday,	Stopped 3 hours with snow
~~Plumbers~~, *Labourers*	46	Wednesday,	Good
~~Plasterers~~, *Cutters*	18	Thursday,	Do
~~Slaters~~, *Engineers*	3	Friday,	Do
Smiths,	1	Saturday,	Do
Total,	174		

STATE OF THE WORK.

Pavilion N° 3. The walls of pavilion leveled for ground floor beams.
Do. N° 4. The iron beams on for ground floor and commenced to build on top of same.
Do. N° 5. The side walls of pavilion leveled for asphalte.
Servants Home. Part of under building up to ground line.

× Drawings required. Plans also details for base of servants home.
× " — " Roof plan of pavilions
× " — " Plan of main ventilating flue for pavilions

GENERAL REMARKS.

The progress of the works is still very much delayed principally owing to want of stone.

Geo Ballingall Clerk of Works.

Weekly Report on Works in Progress, No. 31, 5 March 1898. Mr Ballingall records his irritation at Mr Lownie's failure to provide enough stone. (By courtesy of Edinburgh City Archives)

In the meantime Mr Brebner, the sub-contractor for drainage works, complained that Mr Lownie's men had left stone about which interfered with the progress of his work. Mr Ballingall's Weekly Reports showed building work had stopped for three weeks in February 1900 because of frost and snow but there appeared to be no justification for Mr Lownie when Mr Ballingall reported on 22 September 1900 'No progress has been made with the mason work since 6th June'.[31] Attached to the Weekly Report No. 199 of 25 May 1901 is a letter from Mr Lownie to Mr Ballingall:

> Dear Sir – I have just learned that the angle tiles for the staircase at Colinton Mains have again come in too short. I propose coming out tomorrow forenoon to see you regarding this matter. Yours faithfully.

Pencilled at the foot of this letter is Mr Ballingall's comment:

> The above is another example of the blunders we have been having ever since the tiling commenced. G. B.[32]

It is therefore surprising that by the time of the royal opening in May 1903 so many of the buildings in Contracts 1 and 2 were available for inspection by their Majesties. Work was still going on inside these buildings in September 1903 and much of the Contract 3 work was still to be completed, although that was not Mr Lownie's responsibility. It is interesting that Contract 3, partly undertaken by Kinnear, Moodie & Co, was not subject to disputes or delays and, by comparison with Mr Lownie's contract, all went smoothly.

On 20 May 1901 Mr Morham reported to the Building Committee[33] that the probable cost of the hospital would now be £333,861, the cost per bed having leapt from £376 initially to £400, as the higher estimates had been accepted, and now to a massive £556 per bed. He justified this further increase on the grounds of the rough estimates for fittings and furnishings being 'immature in various ways'. The ground for the hospital enclosure had been enlarged, sanitary fittings were to be of an improved design, but at increased cost, and the ventilation system that was eventually adopted was also more expensive than anticipated. Besides, the drainage system was to be dual, for soil and surface water separately, rather than a single system embracing both.

Although the Town Council lamely accepted these increased costs, worse was to come. On 19 May 1902, Mr Morham adjusted the proposed estimates to the total figure of £339,972 3s 6d.[34] Perhaps wisely he did not mention the cost per bed which would now be £566 per bed. This time he blamed the ventilation fans again, fire extinguishers, a reservoir on high ground, the proposed additional boiler power and the proposed permanent access from Colinton Road, the line and arrangement for which were still under consideration. Besides, the accommodation for hospital workers like engineers, porters, male attendants and gardeners on site would add to the original estimates. These sums were exclusive of the cost of the site and of ground accesses (£18,000), City Architect's Department costs (£6,000) and the wages of the Clerks of Works (£5,000). The Town Council were so committed at this stage that there was little complaint they could make.

In addition to these escalating costs, the Council were not yet aware of the likely outcome of the legal proceedings with Mr Lownie. Mr Walker, the final arbiter, acted very quickly after considering the re-measuring, the reasons for delays and the fact that the original arbiter, Mr Ormiston, had not advised taking the work out of Mr Lownie's hands. He found for Mr Lownie and recommended that he be paid £3,051 12s 10d by the Town Council. Mr Walker had:

> satisfied himself that by their acts and omissions, single and cumulative, the Pursuers, the Lord Provost, Magistrates and Council of the City of Edinburgh, had rendered it impossible for the Defender, John Lownie, to complete the Contract within the contract period, which was a period of two years, whereas the Contract occupied a period of at least five years, ...

With interest on the outstanding sum of 5 per cent per annum, Mr Lownie must have considered himself a lucky man. Nonetheless, he was not awarded expenses.[35] So ended this long, tedious, expensive legal process which was finally concluded by Lord Kincairney in his judgement of 1904.[36]

CHAPTER FIFTEEN

A Description of the Third City Hospital

Four useful sources describe the new hospital buildings. The most elegant plans and drawings, with a short introduction by Sir Henry Littlejohn and Mr Morham, are contained in the 'Description and Sketch Plan of Proposed Hospital at Colinton Mains for the City of Edinburgh' published by the Public Works Office in Edinburgh, 5 October 1896.[1] Secondly Bailie Pollard's *The Care of the Public Health and the New Fever Hospital in Edinburgh*, 1898,[2] gives an account of infectious disease management down the ages combined with a detailed description of the proposed new hospital together with plans, architect's drawings and sketches.

The third source *The Edinburgh Fever Hospital – Description with Plans and Photographs*, published in 1903,[3] is a small, red, soft-covered book with a foreword by Councillor W. Lang Todd who succeeded Bailie Pollard as Convener of the Public Health Committee. A green, cloth-covered, hardback edition was also published. Its gold printed front bears the city's Coat of Arms and the title *Edinburgh City Hospital, Colinton Mains, opened by their Imperial Majesties King Edward VII and Queen Alexandra, 13 May 1903*. Apart from including photographs of the main hospital buildings, it is a précis of Bailie Pollard's description of the hospital, without the background information about previous infectious disease management which was such a feature of Pollard's work. Councillor Lang Todd, however, generously acknowledged the contributions of Bailie Pollard and Mr Morham.[4] The photographs by Mr J. C. McKechnie, 31a Castle Street, are good studies for their time. According to Councillor Lang Todd, any profits from the little handbook were to 'be credited to the Toy Fund for the children who have the misfortune to spend some of their time (not always, I know, an unhappy time) within the walls of the Hospital'.

In some respects the fourth source of reference, Mr Morham's 15 page typescript 'Colinton Mains Hospital – Memorandum Accompanying Plans for the Information of the Local Government Board', published on 9 October 1903,[5] is the most useful account as it gives the situation at the time the first patients were being admitted. The Supplementary Note also covers telephones, lighting and the gardens.[6]

A Description of the Hospital 121

The detail of the proposed buildings is given in the Building Specification of 1897[7] which Mr Morham drew up for the invitation of tenders. The hospital site was within reasonably easy access from the city by the improved ambulances. Its elevation at 370–400 feet above sea level would permit good drainage. Initially all the drainage was to have been through the new pipe along the line of the Hospital Road (later named Greenbank Drive) to the main sewer in Comiston Road. Later, as Mr Morham was to point out, and at greater expense, the soil drainage only was conducted by this pipe whilst rain water was drained separately to the south west and discharged into the Braid Burn.

The main access was via the newly constructed, tree-lined, Hospital Road from Comiston Road in the east. Access from the west in 1903 was still by a track from Colinton Road which was eventually made into a permanent road. It then continued north eastward to the principal entrance midway along the northern aspect of the hospital site. Separate gates were also made at the eastern end of the north side for access to the mortuary and 'for cartage of Coals etc. to the Laundry Buildings, and for general garden purposes'. A permanent west gate was initially not planned, possibly for security reasons and to prevent unsupervised traffic. Moreover, as Mr Morham pointed out in his Memorandum of 9 October 1903,[8] the temporary smallpox hospital was in the way.

Gas lighting was finally decided upon for the approach roads although electricity was used for outdoor illumination within the hospital grounds. Electricity also powered all the interior lighting (except for the cottages), the ventilation system and laundry. Gas, however, was supplied to the kitchens and laundry (as well as electricity), hot closets and the small ward kitchens, and was available at strategic positions in the wards in case the electricity supply failed.[9]

The gardens were to be laid out so that a double line of fencing with hedges between would separate the pavilions with different types of infection from one another. Airing grounds between the pavilions were laid out and also: 'Protective plantations', clothes greens and a vegetable garden. Some of the beech hedges still remain. The protective plantations of Corsican pines were chosen for their aromatic scent, which was refreshing for the patients and staff and helped to disguise unpleasant hospital odours.[10] The perimeter fence to the south was 5 feet high with metal spikes dug 1 foot below the ground, Not even this was able to deter children from Oxgangs who, hearing of free ice cream being served at one of the hospital fetes, managed to get in by digging underneath.[11]

In response to Professor Koch's enthusiasm for the germicidal properties of sunshine, Mr Morham would have oriented the new pavilions at the old Infirmary site on a north–south axis had the redevelopment there gone ahead. At Colinton Mains the 130 foot long ward pavilions were also oriented north–south and built sufficiently far apart so as not to overshadow each other:

> the southern ends being kept free as far as possible for the admission of Sunlight; and the bedrooms in the Staff quarters are so arranged that each may at some period of the day receive a share of whatever sunshine may be going.[12]

The site, gently sloping to the south, also faced the sunshine. To the north the two Craiglockhart Hills gave some protection from the wind.

The maximum bed capacity was 600. Each class of infection was treated separately in one or more pavilions. The cubic capacity of space per bed, then considered very important, ranged from 1,774 cubic feet for measles, chickenpox and whooping cough to a maximum of 2,925 in Ward 22 in the south west corner which had 10 beds for typhus fever. The chickenpox, whooping cough and typhus blocks, the reception and discharge blocks and isolation cottages were all single-storey. Other patient accommodation was in two-storey pavilions. The 320 scarlet fever beds[13] occupied the east of the hospital including Pavilions 2–8, Isolation cottages 9–12 and the reception and observation wards. The site of the scarlet fever observation wards later became the new kitchen and staff

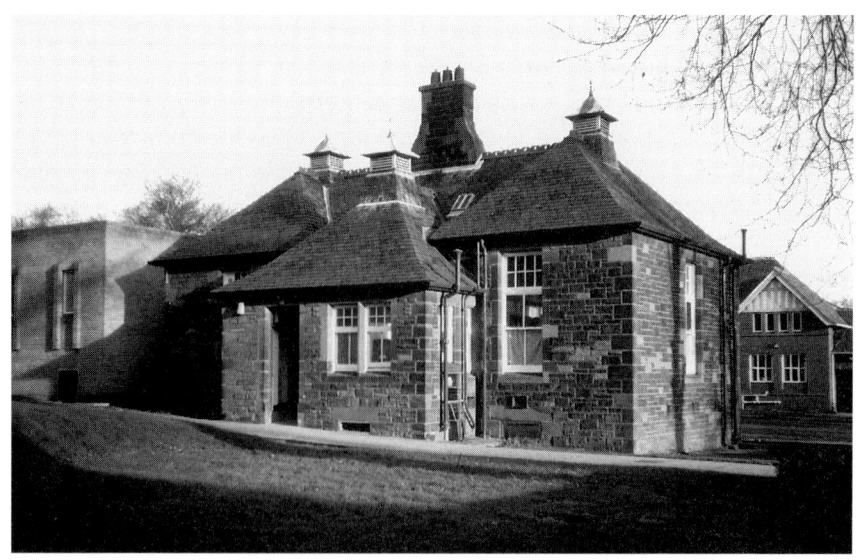

Isolation cottage 10. Note the soiled-linen chute between the facing windows. Behind on the right is one of the two mock-Tudor gables of the laundry. (Photo: J. A. Gray)

dining room in 1971. To the west of the general offices, stores and kitchen was another reception and observation ward where the general stores and pharmacy now stand. Immediately west of these was Pavilion 14 for diphtheria. It was purposely situated near the gate and equipped with an anaesthetic room and operating theatre where emergency tracheostomies could be done on infants arriving with asphyxiating laryngeal diphtheria. Pavilions 15 and 16 housed typhoid patients and the smaller Pavilion 17 with 30 beds accommodated erysipelas. Cottages 23–26 were used for isolation. Pavilions 18 and 19 (possibly with Cottage 25) had 80 measles beds, Pavilion 20 had 19 chickenpox beds and Pavilion 21 had 19 beds for whooping cough.

The scarlet fever pavilions had a single discharge area common to all the wards (situated across the road and north of the scarlet fever reception area). The other pavilions had their own discharge room or rooms, at the north of each and separated from the ward by the main hospital corridor. In the same site was the nurses' toilet, hand lift, ward kitchen and pantry. The staircase to the upstairs ward was also in the north part of each pavilion. It led directly off the service covered way so that it did not communicate with the ground floor ward. There was a service hand lift (erroneously called a patients' lift) in the well of each staircase and at the southern end of each pavilion a 'panic stair' in case of fire.

An exception to this general arrangement was the entrance in the middle of the eastern aspect of Pavilions 20 and 21 (chickenpox and whooping cough respectively) which was reached by a separate covered way running southwards as a tributary of the main east–west covered way.

Again, with the exception of Pavilions 20 and 21, most wards were entered off the covered way through a short corridor with usually a two bedded 'separation room' on the right (west) and opposite on the left (east) a single bedded private room and then the patients' toilets and baths. Beyond the 'separation room', which could be used for patients with complications and the seriously ill, lay the doctor's room. The side wards, doctor's room and the centre of each ward were given extra heating by coal fires, but steam pipes and radiators supplied most of the background warmth. Pavilion 14 had six small separate bays at its southern end close to the tracheostomy theatre. Until recently Ward 14A (upstairs) had a walk-in cupboard filled with Heath Robinson-like steam coils and a boiler, controlled by pressure gauges with large dials, to supply humidified air to the tracheostomy rooms. Apparently this ingenious contraption proved unsatisfactory owing to the excessive condensation of water vapour in the pipes.

The sanitary towers, for which Mr Morham had such difficulty in obtaining glazed tiles from the contractor, were usually on the east side

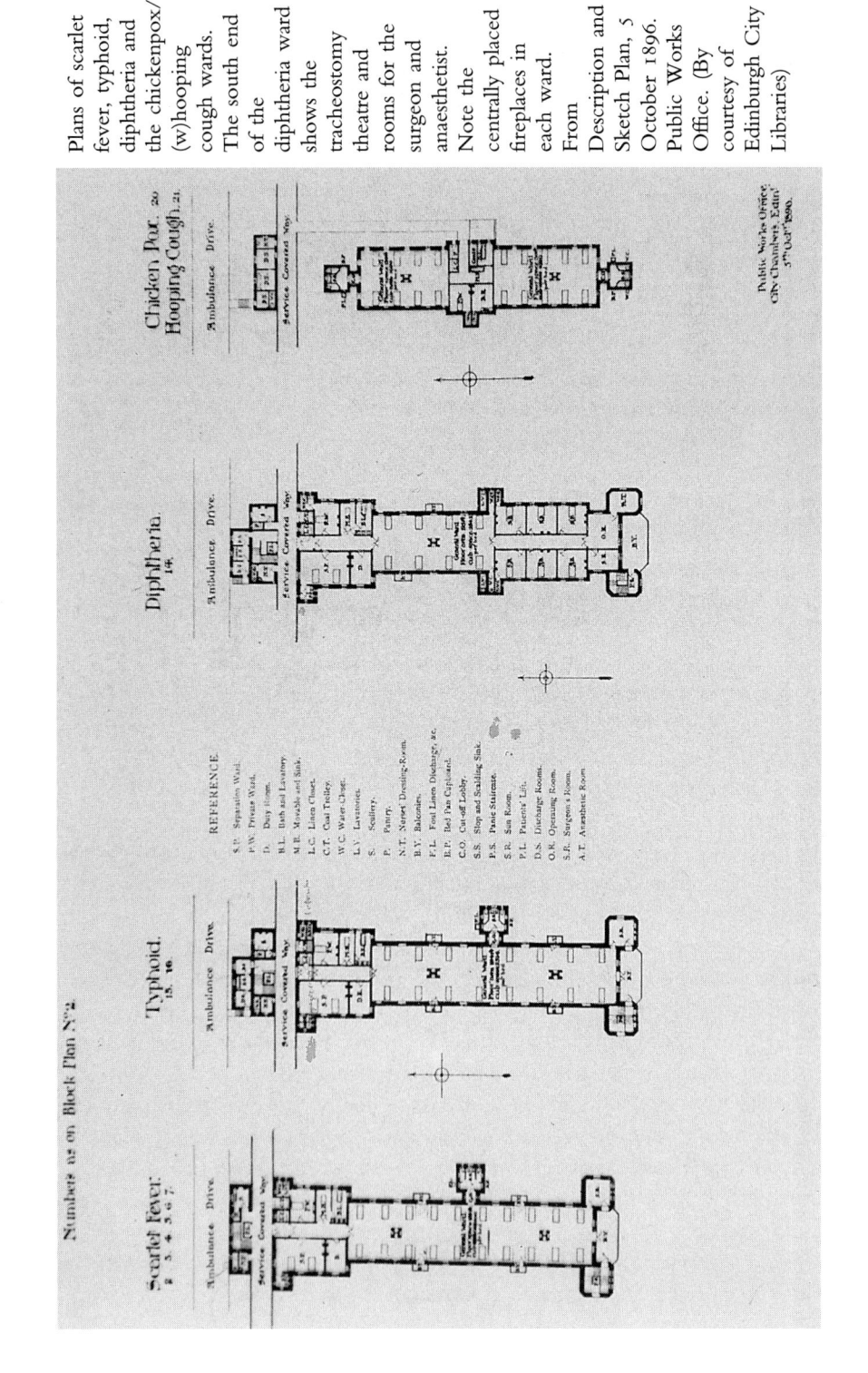

Plans of scarlet fever, typhoid, diphtheria and the chickenpox/(w)hooping cough wards. The south end of the diphtheria ward shows the tracheostomy theatre and rooms for the surgeon and anaesthetist. Note the centrally placed fireplaces in each ward. From Description and Sketch Plan, 5 October 1896. Public Works Office. (By courtesy of Edinburgh City Libraries)

A Description of the Hospital

Glazed tile-lined soiled-linen chute, Cottage 10. Note the carbolic tank, with brass tap and plug and vermin proof netting. (Photo: J. A. Gray)

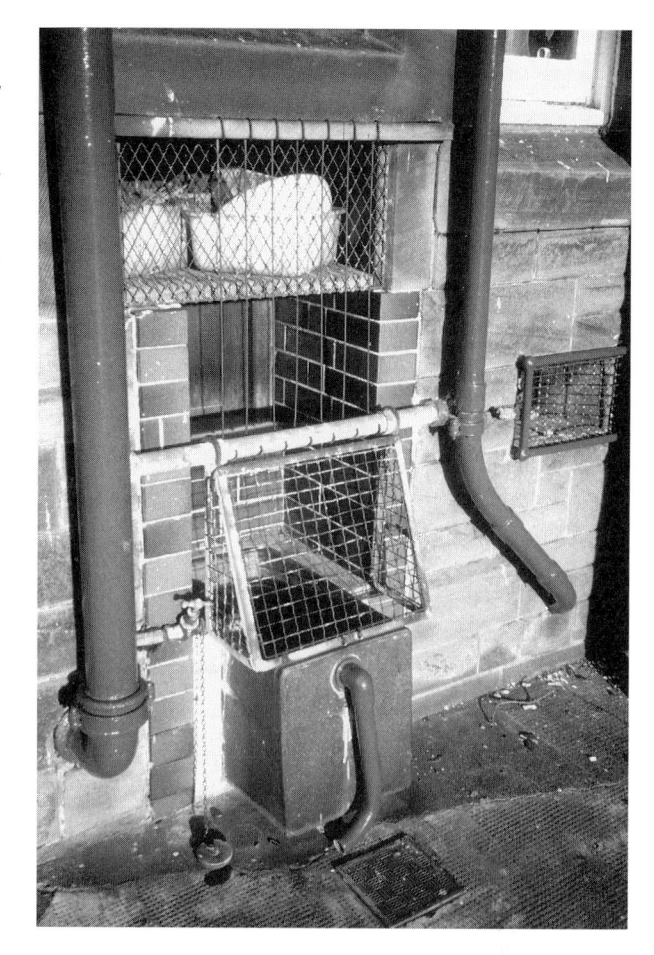

and half way down the pavilion except in the chickenpox and whooping cough wards where they were situated at the southern end. These areas were usually approached by a lobby cut off from the ward. They contained two water closets and a 'slop' and 'scalding sink' for emptying and cleansing the metal bed pans which were then dried in adjacent ventilated cupboards. Foul linen was disposed of down open, brown, glazed tile chutes into carbolic tanks connected to a flushing system from a cistern in the upper part of the sanitary tower.

To obtain the maximum sunshine, most pavilions had small balconies on either side and a sunroom in the south eastern turret opposite the panic stair. A large open balcony was a feature at the southern end of most pavilions. Besides catching the sun, especially in the upstairs wards, these balconies afforded a spectacular view of the Pentland Hills.

On the plans and drawings,[14] the isolation cottages and observation wards (Nos. 9–12 and 23–26) appeared more sophisticated than they eventually turned out to be. Originally there was to be a separate annexe with scullery and nurses' toilet across the service way from the entrance to the ward. This then led into a short corridor and the day room at the rear of the ward of west-facing cottages off which were two, two bedded observation rooms each with a separate cut-off lobby and water closet. In the centre, to the east of the day room, was the coal store and, separate from it, the linen room and bathroom.

Taking Cottages 23 and 24 as examples of east-facing cottages, the main entrance gave directly onto the bathroom/lobby (which must have been cold and embarrassing for patients when the outside door opened); this led to a short corridor with coal store and linen room opposite. Behind this was the nurses' day room with glazed observation panels which allowed the staff to see into the two bedded rooms on either side without them having to change into their gowns and enter the rooms. To the left of the entrance lobby was a toilet and sluice with a chute leading outside to the carbolic tank which received soiled linen. Neither the separate annexe across the service way nor the cut-off lobby and water closet off each observation room that had appeared in the original plans materialised in the final buildings.

Although popularly named 'smallpox cottages' these isolation and observation wards were not often used as such; the temporary wooden wards to the north west of the hospital were used for smallpox. However, in the last Edinburgh smallpox outbreak in 1942 when 36 patients were notified, some of the 'smallpox cottages' accommodated female patients as an overflow from the temporary hospital.[15] In 1973 a small family recently arrived from Asia was isolated in Cottage 25 for three days under suspicion of smallpox but happily an non-infectious skin eruption was diagnosed instead.

The Building Specification[16] detailed the cavity walls – stone outside and brick within – with a 2½ inch gap for insulation and, also, the widespread use of 'double glazing' or what today would be called secondary glazing. Another highly modern feature was the open-sided, slate-roofed, covered ways. These connected wards and other buildings and thoroughly aerated the staff as they moved about the hospital. Many former employees and patients will remember how on wintry nights the snow seemed to blow straight off the Pentlands across these passages. Much later the side walls of these covered ways were glazed and the corridors boxed in. With the centrally placed kitchen, the covered ways allowed the quick delivery of food that was still hot even to the more distant wards.

Below the covered corridors were subways for supplying steam, gas, hot water and electricity. Small carts also used these subways for supplying coal to those wards that had open fires. Mr Welstead[17] recounts that when he took up the post of Group Secretary in 1952, a house physician told him that it was possible to walk underground from the medical residency to the nurses' home (or indeed to any of the wards or major buildings). He refused to elaborate further on any unplanned use for these subterranean passages!

Mr Morham was proud of the ventilation in the wards and offices.[18] Where possible this was natural via gratings in the walls opposite the steam coil radiators and cross-draughts from opposing windows on either side of the wards. Glazed flues within the walls assisted downcast extract ventilation from the central fireplaces in the two-storey pavilions. This connected with ventilating fans in the basements at the foot of the chimney stacks which helped the vitiated air to rise and be discharged. Upcast ventilation in the single-storey wards without central fireplaces was again through flues within the walls continuing into trunks along the roof where rotary fans would discharge the vitiated air through ridge ventilators. Despite their sophistication, it is doubtful whether these fan-assisted ventilation systems were effective. Certainly some wards were occupied in late 1903 and even in 1904 without mechanical ventilating systems because appropriate motors and switch gear had not been supplied in time.[19]

The central, administrative buildings (general offices on the plans) faced the principal gate in the middle of the northern aspect of the hospital grounds. To the west was the Medical Superintendent's house. The general offices comprised on the ground floor the doctors' room, Matron's and clerk's offices, waiting room, mess room for the assistant medical staff, a committee room and an instrument room. Upstairs there was a sitting room and three bedrooms for the assistant medical staff, a small spare room and a room for the Chaplain.

The Medical Superintendent's house had a dining room, sitting room and kitchen on the ground floor, a drawing room, two bedrooms and a bathroom on the first floor, and a servant's room in the attic. Originally designed as a family home, it was temporarily converted to bachelor accommodation when the marriage engagement of one of the Medical Superintendents was broken off. Happily everything turned out well a little later on, the wedding took place, and the house was converted back to family accommodation. This sequence of events came to light when dry rot was found in the house in the 1950s. It was apparently due to a ventilator, blocked up during the conversion to bachelor's quarters, not having been satisfactorily unblocked when the house was restored again as a family home.[20]

The store block provided storage for dry food, soft goods, crockery and hardware. Drugs were also dispensed from here through a dispensary.

The store room for mattresses on the ground floor had a sewing room above. In the central block, there was also the kitchen with sculleries and larders, and other offices. There were separate entrances to the servants' and nurses' dining rooms. The nursing staff refectory was divided by a glass screen into a scarlet fever nurses' dining room and one catering for other nurses. Both of them had separate entrances and serveries. Outside was a shed for dinner trolleys.

In the two-storey servants' home with central attic, accommodation for 60 domestics was provided by 15 cubicles in each of the four large wards. The four head servants had their own bedrooms. Also provided were a sitting room, recreation room, sick room and requisite baths and 'lavatories' (for washing) and WCs.

The male staff were accommodated in rooms above those of the assistant doctors in the general offices. Workmen stayed in the East and West Cottages and in the lodge at the Comiston Road end of Hospital Road.

In the four-storey nurses' home, separate rooms were provided for 150 nurses. Matron's house was on the first floor in the south east wing. Five day rooms were provided for off-duty nurses. There were two sick rooms with small kitchens and offices attached. The main sanitary accommodation was in towers in the north east and north west with baths, lavatories, water closets and slop sinks. The two main staircases were at each end of the main building with additional winding stairs at the south end of each wing. A portion of the roof over each wing was protected with an iron railing to give 'an open-air promenade'. The main attraction of the nurses' home was the 50 feet × 30 feet central recreation hall, big enough for badminton. Mr Morham stipulated carefully the quality of wood for the flooring, gallery and wall panelling. This made for an interesting, if rather gloomy, interior despite the large bay windows at the southern end looking out over the gardens and up to the Pentland Hills.

An internal telephone system working from a central exchange in the general offices connected the more important parts of the hospital and offices with extensions to the cottages beyond the hospital enclosure, east and west.[21] A private wire connected the hospital to the Central Police Office with branches to the chambers of the MOH and City Superintendent of Works. A further wire was introduced on the National Telephone Company's exchange to allow communication between the general offices and the stores, doctors' and Matron's houses. Within the nurses' home there was yet another system connecting separate parts of this large building.

The laundry and boiler house with disinfector and incinerator were

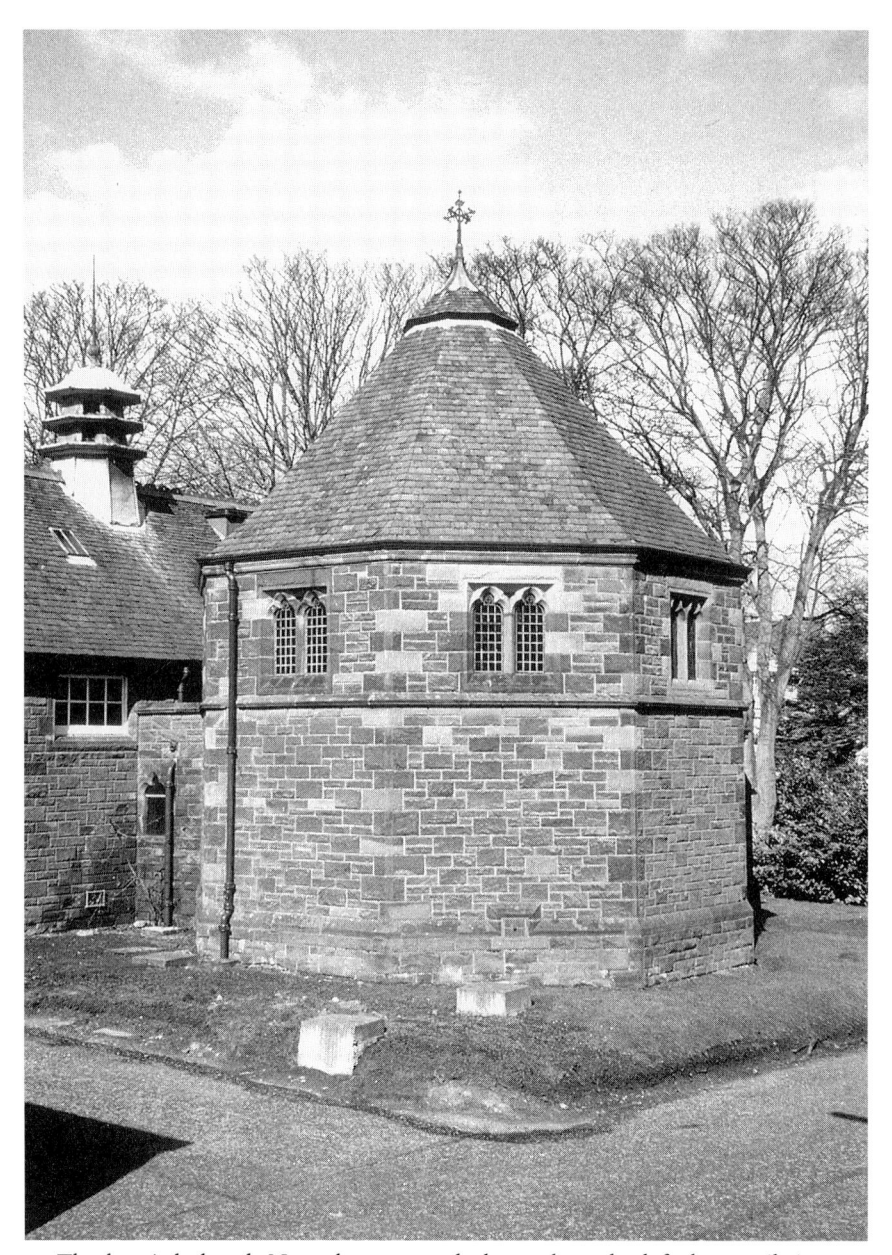

The hospital chapel. Note the octagonal plan and on the left the ventilation turret over the mortuary, the design inspired by architecture in Fatehpur Sikhri in the Punjab. (Photo: J. A. Gray)

situated east of the scarlet fever pavilions. In the laundry, washing of patients' items was kept strictly separate from those of the staff. The boiler house had 'four large Lancashire Boilers with Mechanical Stokers, Economisers ... Hot Air Batteries and Drying Chambers'.[22] Super-saturated or super-heated hot air or steam was available for selected items in the disinfector depending on requirements. The flues from the furnaces in the boiler house were fed directly into the incinerator where refuse and obnoxious matter was destroyed. Several coal stores were situated in the hospital. The largest, an open area, was adjacent to the boilers.

At the north east corner of the grounds towards the ambulance yard was a complex comprising the mortuary, post-mortem room, octagonal-shaped gothic chapel and workshops. A viewing room with glazed panel on one side of the chapel separated grieving relatives from direct contact with the deceased. The education block for the instruction of nurses and medical students, had a small semicircular lecture theatre, lecturer's room, laboratory and bacteriology museum with appropriate offices.

The lodge at the main hospital entrance opposite the Medical Super-intendent's house was home for the gatekeeper. It had a visitors' waiting room attached. Finally the ambulance yard in the far north eastern corner is shown as a hollow plan building surrounding a courtyard with entrances north and south; that to the north led to the north east gate, which presumably was also used by the mortuary staff for the discreet removal of the deceased. Like the gatekeepers' lodge, there are no plans or drawings in the four sources mentioned to describe the ambulance yard. It is thought some male staff were accommodated in upstairs rooms there, in addition to the attic bedrooms of the general offices and in the East and West Cottages.

Apart from its utilitarian function, Colinton Mains Hospital incorporated many modern features resulting from the researches Bailie Pollard and Mr Morham had carried out on their visit to the continent. It was fortunate to have such a superb, elevated site and gentle southwards slope. In those days there were lovely views of the Pentland Hills, uninterrupted by the present housing estates which have engulfed the original Colinton Mains Farm. The 50 acres not built upon were devoted to pine-planted woodland interspersed with glades which made a gracious setting for Mr Morham's designs. The cosy warmth of the Dumfriesshire red sandstone buildings surmounted by grey slate roofs finished with red ridge tiles remains pleasing today and reduces some of the institutionalised atmos-phere. The pagoda-like towers for the ventilation apparatus are reminiscent of Fatehpur Sikhri in the Punjab.[23] They punctuate the roof ridges and, silhouetted against a setting winter sun, add a touch of eastern romance.

Despite the more recent building of operating theatres, teaching rooms and the Rayne Laboratory on the airing grounds in between some of the original pavilions, nothing can take away from the openness and sense of freedom that the site inspires. Patients incarcerated for several weeks with virtually no communication from visitors for the duration of their hospital stay must have derived comfort from the open vistas and the fine views of the hills.

Yet some disagree with these sentiments. Architects writing about the City Hospital in *The Buildings of Scotland* have this to say:

> Except for the central administration block and some ancillary buildings (e.g. the mortuary and octagonal Gothic chapel to the NE) the effect is industrial, a Japanese distillery to judge by the big pagoda ventilators. Japan is also evoked by the covered walkways with prettily fretted wooden canopies.[24]

There can be no accounting for differences in taste, not even in architecture!

Concluding his description of the proposed new hospital,[25] Bailie Pollard shows the source of inspiration which he and his Public Health Committee must have drawn upon. He quotes from Professor Bümm who was describing the splendid new hospital that had just opened in Basel:

> The most suitable buildings, the most efficient arrangements, the finest furnishings do not alone suffice for the proper working of a hospital. To these there pertains some other thing, something intangible and of endless importance. That something is the spirit that must hold sway throughout the whole house – the spirit of Humanity, of Duty, and of Order. May each one occupied in this place – the teacher and the learner, they who nurse the sick and they who do the most menial work – may each and all constantly seek to own a consecrated earnestness in their calling, may each fulfill his and her part with complete devotedness and cheerful self-sacrifice. Then will the blessing of God not be wanting.

CHAPTER SIXTEEN

The Royal Opening, 13 May 1903

A State Visit to Edinburgh and Glasgow by King Edward VII and Queen Alexandra when only in the third year of their reign had to be something of an occasion. *The Scotsman* of Saturday 28 March 1903,[1] records that the Edinburgh Town Clerk had received the previous day the official intimation of the visit which was to start on 11 May 1903. This announcement had 'occasioned the liveliest of satisfaction both in the East and West of Scotland'. Although *The Scotsman* sounded reassuring that a recent drainage problem at the Palace of Holyrood House had been corrected, the Town Council must have been disappointed that the royal party decided to stay in Dalkeith and not at Holyrood. This precluded evening functions during the visit for His Majesty had been advised to avoid risking a chill in driving back to the country at night.

The Scotsman of 28 March 1903 continues:

> It has also been suggested that the King during the course of his visit might be graciously pleased to open the new City Hospital for infectious diseases, built at Colinton on the outskirts of the city, at the cost of over a quarter of a million sterling.

The cost had already escalated to nearer £350,000 but this was not going to deter the civic dignitaries from a royal occasion. On the contrary, the munificence of the Town Council, by providing such a fine and very expensive institution for its citizens, was more a matter of pride and self-congratulation. The bills could come in later.

On the morning of Wednesday 13 May 1903, in the park at Dalkeith House the King and Queen presented war medals for the South African campaigns.[2] The *Edinburgh Evening News* columnist[3] sounded peeved that the King, who was to visit Edinburgh Castle later that day, had not presented the Black Watch with their medals on the Esplanade so that the citizens of Edinburgh could have been more closely associated with their regiment, the 'Gallant Forty Two'.

The royal couple next went by special train to Waverley Station, thence by carriage through streets thronged with applauding spectators to Holyrood House. There, before lunch, the King inspected the Royal

Company of Archers and a parade of veterans of the Crimea and of the Indian Mutiny.

There was a public holiday in Edinburgh for the royal visit, though some merchants stayed open.[4] Special trains were run from Perthshire and the west to convey well wishers to the capital for the occasion. The city was festooned with decorations. Ceremonial arches over the streets proclaimed 'Honour and Welcome', 'Loyal Caledonia's Welcome' and 'Long Live Your Majesties' while troops in scarlet, blue and 'more drab' uniforms lined the routes.

The public's warm welcome to their King and Queen seems to have been genuine and the royal couple responded accordingly. Yet nationalists of today who refuse to call our present Queen, Elizabeth II, may be interested in the comments in *The Scotsman* of 14 May 1903. Here the newspaper mentions 'the pathetic clinging to the title British, and the refusal to give our Monarch his English numeral'. A postcard from Glasgow declared that Scottish people 'would not allow advertisements in publications that placed the sign "VII" after the name of King Edward or that speak of the Empire as "English"'. *The Scotsman* felt it was likely that the postcard's author 'dreams a dream of the restoration of the ancient glories of our city, of the return of the Court of Holyrood, of a Scottish Parliament to the High Street ...' Unlike post-Referendum Scotland in 1997, this was a minority view in 1903 for *The Scotsman* records of the royal visit:

> Enthusiasm reigned supreme, and at every stage in the long route a wave of vociferous cheering ran in front of the Royal carriage, while from house windows and stands the gay flutter of handkerchiefs waved welcome to their Majesties.[5]

After lunching at Holyrood House, their Majesties drove through more applauding crowds to the Royal High School, the Castle and St Giles' Cathedral. Speeches were delivered, replies given, keys proffered to the King, acknowledged and returned, and bouquets presented to the Queen. According to *The Scotsman*,[6] however, 'the crowning ceremony of the Royal visit to the Scottish capital' and also the last ceremony the King and Queen were to perform on this visit was the opening of the new City Hospital.

At the City Hospital all the preparations had been made for the royal visit and excitement was running high. The weather was the only thing that could not be guaranteed. Wednesday 13 May had started off dull with an occasional slight drizzle. A thick Scottish mist had swept across the Pentlands driven by a cold, raw, south westerly wind. In the end, the threatened rain held off and the ceremonies at the City Hospital in the late afternoon were blessed with some bright sunshine.

Both *The Scotsman* and the *Edinburgh Evening News* of the 14 May 1903 gave colourful accounts of the previous day's proceedings as follows. Councillor Brown and Mr McHattie, the hospital gardener, were responsible for the decorations. The royal standard, union jack and other flags adorned the top of the general offices. There was bunting everywhere. A crimson draped platform was built before the offices and embellished with 10 foot-high potted palms. The window sills of the royal rooms were also decorated with palms, cineraria, spireas and creeping plants. The entrance hall was tastefully ornamented with lilies. On either side of the platform were stands each accommodating 600 people and an enclosure on raised ground to the right of the entrance held a further 800 spectators. The whole Avenue (now Greenbank Drive) from Comiston Road was bedded with hardy shrubs, flowers and rhododendrons.

The royal rooms themselves were lavishly decorated. For the King, antique tapestries adorned the walls, and the furnishings in Queen Alexandra's room were in the style of Louis XV and XVI. So delighted was Her Majesty with her surroundings that she enquired if the furniture had come from London. How the Councillor responsible, Judge Brown,

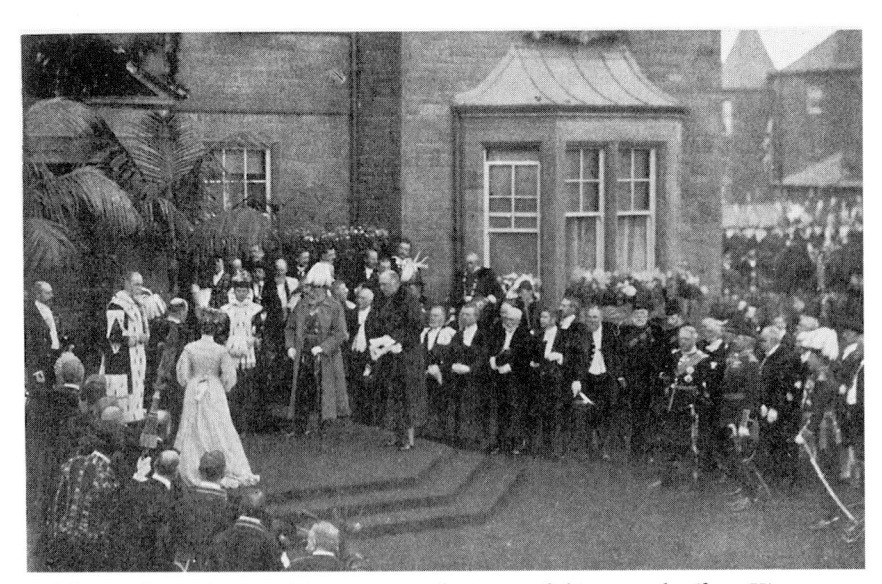

The royal opening, 13 May 1903 on the steps of the general offices. King Edward VII in greatcoat and plumed hat with Queen Alexandra on his right. Lord Provost James Steel in ermine-trimmed robe is on the left. (Reliable Series Postcard by courtesy of Dr K. S. Liddell. Crown Copyright: Royal Commission on the Ancient and Historical Monuments of Scotland)

The Royal Opening, 13 May 1903

must have enjoyed replying that the furnishings for the King's rooms were by Mr W. Adams and those for the Queen's by Messrs J. Ciceri & Co, both of Edinburgh.

Mr William Adams, a woodcarver to trade, had built up a huge reputation in antiques and *objets d'art*. He frequently travelled to the Continent to find elegant furniture, bronzes, ceramics and old master pictures which were displayed in the six spacious floors of his emporium in Shandwick Place.[7] Mr Joshua Ciceri came from north Italy to Edinburgh as a young man. He entered the business of his uncle manufacturing embossed and engraved mirrors and collected beautiful pictures and antiques for his showroom in Frederick Street. He had already enjoyed the patronage of the King, when Prince of Wales, so he knew what was wanted for the furnishings that he arranged for Queen Alexandra at the opening of the City Hospital.[8]

The opening ceremony was scheduled for 5.30 p.m. and the hospital gates were not to be opened to admit spectators until 2 p.m. Yet so popular was the event, that people began to arrive as early as 9 a.m. to get a good vantage point. By midday there was a 'constant throng of vehicles and foot passengers all making their way to the scene of the day'.[9] By 4 p.m. almost everyone had arrived.

Besides the two stands each holding 600 spectators and the 800 accommodated in the main gate enclosure, 3,300 more packed into the corridors of the western pavilions and hundreds more occupied the windows of the wards. In the south western pavilions were 1,900 more and a total of 4,000 in the scarlet fever pavilions to the east of the general offices. Estimates of the crowds within the hospital grounds vary between 10,000 and 12,000. The Edinburgh High Constables, who ushered the spectators to the best vantage points and yet avoided dangerous overcrowding, were accorded special mention. Some people secured seats on benches provided in the corridors and the time passed quickly with entertainment by Pipe Bands of the Police and Dr Guthrie's School. Although few of these spectators saw the actual opening, they had a splendid view of the royal carriage which completed a circuit of the hospital grounds just before the official opening took place.

The event had been planned with great care but the enthusiasm of the crowds, not only to be present at the opening but to get there early and enjoy the provisions arranged for them, had been much underestimated. The embarrassing sub-heading in *The Scotsman* read 'Paucity of Refreshments'. The tickets for admission were coloured differently for the different sections and to each was attached a coupon entitling the holder to tea and cake between 3 and 5 p.m. Of course those who arrived early clamoured for their refreshments before 3 p.m. In a moment of weakness someone opened the doors too early so by the time 3 p.m arrived 'the tables had literally been swept of all vestige of food'. One of the attendants attested 'upon his solemn oath he saw one party having four helpings whilst another said that some of the parties seemed to have had no food for weeks'. There were numerous complaints. One man who did get something to eat told his friend the biscuit was only about one inch in diameter. Near the main gate there was a select marquee with an ample supply of food and beverage and, for those privileged to be in the stands on either side of the platform, tea and cake were served in the nurses' dining room by 30 nurses detailed for this duty.

A guard of honour of Argyll & Sutherland Highlanders was waiting at the gate, and the route from Comiston Road was lined by Seaforths and Volunteers of the Second Regimental District. At 3 p.m. the members of the Corporation drove to the hospital with attendant halberdiers and the bearers of the Sword and Mace. They wore court dress or uniforms below their civic robes of office. The Lord Lieutenant of the County, Lord Rosebery, was cheered on his arrival about 5 p.m.

This suggested the King and Queen would soon be arriving, but first came a detachment of the Lancers which would escort the King and Queen back to Dalkeith Palace. The platform welcoming party included Lord Provost James Steel, with Lady Steel, Lord and Lady Balfour of Burleigh, the Duke and Duchess of Buccleuch, the Earl of Rosebery, Councillor Lang Todd, Convener of the Public Health Committee with Mrs Lang Todd, and Mr Morham in court dress, together with the City Magistrates and Councillors wearing scarlet robes and cocked hats. Also present were Sir Henry Littlejohn and the Lord Provosts of Aberdeen and Dundee. The nurses, in their neat and becoming white dresses, stood in front of the Medical Superintendent's house.

On the journey to the hospital the royal carriage paused momentarily in Morningside at the Bore Stane. A particularly warm welcome was given as the procession neared the hospital. This cheer:

> went up with great lustiness from the throats of the little boys and girls in the adjoining Poorhouse ... and their Majesties recognised the welcome given to them from that humble quarter.[10]

Continuous cheering greeted the procession as it turned left through the hospital gates at 5.25 p.m. The royal carriages were preceded by mounted police and escorted by the Life Guards. They rode via the Ambulance Drive at a good pace around the pavilions then drew up in front of the general office at precisely 5.30 p.m.

As the King and Queen alighted from their carriage, the sun obligingly broke through and lit up the platform party. The King was greeted by Lord Provost Steel and Lady Steel with whom he shook hands, the Queen acknowledging them with a bow. The King and Lord Rosebery next shook hands and chatted. Lord Balfour then introduced Councillor Lang Todd who addressed the King. He reminded the King that, when Prince of Wales, he had laid the foundation stone of the new Royal Infirmary at which time the Corporation took over the management of fever patients. When the old Infirmary site was found inadequate the Town Council had purchased Colinton Mains Farm. With the enthusiasm of the late Bailie Pollard and to the design of Mr Morham they had built for £350,000 a hospital 'second to none in your Majesty's Kingdom'. He then respectfully called upon the King to declare the hospital open.

The King replied briefly congratulating the Corporation on the completion of this great building. He felt confident it would improve the sanitary administration of the city and he trusted it would realise all the anticipations of benefit which led the Corporation to undertake so large a work. It was a pleasure for him and the Queen to visit the city at a time that enabled him to open the hospital.

Councillor Lang Todd then presented the King with a ceremonial gold key made by the Edinburgh jewellers, Hamilton & Inches.[11] The bow of the key was a quatrefoil inscribed with *Nisi Dominus Frustra* surrounding the Arms of the City, below which was the date *13th May 1903*. The stem had an elevated spiral carving inscribed *Edinburgh City Hospital* and the bit was a complex X-shape.[12] The King then unlocked the door and entered the reception room to loud cheers from the spectators.

Both of Charles J. Smith's books[13] covering the opening ceremony describe the hesitation which followed the opening of the door. The King invited the Lord Provost to go in first, but the Lord Provost deferred to the King whereat the Lord Provost in his broad Scots accent is reputed to have exclaimed 'Hoots, man, we'll baith gang in the gither!' This cannot have been taken amiss by King Edward for he elevated the Lord Provost to Sir James Steel of Murieston a few minutes later. His baronetcy was confirmed shortly after by letter.[14]

James Steel was an extremely wealthy man. Born in 1830 of farming stock, he came to Edinburgh in 1866 and set up business as builder and quarrymaster. He was responsible for some of the fine terraces at Edinburgh's West End, much of the development in Dalry and flats in Comely Bank. He became a town councillor in 1872 and contributed generously to the building of the present Braid Church. He died in September 1904 shortly after he relinquished office as Lord Provost.[15]

In the reception room, in addition to conferring a baronetcy on the

Lord Provost, the King had presented to him: Lord Balfour of Burleigh; Sir Henry Littlejohn, the MOH; Dr Affleck, Consulting Physician; Dr Ker, Medical Superintendent; Mr Morham, City Architect; and Miss E. L. Sandford, Lady Superintendent. Miss Sandford gave a bouquet of pink roses and lily of the valley to the Queen who chatted with her about the hospital and the nursing profession. Mrs Lang Todd presented the Queen with a specially bound copy of the booklet about the hospital.[16]

The Queen was then escorted by Lord Rosebery to the east of the general offices where, with the help of Mr McHattie, the hospital gardener, she planted an English elm with a silver spade. She declared it to be 'a bonnie tree' and requested that Mr McHattie look after it well. The King's turn came next. He planted a Scottish elm to the west of the general offices, but did so less efficiently than the Queen. Indeed so leisurely was the King's shovelling of soil about the roots of his elm that a few moments later it nearly toppled and had to be steadied by Mr McHattie. The King retrieved the silver spade with good humour and, while the spectators cheered loudly, he added three more shovels full of soil which kept the tree upright.[17]

The King and Queen then entered their carriage at 6.00 p.m. and, escorted by the 17th Lancers, drove off to Dalkeith Palace. So the great day ended. In that brief but momentous half hour, the new City Hospital could not have had a more auspicious and ceremonial opening. It was a day that everyone would remember.

PART FOUR

Dr C. B. Ker's Superintendentship 1903–25,
the City Hospital and Tuberculosis,
and
Dr W. T. Benson's Superintendentship 1925–36

CHAPTER SEVENTEEN

Dr Ker's Early Years and the Temporary Smallpox Hospital

The City Hospital at Colinton Mains has been fortunate in its four Medical Superintendents. The first of these was Dr C. B. Ker whose obituary in 1925 justifiably praised the excellent service he gave.[1]

Claude Buchanan Ker, son of a general practitioner, was born in Cheltenham in 1867. When still a schoolboy at Malvern College, he became interested in the armed forces and commanded an artillery battery in the local Volunteer Corps. Following family tradition, the Indian Civil Service seemed his appropriate calling but illness prevented him from completing the entrance examinations. He therefore decided to become a doctor and qualified in Edinburgh in 1890. After appointments as house surgeon in the Royal Infirmary and Simpson Memorial Hospital, his interest in infectious diseases was stimulated when he became a clinical clerk to the City Fever Hospital. He rose to be Assistant Medical Officer there and won a gold medal in 1896 for his MD thesis on 'The General Treatment of Enteric Fever'.[2]

In 1896 Dr A. F. Wood died and Dr Ker was appointed to succeed him as Medical Superintendent of the City Hospital at the age of only 30 years. He passed the Membership examination of the Royal College of Physicians of Edinburgh in 1898 and was elected a Fellow in 1901. He had assisted Bailie Pollard, Convener of the Public Health Committee, in planning the new fever hospital and, as the new Medical Superintendent, was responsible for the move to Colinton Mains from the old Infirmary site.

Dr Ker's superintendentship at Colinton Mains covered the first 22 formative years of the new hospital. He combined clinical duties, teaching and administrative skills with hard work and was highly respected, his staff affectionately referring to him as 'CB' His opinion was often sought by his peers in difficult cases of diagnosis and management.

His leadership qualities partly stemmed from his interest in military history and the organising skills of Napoleon. Memorabilia, pictures and books about the little Emperor adorned his sitting room in the Medical Superintendent's house. The writer of his obituary[3] believed Dr Ker had the qualities of a general. Had he not pursued a medical career he

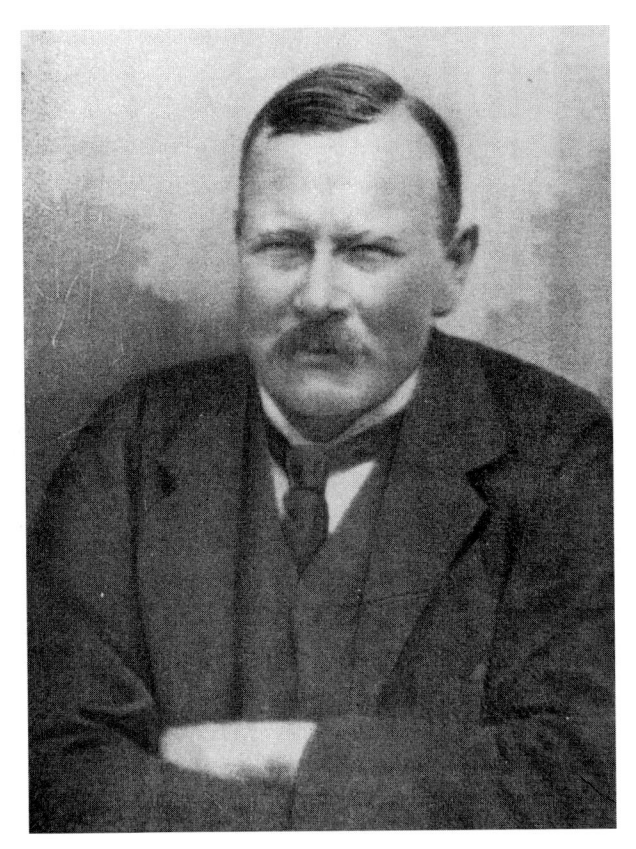

Dr Claude Buchanan Ker, Medical Superintendent, 1897–1925. (Photograph first published in the *Edinburgh Medical Journal*, 1925;23: 265–9 and now reproduced by kind permission of the *Scottish Medical Journal*)

would have been very successful in the Army. Dr Ker's leisure interests also included Latin and Greek in both of which he was fluent. Despite his poor vision and consequent non-participation in sports, he was Honorary Vice President of the Edinburgh Athletic Club and a keen supporter of rugby football, regularly attending the international matches at Inverleith.

In 1898 he was commissioned Surgeon Lieutenant in the Queen's Brigade of the Royal Scots and appointed to the Medical Bearer Company of the 4th Infantry Brigade. Later, in 1908, he was promoted to the rank of major in the Royal Army Medical Corps (RAMC) Territorial Defence Scheme. During the First World War he served at North Queensferry and later commanded a prisoner of war camp. His poor eyesight debarred him from active participation in athletics and from military service overseas, in both of which he would have wished to have played his part. He was, therefore, discharged from the armed forces during the First World War back to his duties at the City Hospital.

Dr Ker served on the Board of Management of the Royal Infirmary of Edinburgh and the Board of the Royal College of Nursing. In 1924, the year before he died, he became a Member of the Council of the Royal College of Physicians of Edinburgh, a Member of the Faculty of Medicine of the University and President of the Fever Hospitals Medical Service Group of the Society of Medical Officers of Health.

Dr Ker's contribution to the medical literature included original work on naphthol treatment in enteric fever and, with Dr Harvey Littlejohn, son of Sir Henry Littlejohn, a description of the typhus outbreak at the turn of the century.[4] He wrote review papers on Fourth Disease and on incubation and quarantine periods. He was the author of a 300 page *Manual of Fevers*[5] published in 1911 and intended for medical students. His highly successful *Infectious Diseases – A Practical Textbook* was first published in 1909, with a second edition in 1920. A posthumous third edition, revised by Dr Claude Rundle of Liverpool, appeared in 1929.[6]

Sadly, in 1925, when aged only 58, Dr Ker died of influenza, complicated by pneumonia. He left a widow and children and a very wide circle of personal and professional friends. He seems to have been a man whom everyone liked and respected. Certainly the City Hospital owes him a major debt for having steered it through the first 22 years at Colinton Mains and for having established its reputation.

The move from the old Infirmary site and the early years at Colinton Mains must have been difficult but at the same time exciting and challenging. As Dr Ker had spent many hours with Bailie Pollard and Sir Henry Littlejohn planning the new hospital, he must have been delighted when the new buildings fulfilled their intended function so satisfactorily. Yet after he had been presented to the King at the opening ceremony in 1903, all was not going to be plain sailing for Dr Ker.

Mr Ballingall's Weekly Reports on Works in Progress from the office of the Clerk of Works show that even at the time of the royal opening there was still much work to be done in the hospital. On 9 May 1903, Mr Ballingall stated 'All workmen principally engaged preparing for the Royal Visit in Pavilions 2–8 ... also Nurses' and Servants' Homes'.[7] Two weeks after the royal opening there were still joiners and plumbers in Pavilions 6 and 7 whilst the painters remained busy in Pavilions 4–8, the general offices, doctors' house and nurses' home. It is likely therefore that their Majesties only saw the outside of the pavilions, the nurses' home, servants' home and doctors' house. The general offices, however, where the King and Queen were received, must have been completely ready, at least in the downstairs rooms which were so lavishly decorated and furnished for the royal opening.[8]

Most of the work in Contracts 1 and 2 was probably nearing completion by 19 September 1903 apart from some painting, plumbing, staining of floors and fitting of locks.[9] At about this time Mr Ballingall assumed responsibility as Clerk of Works for Contract 3 as well which included 'Pavilions' 9–14, the education block, chapel, mortuary, laundry and east and west cottages. On 24 October 1903 he commented:

> Wards 1, 2, 3, 4 are occupied (without ventilation systems owing to motors and switches not being in working order). East Cottages and Comiston Lodge occupied.[10]

The next week Mr Ballingall reported the occupation of Wards 5 and 7, but still without mechanical ventilation. In Reports 337 and 230 (6 February 1904),[11] Wards 19, 20, 21, 25 and 26 were stated to be ready for occupation, but they still lacked ventilation systems. Even in his final Report of 19 March 1904, there had been no further progress with the mechanical ventilation and it is doubtful if it ever really worked.[12]

Presumably from the autumn of 1903 either a few patients were being transferred from Infirmary Street to Colinton Mains or, more probably, as the new wards became available at Colinton Mains, starting with the scarlet fever pavilions, it became possible to close wards at Infirmary Street when the last patients there were discharged. After the transfer was complete, some of the new wards were to be kept vacant to cope with outbreaks and also to allow for the proper disinfection of wards in rotation. For these reasons, infectious diseases wards even today show a relatively low bed occupancy compared with the wards of other specialties.

Smallpox patients were not admitted to the pavilions but were accommodated in the temporary buildings north west of the hospital and below the old quarry on Wester Craiglockhart Hill in the area now occupied by Wester Hill housing estate. After the public outcry about temporary wards in the Queen's Park during the smallpox outbreak of 1892–95, some of the wooden structures that had not been used there were removed to Colinton Mains in November 1895.[13] These formed the nucleus of the new 'temporary' smallpox hospital shown on the Sketch Plan of 1896.[14] The Post Office Plan of Edinburgh and Leith, 1899–1900,[15] gives no indication of these buildings perhaps because they were wooden or because it was presumed they would be demolished when the new fever hospital opened. The Post Office Plan, 1905–1906, however, shows four rectangular buildings in the site, labelled 'Temporary Smallpox Hos'. One of these, the administrative block, runs on an axis west by south west and east by north east; immediately south of it are two wards, which lie parallel to each other and on an axis at right angles to the administrative block. On this same axis but at the western extremity of the site lies another longer building which may also have been staff quarters.

An early but undated Valentine Series postcard[16] shows three wooden buildings in the foreground of the picture of Colinton Mains Fever Hospital viewed from the north west near the summit of Wester Craiglockhart Hill. Each block has two chimneys dividing the roof into approximate thirds. In the south west corner of the temporary hospital compound stands a tall, isolated chimney, probably belonging to an incinerator. The whole site is surrounded by a formidable wooden paling fence strongly buttressed on the inside. Miss J. K. Taylor (Matron 1965–69) photographed the hospital from an almost identical spot in the late 1940s. Her picture clearly shows two of the wooden buildings, possibly in a dilapidated state, the tall chimney and part of the buttressed boundary fence. All four of the original buildings of the temporary smallpox hospital continued to be shown on maps still obtainable in the late 1950s.[17]

Smallpox continued to be a problem over the turn of the century. Following the outbreak of 1892–95 which affected 701 patients, no further cases occurred for two years. Seven cases of smallpox were notified in 1898, none in 1899, but a further five occurred in 1900.[18] Knowing that there was smallpox in various parts of the country, Sir Henry Littlejohn kept the temporary hospital at Colinton Mains 'in constant readiness' towards the end of 1899.

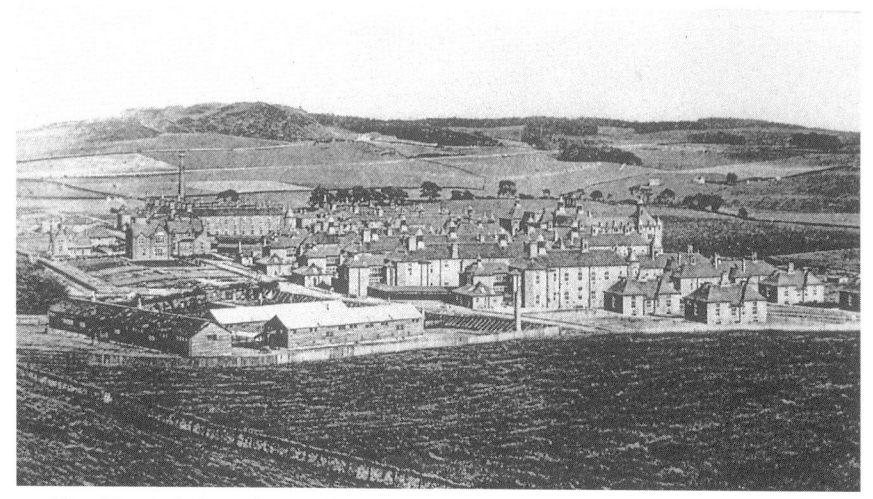

City Hospital from the north west. An undated Valentine Series postcard, ca. 1910. The three wooden blocks of the temporary smallpox hospital with its buttressed fence and incinerator chimney are in the left foreground. The absence of surrounding houses shows how much the hospital was then isolated from the rest of the city. (By courtesy of Dr K. S. Liddell. Crown Copyright: Royal Commission on the Ancient and Historical Monuments of Scotland)

The first of the five patients with smallpox in 1900 was admitted on 12 January from the Morningside Asylum. This patient had sailed from Buenos Aires to Southampton, probably acquiring smallpox *en route* in Lisbon on 29 December 1899. From Southampton he travelled to London and thence direct to Edinburgh where he arrived on 3 January 1900, spending the night in a house in the New Town. The next day he was arrested on a minor assault charge and placed in police custody. Thought to be insane, he was moved to Morningside Asylum on 5 January. A week later when signs of smallpox appeared, he was transferred to Colinton Mains (temporary smallpox) Hospital. Thanks to Dr Thomas Clouston's prompt revaccination of all contacts in the asylum, disaster was averted and no further cases developed.[19] The four other patients notified with smallpox in 1900 were unconnected with this incident.

In the winter of 1903, some labourers at the Talla Waterworks contracted smallpox which spread quickly to Edinburgh. Sir Henry Littlejohn reported 168 cases occurring mostly in lodging houses in the Grassmarket and Cowgate.[20] This was the biggest smallpox outbreak for ten years. The civic authorities were almost caught out again with insufficient isolation facilities, as they had been in 1894. Mr Ballingall's Weekly Report on Work in Progress of 20 February 1904[21] records the panic building of a New Smallpox Ward for which he had 61 men working that week – 38 joiners, 13 plumbers and 10 labourers. The following week 89 were employed, including 20 roadmen. Mr Ballingall recorded almost breathlessly:

> The joiner work of ward now finished on Thursday. The plumber work, putting up fences. Roads and drains completed on Saturday – and the ward occupied the same day.[22]

It is not stated if admissions were delayed till the building was finished and, if so, where patients were accommodated in the meantime.

Dr Ker managed a total of 170 patients at Colinton Mains during this outbreak. Fifteen died, giving a mortality of 8.8 per cent.[23] Despite the prevailing westerly wind blowing towards the new fever hospital and Craiglockhart Poorhouse only 200 yards away he commented with relief there was no evidence of aerial spread from the temporary smallpox hospital. He subsequently used this experience to suggest the Ministry of Health's regulations were too strict in forbidding smallpox hospitals to lie within half a mile of a population of 600, any fever hospitals, poorhouses or similar institutions.[24] Dr Ker also correlated the severity of illness and mortality with the absence of previous vaccination and noted that the milder cases occurred in patients with more than one vaccination scar. The fact that 144 of his patients had been vaccinated in infancy suggested to him that immunity waned over the years. He later strongly advocated routine revaccination.

Dr Ker regarded with a 'melancholy reflection ... the extraordinary attitude of this country towards vaccination' which made smallpox hospitals a practical necessity and not 'merely academic'.[25] Having discounted the risks of aerial transmission of smallpox between buildings, he favoured having temporary smallpox isolation facilities close to permanent fever hospitals. In that way the most experienced and trustworthy staff could be recruited for smallpox hospital duty whilst vacancies created in the permanent hospital could be filled for the time being by less well trained staff.

Dr Ker's military background made him a stickler for discipline. He insisted that the fundamental rule in administering a smallpox hospital was:

> so far as possible, to prevent all coming and going. To secure this, I do not allow the nurses ever to leave the hospital grounds. They are sent over from the permanent hospital in their uniforms, are allowed to take no outdoor dress, and understand that they must be prepared to stay for at least six weeks. The grounds are spacious enough to secure ample facilities for exercise, and a week's holiday, after the term of service is over, is sufficient recompense for the imprisonment. In this way nurses, at all events, cannot spread the infection.[26]

The same rules applied to domestic staff and porters so reducing the:

> dangerous staff to the visiting physician and the ambulance attendants, of whom probably the latter constitute the only real danger.[27]

Overalls were to be worn by anyone entering the wards and their hands were to be carefully disinfected on leaving. The only other visitors allowed were such 'clergymen as will submit to the regulations, and relatives of absolutely hopeless cases'.[28] All staff and visitors were vaccinated. Food and stores were deposited at the outer gates of the temporary hospital and then transported to the wards by smallpox hospital designated porters.

A 'Report as to Smallpox Accommodation' of 1910[29] submitted by the Medical Officer of Health, Dr A. Maxwell Williamson, Dr C. B. Ker, and Mr J. A. Williamson, City Superintendent of Works, showed that the present site and the condition of the buildings were satisfactory. Reservations were made, however, about the cinder track running east–west to the south of the temporary hospital and north of the permanent hospital, so an additional wooden paling fence was built within the one already standing, just to be sure no one walking along the cinder path could become infected. On the south side of Wester Craiglockhart Hill a barrier was to be constructed to enclose the north side of the temporary hospital. Dry earth or sand closets were recommended for patients, but there were water closets in the administrative and staff quarters.

The smallpox hospital could then hold 50 patients or, in an emergency, up to 70 which was considered adequate provided the public complied with vaccination and revaccination programmes. The Report[30] bemoaned the fact that, unlike the German Empire where vaccination and revaccination were enforced, smallpox hospitals were still required in the United Kingdom. Mainz was the only town in Germany where separate provision for smallpox was made; in other German cities, because of 'the population being perfectly protected by their vaccination and revaccination, at school age and military service age', it was safe to treat smallpox in general hospitals.

Although vaccination sometimes caused adverse effects, British medical authorities strongly disapproved of people avoiding vaccination and revaccination 'on the grounds of conscience'. Generalised vaccinia, a widespread skin eruption with subsequent scarring and, rarely, fatal encephalitis, might occur occasionally after vaccination, especially in children with eczema. Nevertheless these complications should not excuse the general public from complying with the vaccination laws.

Smallpox was of course a major problem when it occurred, but the City Hospital was largely concerned with the management of patients with other diseases, particularly streptococcal infections. Of the 2,817 patients admitted to the City Hospital in 1904, 942 had scarlet fever of whom 27 died and 136 had erysipelas of whom 3 died. Dr Ker recommended bed rest for the first three weeks to tide scarlet fever patients over the 'mostly likely nephritic period',[31] which was thought to be induced by chilling. This policy kept bed occupancy high and justified the provision of at least 320 beds for scarlet fever. Intramuscular or, in toxic cases, intravenous, horse-serum-derived scarlet fever antitoxin was injected early but (fortunately) was rarely required to be given more than once. In pre-antibiotic days antitoxins were regarded curative and likely to reduce complications.[32] Today one wonders how much of the alleged post-streptococcal arthritis was more a manifestation of iatrogenic serum sickness.

More than with other infections, except smallpox, the scarlet fever nursing staff were segregated from their colleagues. Scarlet fever nurses worked in the 'red' corridors and wore pink uniforms whilst those in the 'blue', non-scarlet fever corridors appropriately wore blue. Even in the nurses' dining room, the scarlet fever nurses were segregated from the other staff by a glass partition.[33] These rules were strictly enforced.

Any nurse apprehended in a corridor or ward other than her own without permission could be dismissed instantly.[34]

Forty-one of the 579 patients admitted in 1904 with diphtheria died, giving a mortality of 7.1 per cent.[35] Much faith was later placed in horse-derived antitoxin despite the frequent sequelae of anaphylaxis, serum sickness and the rashes, photographs of which appear in Dr Ker's textbook.[36] Yet most of the early deaths (11 within 48 hours and a further 12 between 48 hours and 7 days of admission) were more likely due to asphyxia from laryngeal obstruction and early myocarditis rather than due to later heart failure and paralyses. Laryngeal diphtheria was treated in a tent with steam kettles or, as in Ward 14A, with steam from the boilers supplied at reduced pressure through pipes on swinging brackets on each side of the patient's cot.[37] In children with incipient laryngeal obstruction, Dr Ker initially attempted intubation with a vulcanite tube, with the tracheostomy instruments standing by in case of failure. Only when the patient was *in extremis* would he advise tracheostomy before intubation.

Other killer diseases were whooping cough with a mortality of 19.2 per cent in the 125 admissions during 1904 and measles with a 4.2 per cent mortality in the 587 admissions that year. Typhoid, 'relapsing fever and continued fever' together accounted for 174 admissions in 1904 with 18 deaths, a mortality of 10.3 per cent. A mysterious eight deaths were recorded in the 73 patients admitted for observation. Although not analysed separately, at least five were due to tuberculosis of which three were caused by tuberculous meningitis. The 14 patients admitted with chickenpox and the six with 'typhus' all survived.

There were in all 163 deaths among the 2,817 patients treated in 1904, a mortality of 5.78 per cent. The daily average number of occupied beds was 321 at a cost per occupied bed per annum of £54 13s 3d.[38]

The City Hospital Bacteriology Department opened in October 1904. This provided a more scientific diagnosis in doubtful cases of diphtheria, scarlet and typhoid fever. It also facilitated the more rational discharge of patients with diphtheria and scarlet fever so as to reduce the risks of cross-infection.[39] In the next year, 3,402 specimens were examined of which 2,675 were on diphtheria cases and the remainder on scarlet fever/ diphtheria differential diagnosis problem patients and in those with typhoid fever. Dr J. Halley Meikle, Dr Ker's Senior Assistant, was in charge of the laboratory but left to become Medical Officer to the Edinburgh School Board in 1906.[40] He was followed by Dr T. Lauder Thomson and, in July 1908, Dr John Ritchie was the Senior Assistant and Bacteriologist.

From 1907 onwards, a daily bulletin about the progress of patients at the City Hospital was published in the *Bulletin, Evening News* and *Evening Dispatch*. Each patient was given an identification number on admission which preserved anonymity but could be easily referred to by relatives. This system gave up-to-date information to relatives who had neither a telephone nor transport for visiting the hospital. In fact, the visiting of infectious patients was strongly discouraged and the only direct contact permitted between patients and visitors was a wave from an ambulant patient to a visitor on the airing ground outside the ward. A typical bulletin from the *Evening News* of 16 January 1912[41] would be as follows:

EDINBURGH CITY HOSPITAL
TODAY'S BULLETIN

Dangerously ill; friends requested to come out,	[1 identification number given]
Seriously ill, no immediate danger,	[14 identification numbers given]
Ill, making satisfactory progress	[105 identification numbers given]
Not quite so well, no cause for anxiety	[8 identification numbers given]

It may be inferred that all the patients whose numbers are not referred to in this Bulletin are making satisfactory progress.

The latest report in regard to patients may be obtained during the day by applying to the Public Health Office, City Chambers. Inquiry may be made there by telephone No. 812 (Central) or directly to the City Hospital No. 772 (Central) between 5 and 5.30 pm.

(In the newspaper, the individual identification numbers are listed for each category of severity of illness. See illustration opposite.)

These daily bulletins continued until 1961 when visiting became more relaxed, and there was better public transport and more telephones. By that time relatives were allowed to accompany patients, especially children, in the ambulance taking them to hospital.

In bygone days safe transportation of fever victims to hospital could pose problems. In William Adam's Royal Infirmary the central staircase was wide enough for sedan chairs carrying patients to reach all the floors.[42] So convenient was this method of transporting patients to hospital over short distances that it may have only slowly given way to horse-drawn ambulances. The St John Ambulance Association, which started in London in 1878, soon extended to several Scottish cities including Edinburgh. It was gradually replaced in Scotland by the St Andrew's Association formed in 1882 by Dr George Beatson.[43]

> **EDINBURGH CITY HOSPITAL.**
>
> TO DAY'S BULLETIN
>
> Dangerously ill: friends requested to come out: 517.
>
> Seriously ill; no immediate danger: 162, 285, 298, 312, 320, 482, 457, 470, 473, 505, 616, 519, 863, 935.
>
> Ill; making satisfactory progress: 51, 114, 210, 211, 250, 286, 295, 309, 316, 319, 321, 323, 323, 324, 326, 348, 349, 353, 370, 374, 375, 384, 388, 389, 390, 391, 396, 398, 399, 400, 407, 412, 426, 427, 430, 434, 448, 450, 451, 453, 459, 460, 463, 468, 469, 471, 475, 477, 479, 481, 482, 483, 484, 486, 487, 488, 489, 490, 491, 492, 493, 494, 495, 496, 498, 499, 500, 501, 502, 503, 504, 507, 509, 510, 511, 512, 513, 514, 515, 518, 520, 521, 522, 523, 525, 526, 527, 529, 530, 531, 532, 540, 541, 542, 543, 544, 545, 546, 547, 548, 783, 852, 921, 939, 964.
>
> Not quite so well; no cause for anxiety: 57, 68, 308, 533, 534, 848, 901, 954.
>
> It may be concluded that all patients whose numbers are not referred to in this bulletin are making satisfactory progress.
>
> The latest report in regard to patients may be obtained during the day by applying to the Public Health Office, City Chambers. Inquiry may also be made there by telephone, No. 812 (Central), or directly to the City Hospital, No. 772 (Central), between 5 and 6.30 p.m.

Edinburgh City Hospital daily bulletin, 3 January, 1912. *Edinburgh Evening News.*

Dr Tait records that a brougham and a van were available for ambulance duty in 1876.[44] Shortly after 1885, a Mrs Moir of St James Place arranged a contract with the second City Hospital to hire coaches for patient transport and a van for disinfection purposes. Later a makeshift stretcher ambulance was available, converted from a funeral brougham, but what the patients thought of this was not recorded. Mrs Moir twice upset the Fever Hospital Subcommittee by raising the hire charges in 1888 and again in 1890; the Subcommittee's attempts to get her charges down again were only partly successful. It may have been one of Mrs Moir's employees who acquired smallpox transporting a patient to the City Hospital in 1894.[45] Ambulance work was not without its dangers.

After 1900 Mrs Moir provided separate coaches for scarlet fever, diphtheria and typhoid fever and agreed to fit the coaches with rubber tyres for greater patient comfort.[46] Dr Claud Muirhead had objected to the removal of the second City Hospital to the suburbs largely because his seriously ill typhoid patients would be subjected to a longer ambulance journey.[47] However, the improvements in ambulance design and the lower incidence of typhoid fever after the turn of the century fully justified the decision to relocate the hospital at Colinton Mains.

The hire contract arrangement for patient transport ended in 1909 when the Public Health Department bought two motor ambulances, one reserve horse-drawn ambulance and two horse-drawn disinfection vans (one to collect bedding, the other to deliver bedding).[48] The pride of the fleet was a new 18–24 horse power motor ambulance that could hold four persons besides the patient who was conveyed in a basket stretcher. A garage for three ambulances and a stable for two horses was built.[49] The new ambulances cost less to run than the previously hired vehicles and one motor ambulance could take 29 patients to hospital in an ordinary working day. It also conveyed convalescents to Campie House in Musselburgh. In its first eight months' service it covered 12,000 miles.[50]

The faster motor transport was particularly important in getting seriously ill diphtheria patients into hospital quickly especially at night.[51] It also saved nursing time because the fever nurse still had to accompany the ambulance from the hospital to the patient's home and back again (see Chapters 18 and 31).

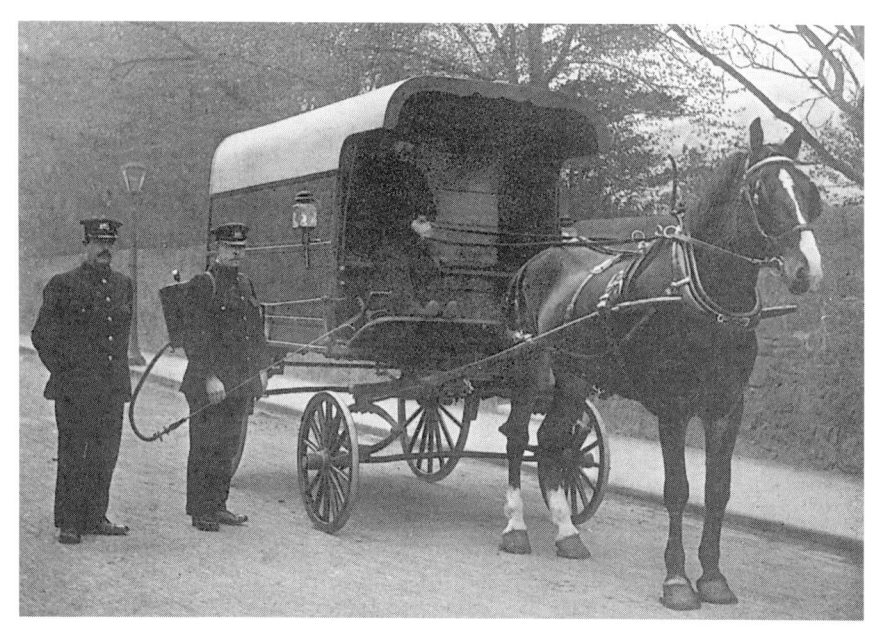

One of the two vans for collecting and delivering bedding. This one was presumably used to uplift infected material because of the attendant's back pack and disinfectant spray. Annual Report of the Public Health Department, 1909, p. 54. (By courtesy of Edinburgh City Libraries)

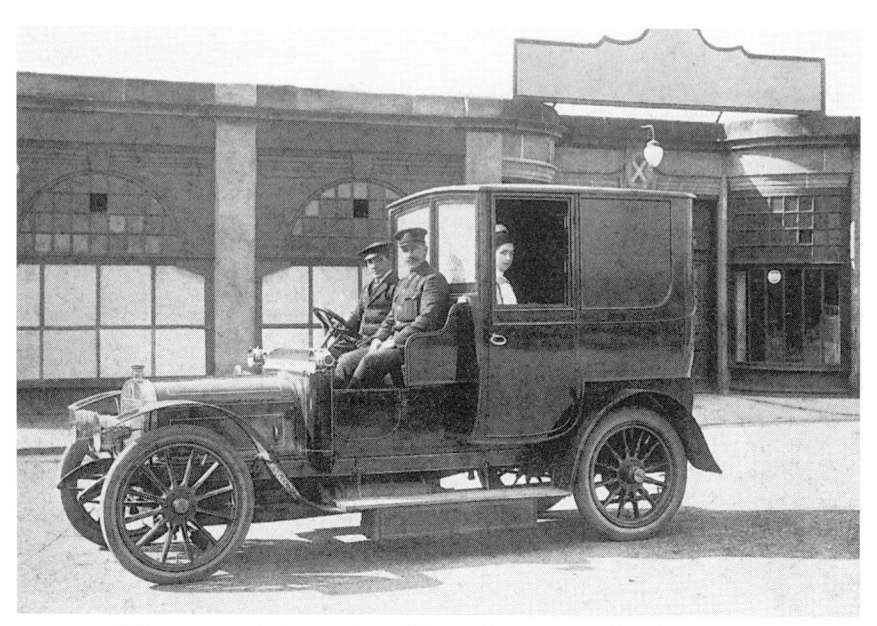

18–24 HP motor ambulance. It could seat four persons besides the patient who was conveyed in a basket stretcher. It uneventfully covered 12,000 miles in its first 8 months of service ca. 1908–09. Annual Report of the Public Health Department, 1909, p. 54. (By courtesy of Edinburgh City Libraries)

CHAPTER EIGHTEEN

Dr Ker's Later Years: The Nursing Staff; Scarlet Fever, Meningitis, Influenza; The First World War

Miss Sandford, Lady Superintendent of Nurses, who had presented the bouquet to Queen Alexandra at the opening ceremony in May 1903, was replaced by Miss I. Thomas later that year. Miss Thomas had come from the second City Hospital on Infirmary Street which the nurses at Colinton Mains irreverently referred to as 'the pest house'.[1] She continued as Matron of the new hospital until 1925, the year Dr Ker died. Like Dr Ker, she was to see many changes during that period, especially in the war years. Together Dr Ker and Miss Thomas were responsible for the smooth running of the hospital.

A Nurses' Roll Call of January 1904 records a total of only 64 nurses, some identified as in first, second and third years of training.[2] Most of these nurses would have come from Infirmary Street except for the probationers. The relatively small number of nurses recorded in 1904 may have been due to the wards either not yet being filled or some not even being open. Although the surviving nurses' registers give details about each nurse, the nursing complement cannot be elucidated from these early records.

A staff photograph[3] taken in front of the recreation room of the nurses' home in 1906 shows Dr Ker in the centre with Miss Thomas in white on his right, three male doctors and 115 nurses. Although this photograph does not take into account those nurses left on the wards while the picture was taken, nor those on night duty, sick or holiday leave, it suggests that the nursing complement at that time was about 150 – matching the number of beds in the nurses' home. A rather stern-looking lady in dark uniform is seated on Miss Thomas' right and may have been the Home Sister or Deputy Matron.

Another photograph taken in front of the general offices in 1918[4] shows 115 members of the nursing staff. Dr Ker with supporting medical staff, or possibly members of the Public Health Diploma course, and one lady in a sari, sit in the centre. Miss Thomas in white uniform is on his right. The probationers, first and second year nurses occupy the

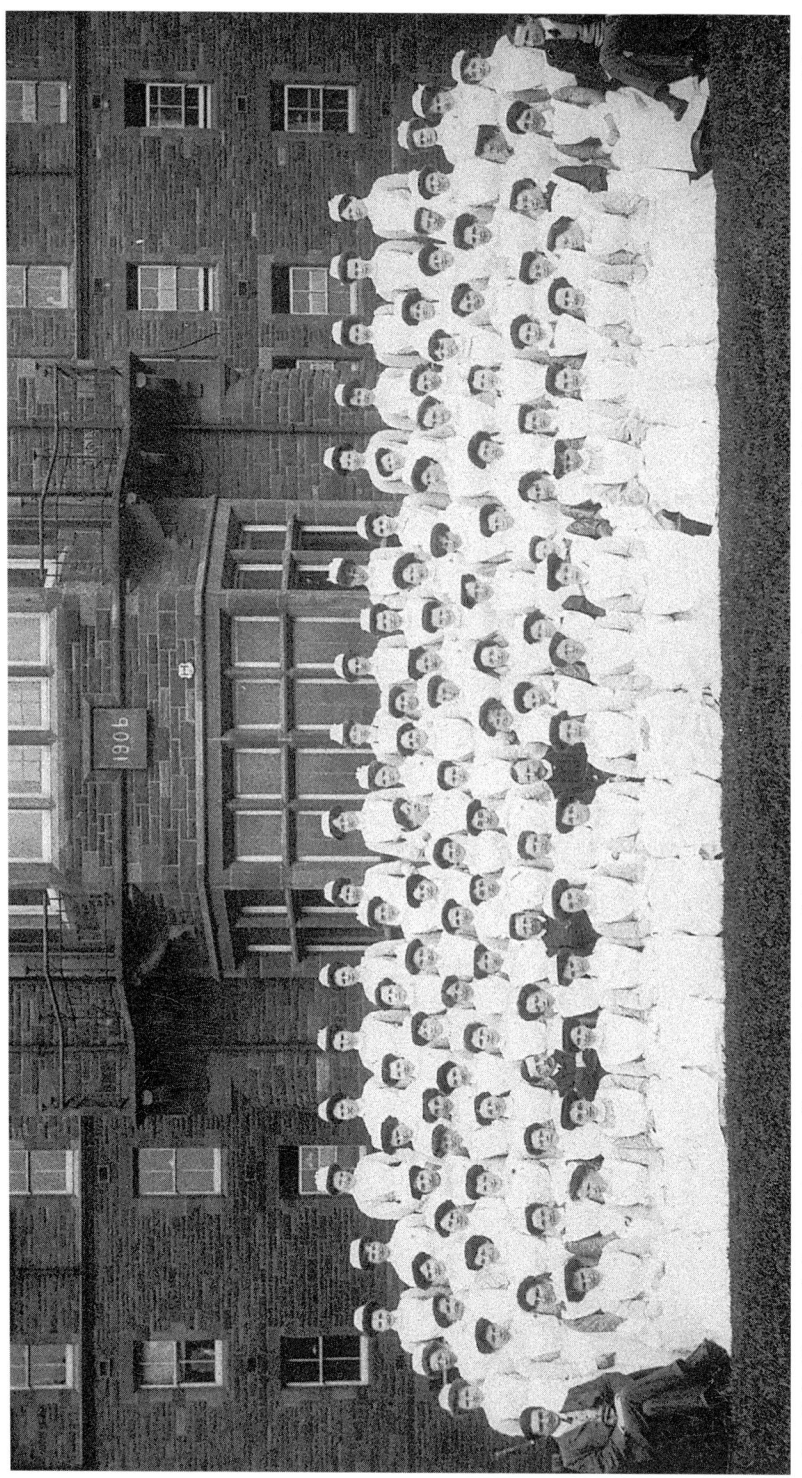

Dr C. B. Ker and the nursing staff outside the nurses' home, 1906. Dr Ker (2nd row centre) has Miss I. Thomas, Matron, sitting on his right side. (Photo: A. Swan Watson, Bruntsfield, Edinburgh)

upper back rows. The third year nurses towards the front of the photograph are wearing hospital badges and a navy blue band on the left upper sleeve. The nursing sisters wore a dark blue uniform with full length sleeves. Nurses in training wore long white detachable cuffs extending from elbow to the wrist over pink or blue uniforms depending on which corridor they were working on.[5]

Ambulance nurses who escorted patients referred by general practitioners into hospital wore an appropriate coloured uniform depending on the provisional diagnosis. According to Miss J. K. Taylor, who was associated with the hospital from 1928 to 1969, this was not a popular duty. It carried a heavy responsibility, for mistakenly to admit a patient with measles to a scarlet fever ward, or vice versa, would have serious consequences.

During 1905 Dr Ker and his resident medical assistants gave courses of lectures to the nurses on elementary anatomy and physiology, hygiene and infectious diseases. In those pre-antibiotic days, management of infection consisted of isolation bed rest, diets, purging and sweating and the occasional application of leeches. In 1911 the Local Government Board instituted a certificate for fever nurses and the first four nurses to be successful were from the City Hospital.[6]

All the sisters were certificated fever nurses (later with Tuberculosis Certificate, RGN and/or CMB). Initially one sister was responsible for a whole pavilion. This explains the relatively small number of sisters compared with the number of wards in both the 1906 and 1918 staff photographs. By 1950, the ratio was one sister to one ward, so that a two-storey pavilion had one sister upstairs and another downstairs.

Scarlet fever patients spent the first three weeks of admission in bed. When febrile, a milk only diet was prescribed with total exclusion of meat and eggs. This regimen continued for two weeks in adults and for three weeks in children. Post-streptococcal glomerulonephritis – inflammation of the kidneys as a sequel to scarlet fever – was supposedly less likely if the patient did not get chilled, hence the prolonged initial bed rest. According to a nurse's lecture notes, glomerulonephritis was treated by giving 'help to the kidneys by acting on the skin or bowel – sweating or purging the patient'.[7] The victim had to endure 20 minutes with two or three hot water bottles (or if insufficient, a hot pack as well) under several layers of blankets. Purging with Compound Jalap was next given to secure a watery motion. Uraemic convulsions were treated with hot packs or 'a few whiffs of chloroform'.[8]

Although the urine of uraemic patients was scrupulously measured and tested for blood and albumin every day, little emphasis was placed on monitoring their fluid intake. Indeed some patients may have been fluid overloaded. Dr Ker's textbook (revised in 1929) recommended that:

> As long as the urine is restricted in quantity, or haematuria persists, ...
> fluids must be liberally supplied in order to assist the elimination of waste
> material by the skin and bowels.[9]

In the management of the vomiting and diarrhoea in toxic scarlatina, however, his book recommended forcing fluids on the patient:

> if his stomach allows it, and if not, they may occassionally be given by the
> bowel. Stimulation, preferably with brandy, or perhaps champagne, should
> be freely resorted to.[10]

According to Catherine Samuel's nursing lecture notes, the diet in post-streptococcal glomerulonephritis was 'Practically pure milk and when the albumin gets down to small quantities and stays that way, eggs are advantageous.'[11]

As a child of nine, about 1921, Professor David Daiches was incarcerated for over two months in the City Hospital with a complicated form of scarlet fever. In *Was – A Pastime from Time Past*[12] he describes this episode with understated humour and wide-eyed childish astonishment. Coming from a polite, middle-class Jewish family he was unprepared for the culture shock of the children's ward where:

> complete pandemonium reigned. Children shouted, threw things, jumped
> on beds, and said rude words ... Their language was astonishing and
> educational.

The nurses seemed to take it all in their stride whilst the doctors 'in white coats lectured over him to students with a pointer'. One or other parent would visit daily and wave to him from the ward door and his GP also attended every day. The children irreverently called the minister who visited the ward on Sundays 'Jumping Jesus' because of the way he bobbed up and down when singing hymns to a portable harmonium.

At Christmas red shades decorated the ward lights. The self-coloured postcards David received as a Christmas gift from his mother, but disguised as originating from the ward, were given to the nurses to post but of course never arrived as they would have been considered infectious and destroyed. All the children were given a simple but thoughtful Christmas present but whether from the hospital or not is unclear. Possibly parents on low incomes were not asked to provide a present whilst young David Daiches' parents were. Inevitably after two months and so much time in bed he required firm rehabilitation to get him walking again. The night before he was taken home in a taxi by his mother, he was given a 'reeking pink carbolic bath'. The intention was to prevent residual infection spreading from him to his family and to limit the number of 'return cases' of which Dr Ker wrote frequently.

Matron's Lectures on Nursing emphasised the importance of a correct professional attitude to work, tidiness and the dusting of wards as well as what would now more properly be regarded as a nurse's responsibilities.[13] Both Dr Ker and Miss Thomas maintained strict discipline. By the second year at Colinton Mains, Nursing Staff Regulations were prominently displayed. They read as follows:

CITY HOSPITAL
NURSING STAFF REGULATIONS

Any Nurse found guilty of NEGLECT, or of CRUELTY to a Patient, PRACTICAL JOKING, INDECORUM, INSUBORDINATION, or who enters a WARD or CORRIDOR, other than her own without direct permission of Dr Ker, shall be liable to instant dismissal and loss of certificate.

Nurses shall receive with Kindness and Consideration all persons who present themselves with a PASS (WITHOUT WHICH NO ONE SHALL BE ADMITTED TO THE WARD) from Dr Ker. They shall see that such Visitors conform strictly to the Rules of the Hospital, and especially that NO FOOD, DRINK, SWEETMEATS, or FRUIT is brought into the Patients. No Visitor is to be allowed to enter a Ward unless wearing the overalls provided for the purpose.

February 1905   By Order

These regulations were necessary to limit cross-infection between patients and to protect the staff and the general public. Nonetheless, and not surprisingly, nurses and domestic staff did sometimes acquire infection. Each Annual Report of the MOH, and later of the Public Health Department (PHD), contains a summary of activities at the City Hospital and from 1905 this was submitted by Dr Ker himself. He described with openness and honesty:

While the health of the staff was on the whole good, a certain number contracted the infectious diseases with which their duties brought them in contact, as under:

	Nurses	Maids
Contracted Enteric	3	0
Scarlet Fever	3	0
Diphtheria	3	0
Measles	1	0
Erysipelas	1	3
	11	3

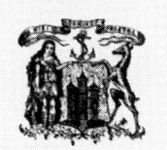

CITY HOSPITAL

Nursing Staff Regulations

Any Nurse guilty of NEGLECT of, or CRUELTY to a Patient, PRACTICAL JOKING, INDECORUM, INSUBORDINATION, or who enters a WARD or CORRIDOR other than her own without the direct permission of Dr Ker, shall be liable to instant dismissal and loss of certificate.

Nurses shall receive with Kindness and Consideration all persons who present themselves with a PASS (WITHOUT WHICH NO ONE SHALL BE ADMITTED TO THE WARD) from Dr Ker. They shall see that such Visitors conform strictly to the Rules of the Hospital, and especially that NO FOOD, DRINK, SWEETMEATS, or FRUIT is brought to the Patients. No Visitor is to be allowed to enter a Ward unless wearing the overalls provided for the purpose.

FEBRUARY 1905.

By Order.

City Hospital nursing staff regulations, February 1905. Either mounted on stiff cards or hung in glazed frames, these were prominently displayed in the wards.

Allowing for changes in the nursing and domestic staffs, it may be said that during the year nearly 230 individuals were exposed to infection. The number of those affected was therefore a little over 6 per cent. All these fortunately made good recoveries.[14]

The following year Dr Ker reported that the seven nurses who contracted scarlet fever, the three with diphtheria, the two with measles and one each with enteric fever, german measles and erysipelas – a total of 15 – all recovered well. Neither in that year nor in 1907 were any of the maids infected, which prompted Dr Ker to suggest that this proved:

> that infection is not much carried from the wards by the nurses, and the immunity in particular of the large numbers of young girls in the laundry is a proof of the thoroughness of the disinfection of the linen before it leaves the wards.[15]

Infection amongst staff continued. In 1913 as many as 21 nurses developed scarlatina, 13 diphtheria, 12 rubella and one of the medical assistants had enteric fever.[16]

Another illness, which was less common than the original eight notifiable infections but which nonetheless carried a high mortality, was 'cerebro-spinal fever', the term often used then for what would be called today meningococcal septicemia or meningitis. It was made notifiable in 1907 along with pulmonary tuberculosis. In the 1909 Annual Report of the PHD,[17] Dr Maxwell Williamson recorded only 28 notifications of cerebro-spinal fever in Edinburgh compared with 53 in 1908 and as many as 206 in 1907 when the death rate in hospital was 78.57 per cent.[18] The mortality, though still high, then fell from 50 per cent to 33 per cent. Dr Ker attributed this decrease to the use of Flexner and Jobling's or the Lister Institute's meningococcal antitoxin which he gave to as many patients as possible whilst supplies lasted. It was injected ideally four times intrathecally[19] over several days in doses of 15–30 ml. Dr Ker believed in giving intravenous as well as intrathecal antitoxin and felt the 77 per cent serum sickness rate which resulted from this treatment was justified by the apparent reduction in mortality.[20]

The war years were particularly difficult for the medical staff as well as the nursing staff. At the outbreak of war, Dr Ker's services were temporarily lost although he returned later to take up his previous post. Dr MacLeod who was in charge of the tuberculosis wards also left, together with two residents and three ward sisters. Dr W. S. I. Robertson, standing in for Dr Ker in 1914, explained how hard it was to obtain replacements.[21] Senior medical students were employed to take up the vacant posts. The laboratory assistant also enlisted, dramatically increasing the problems in a year when the laboratory dealt with 10,639 specimens, more than double the number of 1913.[22]

Dr Maxwell Williamson reported[23] that both scarlet fever and diphtheria were particularly prevalent in 1914. The large military population living in the city under crowded conditions which encouraged throat infections helped to increase the number of admissions to a record of 5,848 patients. By utilising all the wards and cottages, the maximum daily bed occupancy rose to 873, 143 more than the corresponding number in 1913 which itself was 200 more than in any previous year. There was little wonder then that this overcrowding in an understaffed hospital led to more infections among the nurses of whom 24 contracted diphtheria, 18 scarlet fever, 3 measles and one erysipelas. The influenza prevalent that autumn caused a further 18 casualties in the overstretched nursing staff. One resident went off with scarlet fever. Fortunately, all recovered.

Despite all the difficulties in 1914, before Dr Ker had enlisted, both he and Dr James, consulting physician, held classes for 229 medical students and three courses for the public health diploma which were attended by 34 doctors. The nurses too did well, 27 obtaining the fever nurse certificate of the Local Government Board that year. Courses continued for the nursing staff in 1914 on elementary anatomy and physiology, hygiene and infectious diseases. These were given by Dr Ker and his assistants, and lectures on nursing were given by Miss Thomas, the Matron. In 1907 Dr Ker also introduced a short course on medicines by Miss Duncan, the lady dispenser, but these lasted only one year as Miss Duncan then left the hospital. Miss J. K. Taylor[24] recalls lectures on tuberculosis, medicines and diets as part of the nursing training in the 1920s later combined with experience with respirators and in the operating theatre.

Applications for fever nurse training were encouraged. Personal interviews were held by Miss Thomas on Tuesdays, Thursdays and Saturdays between 11 a.m. and 1 p.m. Evidence of successful revaccination was required. Probationers had two hours of recreation daily and, if convenient, a half day off each week. Three weeks holiday was allowed each year.[25] Pay in 1917 was £16 per annum (pa) for first year nurses rising to £19 in the second year and £22 in the third year.

By 1919 the pay for nurses in training had increased to £18, £21 and £24 and it was proposed it should go up further to £22, £25 and £28 respectively for each of the three years of training.[26] At that time, the assistant matron was earning £90 pa, home sister £70, night sister £57 and ward sisters were on a scale from £45 to £70 pa. Staff nurses earned £35–42 pa. The estimated value of the uniform of three dresses and six aprons each year (which were to be returned to the hospital) and the cap and cloak was £3 16s 6d. The hours of duty, excluding meal times, were for ward sisters 55 hours, staff nurses 57 hours, night nurses 72 hours and probationers 66 hrs, for a seven day week.[27]

Miss Thomas had written in May 1919 to Dr A. Maxwell Williamson, the MOH, that 'Owing to the general demand for a shorter working day, I fear we shall be obliged to alter the time-table of our nursing and domestic staff'.[28] The knock-on effect was that an additional 50 staff would be required, straining the limited accommodation 'as we are already greatly handicapped for lack of rooms, and have been obliged to use isolation cottages, as well as sitting rooms, and box-rooms for bedrooms'.[29]

The pay of Edinburgh City Hospital nurses was lower than for nurses in fever hospitals in Aberdeen, Dundee, Glasgow and Motherwell. In some other fever hospitals the Local Government Board examination fees, the cost of books for studying and also a cookery fee were all paid for by the hospital. Not so in Edinburgh. This, together with the overcrowded staff accommodation, led Miss Thomas to point out to Dr Maxwell Williamson:

> You will observe that our rate of payment is the lowest quoted. I find that invariably nursing candidates apply to several hospitals before deciding where to train, and naturally they choose the one where the terms are most generous; this has been especially marked lately, as very many of those who apply do not proceed further with the transaction after receiving our schedule with terms, etc ..., and this change can only be attributed to the better monetary conditions in other hospitals since the war.[30]

The Annual Reports of the PHD were abbreviated from 1915 to 1918 because of the war but very close cooperation was established between the military authorities and the hospital particularly regarding the disinfection of troops and their uniforms. The influenza pandemic of 1918 hit Edinburgh most severely early the next year. In February 1919 the weekly death rate was 48.1 per 1,000 inhabitants and a total of 744 influenza deaths were recorded in the city that year. Sadly three of the City Hospital nurses died of influenza in 1918 and a further two in 1919.[31]

The hospital remained full with 5,302 admissions in 1919. The maximum and average daily bed occupancy figures were 868 and 582 respectively. The American Squadron and the Grand Fleet lay in the Firth of Forth and there were numerous colonial soldiers in the city. The hospital treated 2,005 military and 848 naval personnel even though the Admiralty had taken over East Pilton Fever Hospital for the infectious diseases patients from Leith. On top of a scarlet fever epidemic which kept up the bed occupancy in its own right, there were many cases of measles. Of 5,302 total admissions, however, 340 cases were of tuberculosis and 86 of these fatal.[32] As part of the Edinburgh Tuberculosis Scheme advanced cases of tuberculosis were admitted to the City Hospital (see Chapter 19) and the increased length of stay of these patients added considerably to the pressure on beds.[33]

In 1920 things were beginning to settle down after the war.[34] In all 4,493 patients were admitted, the greatest number in hospital on one day being 702, and the daily average number 529. The nursing staff kept well, or at worst, had only mild infections except, sadly, one newly joined probationer nurse who died of 'an exceptionally virulent attack of Diphtheria'. Twenty-nine nurses satisfied the examiners and gained the first nursing certificate of the Scottish Health Board. The post-war bulge of medical students made it necessary to divide all 307 of them into 10 classes. Sixty-two graduates trained for the Diploma of Public Health (DPH). The appointment of Dr W. T. Gardiner, consultant otologist, was welcomed and he performed 44 ENT operations in the hospital that year. Dr Forrest, Senior Assistant, was replaced by Dr Walter T. Benson who was to become Medical Superintendent on Dr Ker's death in 1925. The cost of an occupied bed had risen to £98 10s 4d per annum but Dr Maxwell Williamson noted that this compared favourably with expenditure in other similar sized institutions. The laboratory analysed 11,502 specimens in 1920.

Twelve patients were admitted to the smallpox hospital in 1920, of whom 9 had the diagnosis confirmed.[35] The attacks were mild which was as well since only one patient had been revaccinated since infancy. All survived. The outbreak could have been serious but for a vigorous revaccination programme carried out by temporary medical assistants vaccinating 'from door-to-door' and the setting up of free vaccination centres in several city police stations. Bills were circulated to every house informing the public about the benefits of vaccination. In all a magnificent total of 80,000 people were either vaccinated or revaccinated. As a result only three additional cases of smallpox occurred despite the presence of the disease in Glasgow and the influx of summer holiday visitors from the west to Portobello.[36]

Later in 1920 a separate, potentially disastrous, outbreak occurred in Craiglockhart Poorhouse, two patients developing smallpox among the 1,000 inmates. Both they and some other suspects were transferred to the temporary hospital and about 900 poorhouse inmates were revaccinated. In all, the outbreak was confined to six inmates. Other contacts were kept under observation in the 20 bedded reception house at High

School Yards. The successful containment of the disease exemplified the effective coordination that now existed between general practitioners, the Public Health Department and the hospital.[37]

In 1921 a major reorganisation of tuberculosis accommodation took place with advanced and early cases being admitted to East Pilton Hospital and the Royal Victoria Hospital respectively so restoring 'all the original buildings of the (City) hospital to the use for which they were designed'.[38] This was particularly important since the boundaries of the city had been extended and every infectious diseases bed was needed to cope with influenza, which became a problem again in 1921 along with a milk-borne outbreak of scarlet fever. In all 4,563 patients were admitted in 1921 with the maximum and average daily bed occupancy being 851 and 558 respectively. Dr Ker congratulated his medical and non-medical staff on their good work and Dr W. T. Benson on the 11,526 laboratory specimens examined that year.[39] Dr Alexander James continued as consulting physician, visiting daily. Dr Gardiner's work on ENT problems further reduced the length of hospital stay of diphtheria carriers and streptococcal cases through tonsillectomy and adenoidectomy. Those with chronically discharging ears were also managed more quickly.

The Annual Report of the PHD for 1922[40] was prepared by Dr William Robertson, the MOH who took over after the death of Dr Maxwell Williamson. Dr Ker[41] reported a quiet year with 4,446 admissions and daily maximum and average bed occupancy of 649 and 471 respectively. It would have been even quieter had it not been for influenza in the early part of the year. The freeing up of the two phthisis pavilions the previous year allowed 450 influenza patients to be admitted, of whom 181 had pneumonia. Among the staff, two nurses died of enteric fever, one contracted on holiday, but the other in the course of duty. Routine Schick testing (for susceptibility to diphtheria) was introduced with a toxin-antitoxin mixture used to inoculate those testing positive (non-immune). Dr Ker hoped that this would protect his staff, 10 of whom had diphtheria that year.

Good results were obtained by the nurses in the Scottish Board of Health examinations: 32 probationers passed the first part and 17 senior nurses passed the final part of the examination. The 339 male and 43 female medical students were divided into 14 sections for teaching, and 22 postgraduates attended the DPH course. Dr Alec Joe, who was later to be the hospital's third Medical Superintendent, worked as Senior Assistant for a few months and Dr Ker 'much regretted' his departure. Dr Joe was succeeded by Dr McGarrity.

1923–24 saw continuing slum clearance as part of the Cowgate/Grassmarket and Leith Improvement Schemes.[42] The source of an increase in scarlet fever causing 43 cases was tracked down to infected milk from a cowshed in Linlithgow. Cessation of supply quickly arrested the outbreak. A further explosion of scarlet fever occurred, however, after stopping that supply, when some of the infected milk was diverted to another consuming district.[43] Dr Robertson hoped that pasteurisation, which was slowly gaining acceptance, would resolve the problem of infected milk for all time.[44] The impact on hospital accommodation was, however, less severe than might have been expected due to the decision to reduce the length of hospital stay for scarlet fever patients from six or seven weeks to only four. Home isolation of scarlet fever patients was now encouraged in cases where it could be carried out safely under medical supervision.

Dr Ker reported 3,965 admissions in 1923 with a maximum and average daily bed occupancy of 600 and 447 respectively. Schick testing of City Hospital nurses followed by immunisation of those positive seemed to be protecting the staff against diphtheria, only five nurses acquiring the disease that year compared with an annual average of 13 during the previous five years.[45] Dr Benson[46] was busy in the community swabbing 113 throats in the investigation of a school outbreak of diphtheria. Finding 24 of the 113 to be carriers, he closed the school a fortnight before the summer holidays were due and no other cases occurred at the start of the autumn term. Dr Benson became involved in encouraging routine Schick testing among school children in Leith. He also made a detailed inspection of water supplies in the city's suburbs.[47] He was, therefore, receiving highly appropriate training to equip him as the next Medical Superintendent of the City Hospital.

In 1924 the highest overall death rates in the city were 19.3 in North Leith, 17.8 in St Giles Ward and 17.7 in St Leonard's Ward, and therefore further improvement schemes were implemented.[48] Again Dr Benson embarked on the country's first large-scale campaign of Schick testing school children with subsequent immunisation of those testing positive. In 26 schools, 3,057 children were immunised with no adverse reactions. The particularly vulnerable pre-school children were targetted next.[49]

In view of the mortality associated with measles and whooping cough, arrangements were made to notify the first case in every household. Two fever trained nurses were supported by a Scottish Board of Health grant to carry out home visits. Interestingly the MOH commented that 'Scarlet Fever and Diphtheria cause more parental alarm, though nowadays less fatal than Measles and Whooping Cough'.[50] Indeed in Dr Alec Joe's Annual Report, as interim Resident Physician, after the death of Dr Ker,[51] he records a hospital death rate of 9.4 per cent for measles and 22.12 per cent for whooping cough compared with a 9.11 per cent and

4.18 per cent death rate in diphtheria and scarlet fever respectively. In the Annual Report of the PHD for 1925,[52] Dr W. T. Benson now recorded hospital death rates for measles and whooping cough at 16.1 per cent and 27.16 per cent respectively and for diphtheria and scarlet fever at only 7.93 and 3.14 per cent respectively. Erysipelas was carrying off 9.19 per cent of those diagnosed in hospital. Dr Benson was hopeful that antitoxin treatment for scarlet fever would reap benefits and that active immunisation would soon follow.

Thus ended the first 22 years of the City Hospital at Colinton Mains. The hospital was working well together with general practitioners and the Public Health Department to combat the classical infectious diseases. Chapter 19 will deal with the important part the hospital also played in controlling the other major infectious scourge, tuberculosis.

There were important staff changes in 1925. Miss Mary Pool came from her post as Matron at the Royal Victoria Hospital to replace Miss Thomas who was completing 22 years service at the City Hospital. Miss Pool would be in charge of the nursing staff for the next 19 years.

Dr Walter T. Benson succeeded Dr C. B. Ker whose untimely death in 1925 after 28 years as Resident Physician or Medical Superintendent was deeply mourned. The plaque in the entrance hall of the general offices at Colinton Mains is as fitting an epitaph as any. Below his bust is written:

> In honoured and affectionate memory of Claude Buchanan Ker M. D., F. R. C. P. E., Medical Superintendent of the Edinburgh City Hospital 1897–1925. His eminence as a physician and his devotion to duty earned alike the gratitude of suffering humanity and the confidence and esteem of his colleagues and fellow citizens.

CHAPTER NINETEEN

The Contribution of the City Hospital to the Control of Tuberculosis: Sir Robert Philip, Sir John Crofton and some Notable Chest Physicians

Edinburgh's important contribution to the control of tuberculosis has already been extensively documented.[1] The Annual Reports of the Medical Officer of Health (MOH) called from 1908 onwards the Annual Reports of the Public Health Department (PHD)[2] also provide valuable information including the statistics for phthisis, as pulmonary tuberculosis was then known. These Reports contain statements by the Medical Superintendent at the City Hospital and, from 1913 onwards, by the Tuberculosis Officer as well. The long but ultimately largely successful struggle to control tuberculosis and the lead given by Edinburgh to the rest of the world in its management are neatly summarised by the late Dr A. G. Leitch, in his article 'Two men and a bug: One hundred years of tuberculosis in Edinburgh'.[3] The two men of vision and determination of whom Dr Leitch wrote were Sir Robert Philip and Sir John Crofton. The bug was the tubercle bacillus or *Mycobacterium tuberculosis*.

Oral evidence about tuberculosis in Edinburgh has kindly been provided by Dr Christopher Clayson, Sir John Crofton, Dr A. C. Douglas, Dr N. W. Horne, Professor J. Williamson and Dr M. F. Sudlow.

To provide continuity, the contribution made by the City Hospital in the fight against tuberculosis is told here up to the early 1970s. To begin with there was controversy about notifying tuberculosis. Dr Robert Philip (1857–1939) had recommended compulsory notification as early as 1890 but this did not then appeal to Dr Henry Littlejohn, the MOH, who told Dr Philip 'Don't throw yourself against a stone wall'.[4] Dr Littlejohn's rather atypical attitude was probably due to his familiarity with tuberculous disease in the autopsies he carried out as part of his forensic work. He had written in 1888 'I hardly ever open a body of a person dying from an injury or disease, but traces of the previous existence of tubercle in the lungs are found'.[5] In other words tuberculosis was incredibly common. Also, until it was far advanced, tuberculosis could be difficult to diagnose before X-rays were available, and Dr

Littlejohn liked accuracy. He probably also felt that the cost of demonstrating tubercle bacilli in sputum, although providing an exact diagnosis, would strain resources. Besides it would only pick out those with advanced pulmonary disease.

By 1900, however, now knighted, Sir Henry was beginning to change his mind about the notification of tuberculosis. In his Annual Report of that year,[6] there still existed, under the heading of 'Constitutional Diseases', the mortality figures for both 'tubercular affections' and cancer, although he felt the former 'should nowadays more correctly have been included under infectious and preventable diseases'. Phthisis alone accounted for 548 deaths in Edinburgh in 1900 or 1.81 per 1,000 inhabitants and most of these deaths were in patients under 45 years of age. A further 270 deaths from non-pulmonary tuberculosis, mainly abdominal and meningeal forms of the disease, brought the total number of fatalities from all forms of tuberculosis for 1900 to 818.[7] With regard to the 'Notification of Consumption,' therefore, Littlejohn said he had been led by 1900 'to the decided opinion that the time has arrived when this important measure should be adopted by the Corporation'.[8] Otherwise he argued it would be impossible to gauge the amount of tuberculosis in the city and to allocate provisions for those patients who should be the responsibility of the Town Council and those who should be treated by the parish authorities. He felt that a mere year's notification would provide enough reliable data and that 1900 was the time to do it.

After the Public Health Committee had presented its report on the prevention of consumption to the Town Council in 1900, the laboratory of the Royal College of Physicians took over the analysis of potentially infectious specimens, including those for tubercle bacilli, all at the city's expense. This removed one of Sir Henry's original objections to the permanent notification of consumption, namely the expense of laboratory testing. By 1903 voluntary notification of pulmonary tuberculosis was introduced but, as fewer cases were reported than expected, compulsory notification was to follow in 1907, and notification of non-pulmonary tuberculosis in 1914.

In the meantime Dr Robert Philip had established the Edinburgh Tuberculosis Scheme which deservedly became a model for the eradication of the disease throughout the world. Dr Edouard Rist, writing from France in 1927, explained Philip's philosophy:

> Two dominant ideas guided him, the first that if the doctor waits until the patient himself seeks advice it is then too late, that it is necessary therefore to go and seek out the patient and take him under care from the earliest beginnings of his illness thus augmenting the chance of recovery and

Sir Robert Philip. (Photo by Drummond Young, Edinburgh, first published in the *Edinburgh Medical Journal*, 1937;44:285 now reproduced by kind permission of the *Scottish Medical Journal*)

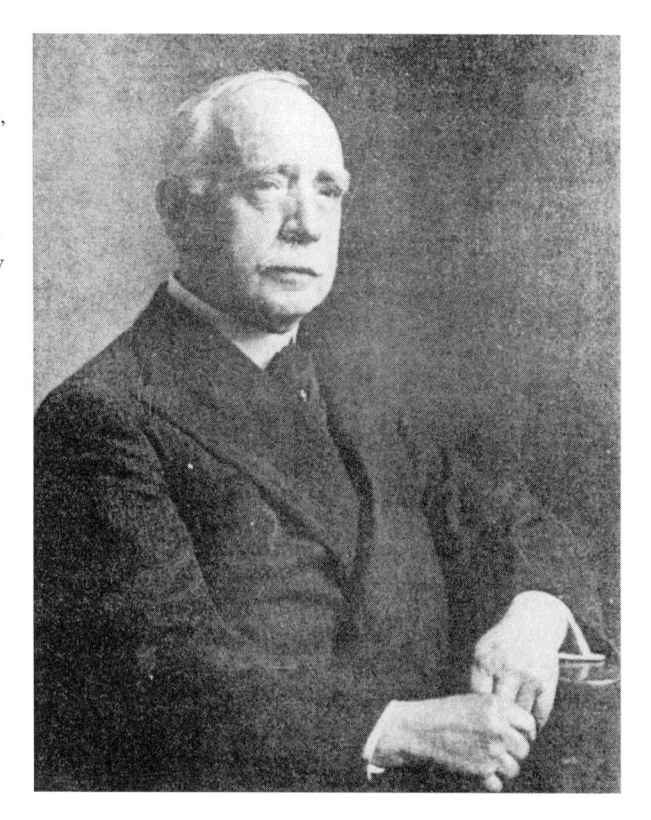

diminishing the risk of infecting others; and the second, that once an individual is declared tuberculous, it is necessary to keep him and his family under observation both medically and socially.[9]

To achieve these aims, Dr Philip set up the first tuberculosis dispensary in the world in 1887 in a three roomed flat in Bank Street in the heart of Edinburgh. Dr Philip, a graduate of the University of Edinburgh, first in Arts and then in 1882 in Medicine, with honours, was well qualified for his role. After working in the Royal Infirmary and studying tuberculosis as a postgraduate in Vienna, he wrote his MD thesis on 'A Study in Phthisis: Aetiological and Therapeutic', which won a gold medal in 1887. After four successful years, the Victoria Dispensary for Consumption proved too small. It moved to 26 Lauriston Place in 1891, where it became the Royal Victoria Dispensary in 1904, then to Spittal Street in 1912 and finally to Chalmers Hospital in 1991.

Under Philip's Edinburgh Tuberculosis Scheme,[10] the Dispensary was the focal point for the visits by doctors, nurses and community workers into patients' homes. From 1894 the former Craigleith House had become the Victoria Hospital for Consumption. It acquired regal status as the

Royal Victoria Hospital in 1903. The farm colony opened at Springfield House, Polton, Lasswade for convalescent patients in 1910 and continued till 1941 when the last patients were discharged.[11] In 1922 the Southfield Sanatorium near the junction of Duddingston Road and Milton Road West started taking in patients. Throughout the MOH monitored the notifications and reported on the progress of the disease which, despite a general decline, showed evidence of resurgence during and after both World Wars.

A vital ingredient in the scheme was the segregation of advanced, and therefore highly infectious cases, at the City Hospital. In 1913 'two single-storey blocks of wood and iron buildings lying to the south of the hospital buildings in the Poorhouse'[12] were used for parish patients with tuberculosis at Craiglockhart under the provisions of the National Insurance Act 1911. By 1921, whether insured or not, all patients with tuberculosis were the responsibility of the local authority. The MOH complained about the difficulty of managing the undisciplined, male, parish inmates who wandered in and out of hospital at will.[13] Even in 1924 there were still 48 beds for patients with pulmonary tuberculosis who should previously have come under the care of the parish council authorities. Whether by this time they were better behaved is not recorded.[14] In 1925, Dr Ker's last year at the City Hospital, 158 parish patients with tuberculosis were admitted, 89 with non-pulmonary disease and 69 with pulmonary disease.[15]

In 1921 considerable pressure was taken off the City Hospital accommodation with the transfer of non-parish patients with advanced pulmonary tuberculosis from the City Hospital to Pilton Hospital and those less ill to the Royal Victoria Hospital. The 63 beds at Colinton Mains were then used for non-pulmonary tuberculosis, mainly disease of the spine, joints, and renal tract,[16] supervised by Mr John Fraser (later Professor Sir John), a consulting surgeon of repute in the city.[17] The sense of relief that much of the burden of pulmonary tuberculosis had been at least temporarily lifted was clear in report on the City Hospital for 1921, the year that Leith was included within the city boundary:

> That the pavilions occupied by the Tuberculosis patients are really necessary for infectious diseases, especially now that the boundaries of the City have been extended, was proved during the milk epidemic of Scarlet Fever in July, and also during that time of Influenza in the current year, as on both occasions every bed in them had to be filled, and a certain amount of overcrowding had to be tolerated in order to meet the rush of cases.[18]

How then did the City Hospital respond to pulmonary tuberculosis during Dr Ker's Superintendentship, playing, as it did, a key role in the

Edinburgh Tuberculosis Scheme by isolating the highly infectious advanced cases of the disease?

The hospital at Colinton Mains first admitted patients with advanced pulmonary tuberculosis on 20 April 1906. At that time the waiting period for admission to the Royal Victoria Hospital was often between 6 and 8 months and there were 65 people on the waiting list.[19] In 1904, 1905, and 1906 there had been respectively 408, 438 and 373 deaths from phthisis recorded in Edinburgh with a range of between 108 and 130 deaths per 100,000 inhabitants.[20] Dr Ker received 121 applications for the admission of phthisis patients in 1906 and accepted 104 of these. Of the 17 deemed inappropriate for admission, 7 were 'unsuitable', 4 were in receipt of parish relief, 2 were withdrawn by relatives, 2 died before admission could be effected, one belonged to Cramond and one was too ill to be transferred. Little wonder then that the death rate among those admitted to the City Hospital was 46.15 per cent. Eleven of the 48 patients who died did so within 10 days of admission. Yet a total of 23 patients were rendered 'non-infectious' and fit enough for discharge. Weight gain of 2 stones was not uncommon and patients were taught:

> the supreme value of fresh air, and the necessity for greater care with regard to their sputum, and the use of pocket spittoons, etc.[21]

In the days before surgical intervention with collapse therapy, phrenic nerve crush, lobectomy, and pneumoperitoneum and, of course long before antibiotics, there was little else that could be done. Yet the protection given to the general public by isolating these highly infectious patients was considerable, the incidence of and mortality from pulmonary tuberculosis being much higher in one- or two-apartment houses than in homes with more spacious accommodation.[22] Hence the removal of even moribund patients from overcrowded houses would have helped to reduce the spread of the disease. A typical advanced case of tuberculosis was:

> When the patient is more or less dependent on others, and is probably confined to bed, when the expectoration is profuse, is teeming with tubercle bacilli, and is apt, despite the patient's best intentions, to be found on the floor, bed, bed clothes, and clothing of himself and the house in which he resides.[23]

By providing a hospital for advanced cases Dr Maxwell Williamson went on:

> ... the city of Edinburgh resulted in accomplishing the very desirable end of increasing markedly the number of 'institutional' as compared with the numbers of 'home' deaths.[24]

In 1905, before the provision of main hospital accommodation, 73 per cent of deaths from phthisis occurred in patients' homes. This figure was quickly reduced to only 51 per cent in 1909 after hospital facilities had become available.[25] Twenty per cent of the infectious patients taken from the community then died in the City Hospital.

Dr Maxwell Williamson also pointed out that such a high admission rate of seriously ill patients with phthisis was less often achieved in other cities largely because a hospital for advanced cases was regarded by patients and relatives alike as a 'home for the dying'. He attributed the successful admission rate in Edinburgh (where there was even a waiting list) to the fact that in the City Hospital:

> the accommodation offered has been of the most superior and attractive nature, and indeed has included all of the apparent essentials and advantages connected with a well-equipped sanatorium for the care of and, if possible, the cure of patients suffering from the disease.[26]

From 1906, with the approval of the Public Health Committee, patients with advanced disease at the City Hospital were accommodated in one of the standard southern pavilions so that there was no external difference between the accommodation for phthisis patients and that provided for patients with routine infectious diseases. Twenty-five female patients were

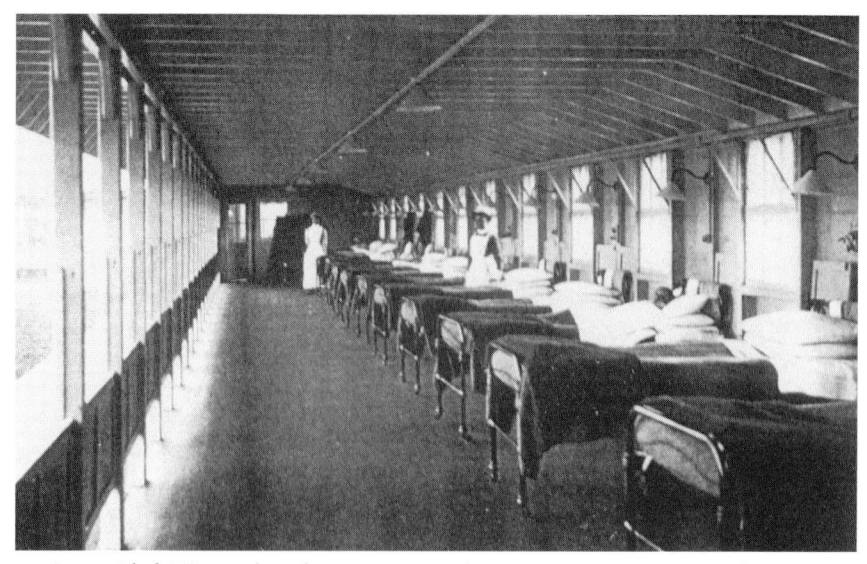

Open-sided TB ward at the City Hospital ca. 1927–28. From Annual Report of the Public Health Department, 1928, p. 34. (By courtesy of Edinburgh City Libraries)

housed in the lower ward and 25 male patients in the upper. In 1908 Dr Ker:

> frankly admitted that the duration of life under the healthy conditions prevailing at Colinton Mains is considerably longer than was originally calculated. Moreover a higher percentage of patients than was expected recover sufficiently to be trusted to resume their employment.[27]

This resulted in the duration of bed occupancy being greater than had been expected so there was always a demand for beds, particularly by men. In 1909 the hospital was criticised over the long detention of one patient for over two years and four others for over one year, but Dr Ker felt to send them out 'would be to sign their death warrant'.[28] Dr Ker indeed made a counter criticism to the effect that, as more than half the deaths occurred within one month of admission, these patients should have been notified and isolated sooner 'if they are to justify the expense of their removal and isolation'.[29]

The greater demand for male beds was partially met in 1909 by providing wooden, open-air shelters for men although Dr Ker admitted that these would:

> still further tend to lower the mortality rate in the wards, and to prolong the life of those of their inmates who ultimately succumb.

The first six two-patient shelters added 12 beds and the subsequent provision of six more shelters raised the total accommodation for phthisis patients from 50 to 74 beds.

The revolving wooden shelters were situated to the south of the tuberculosis pavilion. Dr Maxwell Williamson gave their dimensions as follows:[31]

Diameter of circular concrete base	15 feet.
Width of shelter	10 feet
Height from floor to eaves	6 feet 3 inches
Size of windows	4 feet by 3 feet 6 inches
Floor area	90 square feet
Height of floor over base	9 inches
Depth of shelter, front to back	9 feet
Height from floor to ridge	9 feet 9 inches
Capacity of shelter	720 cubic feet
Shelter can be turned on 6 4-inch diameter rollers	
Cost	£23.

A window was originally placed only at the front but, as the shelter became stuffy, a back window was later fitted as standard so to obtain

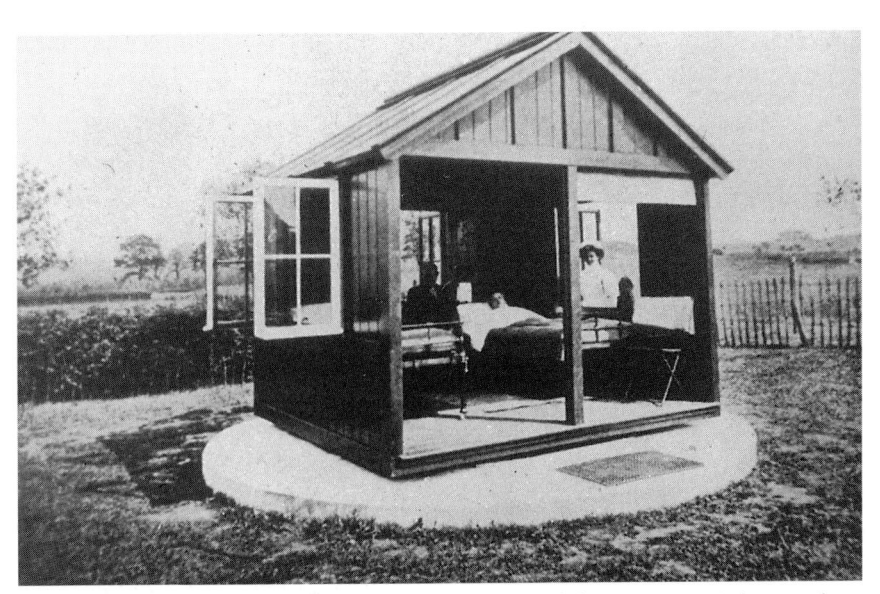

Revolving two-bed TB shelter at the perimeter of the City Hospital grounds ca. 1910. (By courtesy of Lothian Health Services Archive, Edinburgh University Library)

a through draught. A canvas roller blind closed the front, because an earlier experiment with a folding door was unsatisfactory. As lighting with paraffin lamps or candles was considered too dangerous and laying an electric cable too expensive, a small 3 or 4 candle power electric lamp supplied by a battery on the shelter floor and charged once a week proved 'highly efficient in every respect'.[32] The rotation of each shelter allowed it to face the sun at all times of day, to dry out any dampness on the floor depending on the wind direction and kept the whole construction in good repair for much longer than had it been static.

The choice of a compatible 'shelter mate' for the months a patient might expect to be in hospital was not discussed nor whether patients were permitted to change shelters. The shelters were, however, more popular than the wards and proved successful for the moderately advanced cases. They were never used for the severely ill or dying who were considered too frail to brave the elements outside.[33]

In 1910 the Town Council had arranged with the Royal Victoria Hospital to have 10 beds for tuberculous patients allotted there to the Corporation in return for an annual subsidy of £500. Political changes, however, were occurring rapidly. By 1914, following recommendations of the Astor Committee set up in 1912 to consider and report on the problem of tuberculosis in the whole country, the care of all patients with tuberculosis was to be taken over by corporations. As the City Hospital, already a local authority institution, could not possibly provide enough beds, it meant that the Royal Victoria Hospital, the dispensary and the farm colony at Polton upon which they had spent a total of £62,000 would come under the Corporation.[34] With amazingly good grace, the directors of the Royal Victoria Hospital for Consumption drew up Heads of Agreement between themselves and the Corporation. Their Committee, which included the recently knighted Sir Robert Philip, was unanimous in saying it was in the public interest that the dispensary, hospital and farm colony be taken over as part of the 'General scheme of treatment of tuberculosis in the City'.[35] Yet they remained fully conscious of those donors who, over the years, had contributed generously to their cause.

Understandably, Sir Robert Philip, though agreeing to the new arrangement, was suspicious that the Corporation would not pursue the control of tuberculosis as enthusiastically as he had done.[36] Although Sir Robert continued to be consultant and expert adviser to the Corporation, Dr John Guy was appointed Tuberculosis Officer in 1913 as an assistant to the MOH. He also became adviser to the Burgh Insurance Committee. Sir Robert, however, retained his teaching responsibilities in the Royal Victoria Dispensary, Hospital, and Farm Colony and the general direction of the medical care of tuberculous patients in Edinburgh. During the War, however, the Royal Victoria Hospital was taken over, temporarily by the Royal Army Medical Corps (RAMC) as a general hospital, and later by the Red Cross.

All was not lost, however, for Sir Robert. The Minutes of the Victoria Dispensary from 1891 through to those of the Royal Victoria Hospital Tuberculosis Trust in 1965 show how remarkably generous the citizens of Edinburgh had been over the years.[37] As early as December 1892, an auditor was appointed when there was already £2,000 in hand. The Ladies' Committee members collected for the special Christmas Appeal as well as all year round. They arranged fancy fairs and bazaars and a subscription concert to raise funds. Donations and bequests poured in. A healthy bank balance was maintained – more than enough to keep the expanding staff and accommodation required by the Dispensary, to purchase and run Craigleith House as the Royal Victoria Hospital, to buy Springfield at Polton for a farm colony and, much later in 1922, to purchase and run Southfield for use as a Sanatorium. Therefore, when the Corporation took over in 1914, a (very wealthy) Royal Victoria Hospital Tuberculosis Trust was founded.

After negotiating with the University of Edinburgh, the Trust contributed £15,000 towards setting up the world's first Chair of Tuberculosis to which Sir Robert Philip was appointed in 1917. Despite this, in 1921 when the local Insurance Committee was abolished, the Town Clerk did his best to get rid of Sir Robert saying his post no longer existed. Sixty-four doctors, including three past-Presidents of the Royal College of Physicians of Edinburgh and two past-Presidents of the Royal College of Surgeons of Edinburgh, signed a petition to reinstate Sir Robert at the Royal Victoria Hospital. He did then return to clinical practice but to Southfield Sanatorium and not to the Royal Victoria Hospital.[38]

Dr Christopher Clayson, formerly in charge of tuberculosis and chest diseases in Dumfries and Galloway and a past-President of the Royal College of Physicians of Edinburgh, knew Sir Robert well. He respected his vision and drive but was also aware of his stubbornness. If Sir Robert himself had not initiated a scheme, it was unlikely to receive his blessing. As early as 1908, Calmette and Guerin had begun to attenuate bovine tubercle bacilli in France. From 1920 onwards their work came to fruition with immunisation against tuberculosis in France by the Bacille Calmette Guerin (later called BCG) vaccine. In 1928 Calmette had unsuccessfully tried to persuade Sir Robert Philip to encourage the introduction of BCG immunisation in Britain. Dr Clayson vividly recalls one occasion after Sir Robert had planted a commemorative sapling in the grounds of Southfield Sanatorium. Sir Robert told Dr Clayson 'Dear boy when you and I can smoke a cigar together in the shade of this tree we can talk again about BCG'.[39] Sir Robert's intransigent attitude may have delayed the introduction of BCG immunisation in this country until 1949, a full ten years after his death.

In the meantime honours were heaped upon Sir Robert from all over the world. His influence both in his own country and abroad on the control of tuberculosis was immense. From 1887 when he set up the Victoria Dispensary to 1935 (four years before he died) the death rate in Scotland from tuberculosis fell from 265 per 100,000 of the population to only 74 per 100,000[40] – a fitting tribute in itself. Sir Robert died suddenly in 1939. The Chair of Tuberculosis remained vacant until 1944 when Professor Charles Cameron was appointed.

Many of Sir Robert's problems in his later years had stemmed from his incompatibility with Dr Guy, the Tuberculosis Officer, and his successor Dr Herbert C. Elder. This difficulty continued between Professor Cameron and Dr Elder and the unity of the Edinburgh Tuberculosis Scheme was threatened when in-patients and out-patients were followed up by different doctors so destroying continuity of care. Professor Cameron was a very erudite doctor with an extensive knowledge of medicine as well as tuberculosis. It was unfortunate that tuberculosis notifications showed a rise during his professorship, but this was an

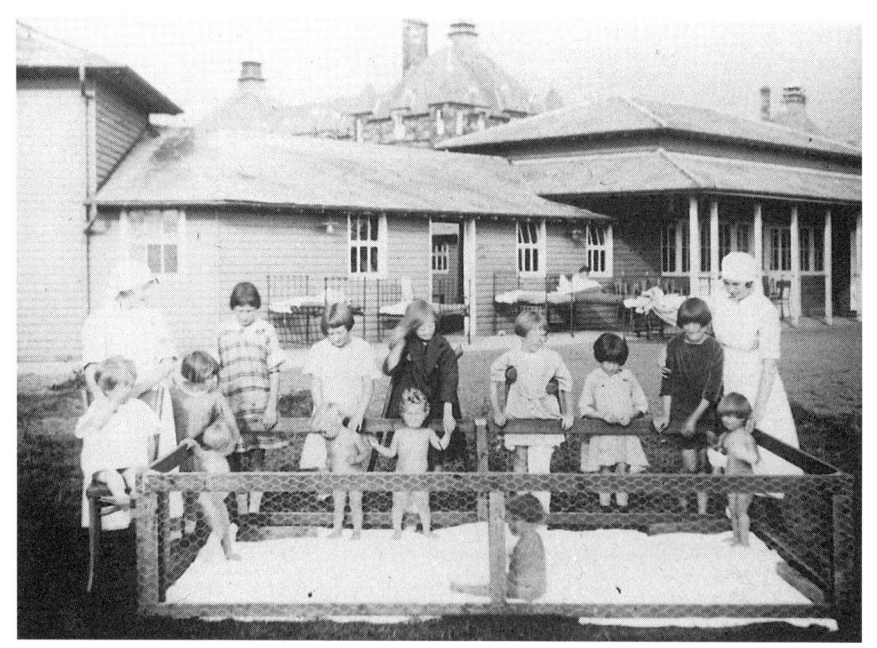

Children's ward for non-pulmonary TB at the City Hospital ca. 1930. (By courtesy of Lothian Health Services Archive, Edinburgh University Library)

inevitable consequence of the Second World War. Professor Cameron retired in 1951 at the age of 65 years.

Professor Cameron was succeeded by the other man of vision and determination, besides Sir Robert Philip: Professor, later Sir, John Crofton. Under him the City Hospital's contribution to the control of tuberculosis was again to the fore. When Professor Crofton was appointed in 1952, he took over more than 400 tuberculosis beds: 201 in the City Hospital, 100 at the Royal Victoria Hospital, 90 or more at Southfield Sanatorium and about 40 at Loanhead.[41] Dr Elder had previously had charge of the tuberculosis patients at the City Hospital (Wards 4, 5, 7, 18 and 19), although 24 of those beds had been looked after by Professor Cameron until he retired.

Professor Crofton was spoken of in somewhat dismissive terms by his predecessor, Professor Cameron,[42] but he was ideally suited for his post in Edinburgh. His medical education was at Sidney Sussex College, Cambridge and he graduated through St Thomas's Hospital, London. He wrote his MD thesis on typhus following experience of this disease in Africa during his military service in the war. After the war he returned to St Thomas's and then worked with tuberculous patients at the Brompton Hospital in London. In 1948 he was appointed a coordinator of the Medical Research Council's (MRC) Streptomycin Trial in tuberculosis. In 1951 he became a Senior Lecturer at the prestigious Royal Post-Graduate Medical School in Hammersmith.

On arrival in Edinburgh, Professor Crofton set about healing the rift between the Corporation and the University. Dr Elder retired in December 1953 and was replaced in 1954 by Dr (later Professor) James Williamson with whom Professor Crofton could work amicably. Professor Crofton insisted on continuity of management with the same doctors looking after the same patients, rather than the previous segregation whereby some doctors did out-patient dispensary duties and out-patient clinics whilst others worked in the wards.

To promote good relations between the hospital and extraneous organisations, including the Public Health Department, Professor Crofton instituted monthly meetings between himself and his close ally, the Hospital Group Secretary, Mr Alec Welstead; the Medical Officer of Health, then Dr H. E. Seiler; a member of the Medical Officer's of Health tuberculosis staff and a general practitioner representative. His team of expert clinicians included Dr A. C. Douglas, Dr I. W. B. Grant, Dr N. W. Horne, Dr Ian Ross and Dr James Williamson. Under this unified service, Edinburgh and Leith were divided into five sectors with one doctor in charge of each, for example Dr Williamson looking after tuberculosis in Leith. The scheme was displayed in the Spittal Street Dispensary on a huge map where different colours designated whether patients were sputum positive, whether they had a cavity and whether there were vulnerable children in their homes.[43]

Results followed rapidly. Within one year the 400 patient waiting list disappeared. From his headquarters in Southfield, Professor Crofton moved to Ward 8 in the City Hospital where he also managed other forms of respiratory disease. The Nightingale pavilion wards were used for tuberculosis together with the wooden accommodation of Wards 28 and 29. X-ray facilities which had started humbly in Cottage 13 in 1948 moved in 1965 to the New Medical Block where they could provide a better service. From an operating suite in Cottage 11 the thoracic surgical team headed by Mr Andrew Logan with Messrs David Wade, Philip R. Walbaum and Robert J. M. McCormack then gave surgical support for the medical tuberculosis team.

By the time antituberculous (antimycobacterial) drugs began to be introduced, therefore, Professor Crofton and his colleagues were ready to carry out sophisticated clinical trials. Backing them strongly were dedicated workers in the Bacteriology Laboratory, namely Dr Archie Wallace and Dr Sheila Stewart and later Drs Margaret Calder and Margaret

Moffat. Funds for research assistants came largely from the Royal Victoria Hospital Tuberculosis Trust.

Apart from trials of Sanocrysin, a form of injectable gold therapy, which had been abandoned because of toxicity in the 1920s, there had been no specific antimycobacterial remedy until streptomycin was developed in the late 1940s, followed by para-aminosalicylic acid (PAS) in 1950 and isoniazid in 1952. Professor Crofton was now ideally placed to study the clinical effects of these drugs in his Edinburgh patients. In 1948 he had coordinated the MRC's study of streptomycin in London followed by a study of the use of PAS singly and then combined with streptomycin. He had become acutely aware of the rapid development of drug resistance when a single drug was used. For this reason he decided to start therapy with the three drugs, injectable streptomycin with oral PAS and isoniazid. Later treatment could continue with PAS and isoniazid alone.

The effect was dramatic. With Professor Crofton's insistence on compliance, cures were effected rather than the initial clinical improvement followed by the disastrous relapses with drug-resistant bacilli that had attended earlier trials with mono-therapy. The rate of tuberculosis decline accelerated from 3 per cent per annum to 15 per cent per annum. Between 1954 and 1957 the number of new cases of tuberculosis reported fell by 59 per cent.[44] There was a transient rise in 1958 when unsuspected new cases were discovered during the successful mass miniature radiology campaign. This was supervised by Dr J. Williamson and Mr A. G. Welstead and advertised widely by the press. Although it caused a temporary increase in notifications, the need for 201 beds for tuberculosis at the City Hospital in 1952 fell to a mere 20 beds by 1958. Moreover the tubercle bacilli were remaining largely sensitive to the three primary drugs.

Dr Andrew Douglas[45] describes the enthusiasm and dedication of the team and the excitement of publishing the results which at first were not always accepted by sceptics elsewhere. Professor Crofton insisted that trial patients were seen daily and their therapy personally supervised by one individual doctor. He rigorously investigated any patient who died or failed to improve on the new drug regimen. Weekly meetings were held to discuss these unfortunate patients and make recommendations. Where cases of resistance did develop, other agents such as viomycin and combinations of high dose tetracycline antibiotics with isoniazid were used. Sometimes thoracoplasty and the surgical removal of diseased lung tissue were necessary in what came to be called 'salvage chemotherapy'. The social implications of the disease were also tackled by almoners and specially trained visitors who assisted families in difficulties because of illness affecting a wage-earner or mother, or where rehousing was required on account of overcrowding or dampness (see Chapter 31).

In his final report to the Royal Victoria Hospital Tuberculosis Trust in 1965,[46] Professor Crofton acknowledged the Trust's generous support of his research over the previous 13 years and thanked his clinical and laboratory colleagues, the MOsH, Drs H. E. Seiler and J. L. Gilloran together with Dr John Mair who had been in charge of the public health aspects of tuberculosis for many years.

Five controlled trials on different aspects of treatment had been carried out by Professor Crofton's team. One of the most important showed that patients with mild tuberculosis who adhered to modern drug treatment could continue safely at work so avoiding economic hardship and interruption to their family and social life by long hospitalisation. Having established the efficacy of triple drug therapy and the importance of reliable laboratory testing for antibiotic resistance, the team investigated the optimum length of treatment with various regimens in patients with differing degrees of disease. Resistance patterns in different countries were studied and the opinion of overseas specialists was sought. Work was also later carried out on non-tuberculous chest disease but, in the context of tuberculosis in Edinburgh, Professor Crofton could report that the death

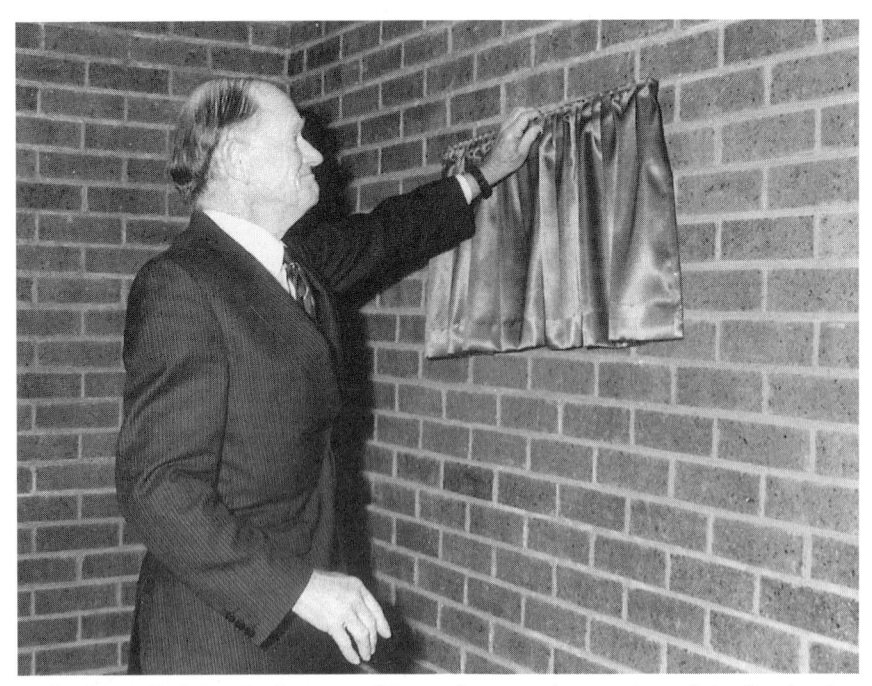

Professor Sir John Crofton unveiling a plaque at the opening of the Regional Virus Laboratory Extension, 16 January 1986 (By courtesy of Sir John Crofton)

rate had fallen from 70 per 100,000 population in 1947 to only 3 in 1964. Besides, the number of new cases reported fell from 165 to 36 per 100,000 population in the decade 1954–64.

Professor Crofton's advice was often sought by the World Health Organisation (WHO) and Health Departments across the world and he travelled widely. Despite the successful campaign in Edinburgh and many Western countries, he warned against complacency. Even the development of new antimycobacterial drugs like rifampicin, pyrazinamide and ethambutol would not contain the disease unless used with the care and circumspection shown by Professor Crofton to the earlier agents, streptomycin, PAS and isoniazid. Suffice to say, the resurgence today of multiply drug-resistant tuberculosis, often together with AIDS, and particularly in developing countries shows how right he was to encourage vigilant surveillance and to urge caution before claiming global eradication of the disease.

Professor Crofton was elected President of the Royal College of Physicians of Edinburgh in 1973, as had the first holder of the Chair of Tuberculosis, Sir Robert Philip before him. Also like Sir Robert, Professor Crofton was knighted, in 1977. Before that Sir John had also served as Dean of the Faculty of Medicine (1963–66) and Vice Principal of the University of Edinburgh (1970–71). In retirement he has remained active and, until very recently, travelled to advise developing countries on their problems with tuberculosis. Many of the patients who were treated at the City Hospital and elsewhere have cause to be grateful both to Sir Robert and Sir John. Countless other millions who never developed tuberculosis, and because of the efforts of Philip and Crofton are now unlikely to do so, must also owe them both an enormous debt of gratitude.

Prominent in Sir John Crofton's team was Dr Andrew Douglas, FRCPEd. He qualified MB, ChB from the University of Edinburgh in 1946 and after service with the RAMC and posts in Edinburgh University's Department of Bacteriology, he joined the Respiratory Medicine team working first in the Northern General Hospital then becoming Senior Lecturer and Consultant Physician in 1963 at the City Hospital and ultimately Reader. He stayed at the City Hospital until 1974. He then moved to the Royal Infirmary where his expertise in respiratory physiology, infections and especially granulomatous diseases like sarcoid, was invaluable. He wrote on tuberculosis, antibiotic toxicity, sarcoidosis and was co-author with Sir John Crofton of the authoritative work *Respiratory Diseases* (1969). He was always a kindly man with great compassion for hard working junior colleagues. Many tired young doctors can recall being greeted late in the evening in the hospital corridor by

Dr Douglas who would say 'How are you getting on? You look weary with well-doing'.

Dr Ian W. B. Grant, MB, ChB, FRCPEd, qualified from the University of Edinburgh in 1941 and was another member of Sir John Crofton's team. He worked both as a Consultant Physician and Part-time Senior Lecturer in Respiratory Medicine at the City Hospital after various posts which included a spell at the Brompton Hospital in London. He wrote extensively on respiratory disorders and contributed chapters and sections in several textbooks. He later became a Consultant Physician to the Respiratory Unit at the Northern General Hospital and was for a time Professor of Medicine in the National University of Malaysia in Kuala Lumpur.

Dr N. W. Horne and Professor J. Williamson whose further activities are described in Chapters 26, 27 and 29 also contributed in a major way to the control of tuberculosis in the 1950s and 1960s.

Dr J. D. (Ian) Ross, likewise was much involved but, after a sudden illness and miraculous resuscitation, worked mainly with Dr Kenneth Reid at the Royal Victoria Dispensary, Spittal Street, and in Wards 5 and 5A in the City Hospital where he had a few beds. Dr Ross was a co-author with Dr Horne of the excellent primer on the treatment of tuberculosis.

Dr A. Barry Kay, a young doctor who worked with Sir John Crofton, later developed expertise in allergies and eosinophils and discovered the role of T-cells in chronic asthma. After senior appointments in the South East Scotland Regional Blood Transfusion Service and in Experimental Pathology in the University of Edinburgh, he became Professor and Director in Allergy and Clinical Immunology at the National Heart and Lung Institute in London. He was elected FRSE in 1993.

Dr David Lamb, who had qualified in University College, London in 1959 and became a Reader in Pathology in the University of Edinburgh, was closely involved in the histological examination of lung tissue for the Respiratory Medicine Unit over many years.

Dr Anthony Seaton, later Professor of Environmental and Occupational Medicine in the University of Aberdeen from 1988, was another brilliant former member of the respiratory medicine team at the City Hospital. He has written extensively on chest disease and atmospheric pollution and is Chairman of the Expert Panel on Air Quality Standards of the Department of the Environment.

The City Hospital's Chest Unit and Department of Respiratory Medicine were both magnets which attracted bright, academic doctors who added lustre to the hospital's reputation.

CHAPTER TWENTY

Dr W. T. Benson's Superintendentship, 1925–36: Serotherapy for Scarlet Fever; Immunisation for Nurses

The story of tuberculosis at the City Hospital has been told from Sir Robert Philip in 1887 right through to Sir John Crofton in the 1960s. In the interim, two Medical Superintendents, Dr Benson and Dr Joe, made their mark on the City Hospital. After the untimely death of Dr C. B. Ker in 1925, Dr W. T. Benson was appointed his successor at the early age of 31.

Walter Tyrell Benson was born at Sibpur, Calcutta, in 1894 where his father, John Benson, was the Harbour Master. Walter Benson's mother was a stern lady with high expectations of her only child. Consequently at the tender age of six Walter was sent home alone to Scotland to further his education. He stayed in Dundee with his maternal grandmother and attended Dundee High School where he was patently unhappy. Perhaps because he was a perfectionist, Walter always found it difficult to make friends, especially with adults, and was therefore regarded as shy. He was, however, in his element with children, later finding his paediatric patients easy to get on with as also his own five children to whom he was a devoted and fun-loving father.

Dr Benson was a true academic. After school he attended the University of St Andrews winning a distinction in Anatomy and graduating in 1915 with a First Class Honours BSc in Physiology. He next entered the Faculty of Medicine of the University of Edinburgh but his studies were interrupted by the First World War. He served in the Royal Naval Volunteer Reserve (RNVR) as a submariner and later as a Surgeon-Lieutenant in the Royal Navy. He was appalled by the living conditions of ratings at sea during war-time and shocked by the death of colleagues who were killed when their ships were bombed. On the cessation of hostilities he returned to the University of Edinburgh and became the most distinguished medical graduate of 1918, qualifying MB, ChB with First Class Honours.

His studying continued and in 1920 he was awarded the Diploma in Public Health (DPH) (Cambridge) with a distinction in Hygiene. In

1922 he was commended for his MD thesis in Edinburgh entitled 'Diphtheria Carriers and their Treatment' in which he showed a marginal reduction in the duration of carriage by patients injected with a detoxicated diphtheria vaccine.[1] In the same year he obtained the Diploma in Tropical Medicine and Hygiene (DTM & H) of London.

Before being appointed Medical Superintendent of the City Hospital and University Lecturer in Infectious Diseases, Dr Benson had been Edinburgh's Assistant MOH and as Senior Assistant Bacteriologist at the City Hospital he was responsible for 11,526 reports emanating from the bacteriology laboratory in 1921. Over the next two years he investigated diphtheria outbreaks in schools and inspected the city's suburban water supplies.

As Assistant MOH in 1924 he gave the Port of Leith Medical Inspection Report and took appropriate action on infections in seamen including malaria and sexually transmitted diseases. He vaccinated the crew of the steam trawler *Lord Rothschild*, one of whose crew had been sent ashore five days previously in Aberdeen suffering from smallpox[2] and happily no cases of smallpox were subsequently reported in Leith or Edinburgh.

Dr Benson passed the MRCPEd examination in 1926, the year after he was appointed Medical Superintendent of the City Hospital. In those days the Membership was not a pre-requisite for consultant status. He was elected FRCPEd in 1928.

Mrs Rosemary Koelliker and Mrs Maureen Ward, two of Dr W. T. Benson's four daughters, have kindly supplied information about their parents. The couple met when they were both on holiday at Crieff Hydro. She was then Dorothy Mathewson, daughter of Arthur Mathewson, an important figure in Dundee's jute industry who built Vernonholme, later to become the headquarters of the Eastern Regional Hospital Board (Scotland). After a whirlwind romance, rather untypical for such a shy man, Walter and Dorothy were married in June 1923. Dorothy was an accomplished artist who had paintings exhibited in the Royal Scottish Academy. Between 1924 and 1937 the Bensons had five red-headed children, four girls and a boy. Their second child, Ken, studied Medicine in Edinburgh and became Professor of Epidemiology in the University of British Columbia.

Dr W. T. Benson was a talented all-rounder, academically brilliant and a perfectionist. He was a superb lecturer and a patient teacher. He played tennis and golf and was the Skip of a curling team. His hobbies included the English language, creating new gardens, motorcycling and tinkering with his beloved Riley and Railton motor cars. He was also a keen fisherman, his self-tied salmon flies often in-corporating some of his daughters' red hair. The Benson family photograph albums show charming

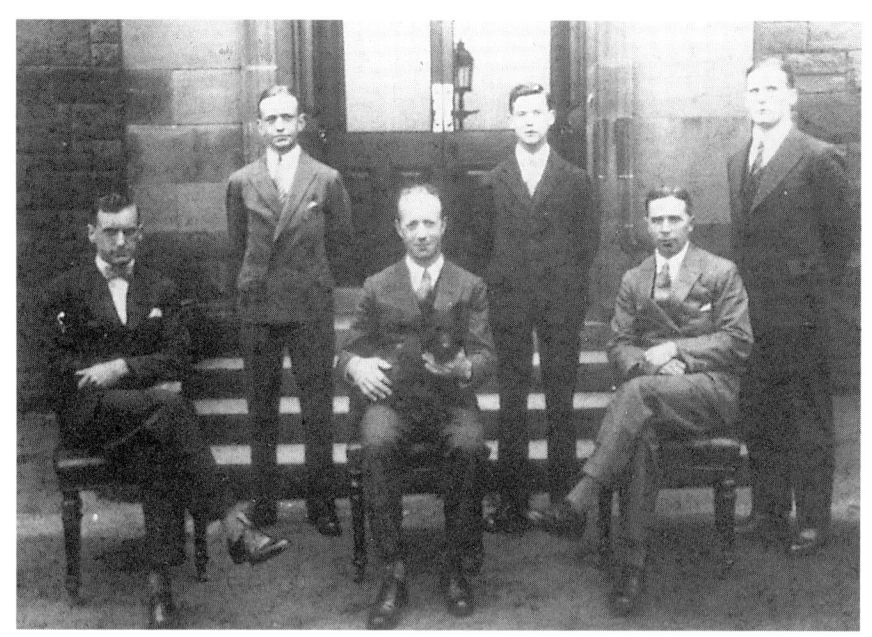

City Hospital medical staff, 1928, in front of the general offices. Standing left to right: Drs Cowan, Dott (later Professor Sir Norman Dott) and Murray Lyon. Sitting left to right: Dr Craig, Dr W. T. Benson (with dog) and Dr Murray. (From Dr Benson's photo album, by courtesy of Mrs Rosemary Koelliker and Mrs Maureen Ward)

holiday snapshots and jolly tennis parties in the Medical Superintendent's garden at the City Hospital, close-up views of natural subjects and, separately, some competent clinical pictures developed and printed by himself. He also collected drawings and etchings and in quiet moments played a mandolin. It is interesting to speculate what greater influence this shy but sensitive and talented man might have had on the City Hospital had he been Medical Superintendent for longer than 11 years. Sadly, having sustained rheumatic fever as a boy, he retired prematurely on health grounds in 1936.

Besides his clinical and administrative responsibilities, Dr Benson was a keen teacher. With his small staff at the City Hospital he provided annually an average of 220 rising to 236 hours of clinical teaching and lectures to medical undergraduates, postgraduates and the nursing staff.[3] In 1935, for instance, 286 medical students received 90 hours of instruction. Although divided into six sections, the class size must have been very large.

Two DPH courses were provided every year each receiving 72 hours of teaching.[4] In 1925, because of a change of entry regulations, only 14 doctors attended but there had been 40 in 1923 and 60 in 1924.[5] After 1925 the numbers picked up again with 32 postgraduates attending the two courses in 1931. Additionally two or more summer courses in postgraduate medical education were held annually.[6]

Each year Dr Benson's Annual Report recorded the number of nurses who completed their three-year fever nurse training, and those who passed the State Examination, the number who went on to general training, and those who became staff nurses. A very few left to get married, attend a Child Welfare Course or enter training for mental health nursing or massage. Each year between 24 and 55 nurses completed training (mean 35.4) and between 24 and 47 passed the State Examination (mean 31.3) Two thirds or more proceeded to general training. From 1925 to 1936 (inclusive), 79 were appointed to staff nurse positions either at the City Hospital or in fever hospitals elsewhere.

Dr Benson wrote the chapter on Infectious Diseases in Dunlop and Alstead's *Textbook of Medical Treatment*. In a paper entitled 'The Control of Diphtheria' he pleaded for the active immunisation of pre-school children against diphtheria.[7] From 1912 to 1934, between 92 and 98 per

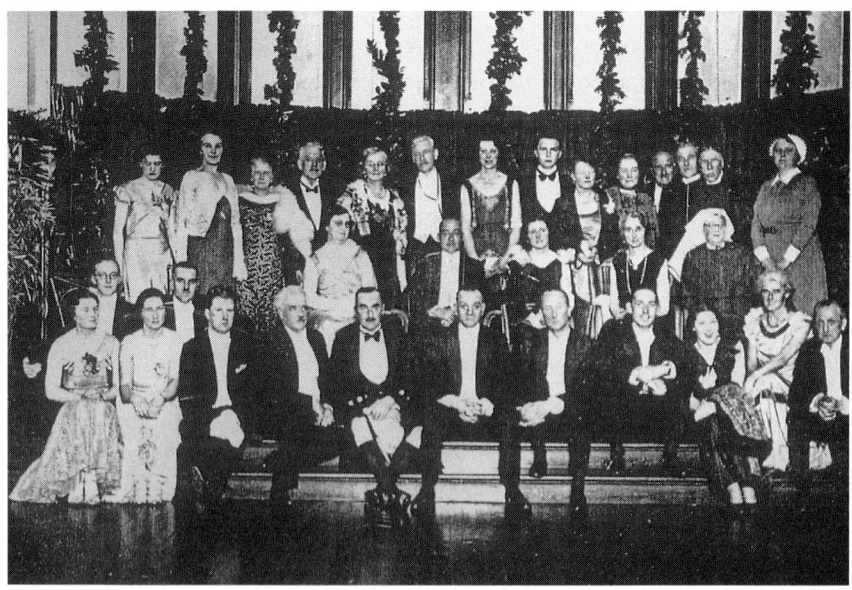

Christmas dance in nurses' recreation hall ca. 1932–34. Front row, sitting 5th from left: Lord Provost Sir William Johnston Thomson-Thomson and sitting 5th from right: Dr W. T. Benson. Middle row, on extreme right in uniform: Miss M. Pool, Matron. The author's maternal grandparents Rev. Bailie A. D. Sloan and Mrs Sloan stand in back row 2nd and 6th from right. (From Dr Benson's photo album, by courtesy of Mrs Rosemary Koelliker and Mrs Maureen Ward)

cent of Edinburgh's notified cases of diphtheria were admitted to the City Hospital showing that the hospital was fulfilling its function appropriately whereas in the decade 1890–99, only 30–50 per cent of notified cases had been admitted. Nonetheless diphtheria carriers, who could be difficult to identify, were at large in the community infecting susceptible children. However, Dr Benson questioned the wisdom of isolating them for, by so doing, he anticipated that the herd immunity would fall. In 1912 the MOH had reported that among 998 diphtheria contacts, the isolation of 58, whose throat swabs were positive, was beneficial to the community.[8] Dr Benson, however, felt that contact isolation was no longer justified.

Dr Benson commented favourably on the protection afforded to the City Hospital nurses by the active immunisation first introduced by Dr Ker in 1922. In the 11 years up to 1934 there was a 95 per cent reduction in diphtheria morbidity in successfully immunised nurses despite their continual occupational contact. In the previous three years only one nurse had contracted diphtheria and it had been a mild attack.[9] Dr Benson also encouraged diphtheria immunisation amongst scarlet fever patients at the City Hospital and, with parental consent, had had 1,000 children between the ages of 1 and 10 years inoculated in one four month period in 1934.[10] This gave an excellent parental consent rate of 80 per cent compared with only 42 per cent in 1924 when he had mounted a campaign in Edinburgh schools to immunise children aged between 5 and 10 years.

Another article by Dr Benson, published in 1938 two years after he resigned his post, describes the contemporary state of knowledge about streptococcal infections.[11] Dr Benson believed that the haemolytic streptococcus was the infecting agent in scarlet fever and not, as others held it, an unknown virus with streptococci merely playing a secondary role. Nonetheless despite the Schultz-Charlton diagnostic skin test and the culture of throat swabs, the diagnosis was not always easy. He correctly surmised that the decline in mortality due to scarlet fever from nearly 5.0 per cent in the immediate post-War years to below 1.0 per cent by 1938 suggested the disease was becoming milder.

Post-streptococcal nephritis was becoming less common. Dr Benson quoted anecdotal evidence which suggested antitoxin injections for scarlet fever patients made little difference to the incidence of nephritic complications. His dietary prescription was much more liberal than that of his predecessors and he felt sure this relaxation of the previously strict diet had not brought about a resurgence of nephritis. He wrote:

> an attack of scarlet fever definitely tends to re-activate rheumatic fever.

That there is some association between haemolytic streptococcal infection and acute rheumatism I feel convinced.[12]

To prevent reinfection and septic complications of scarlet fever, he advocated replacing large open wards with cubicles – or else nursing the uncomplicated patient at home. Severe cases would benefit from intramuscular or intravenous antitoxin given within 48 hours of onset and repeated if necessary. The newly introduced sulphanilamide (Prontosil) and benzyl-sulphanilamide (Proseptasine) 'appear to exert a curative effect on streptococcal infections'. He strongly advocated their use together with antiserum injections in 'the septic form of scarlet fever'. He was already aware that sulph-haemoglobinaemia and met-haemoglobinaemia sometimes occurred in sulphonamide treated patients but noted 'No other toxic effects have so far been observed'. It was early days after all.

Following the severe scarlet fever epidemic of 1933, Dr Benson was forced to discharge convalescent scarlet fever patients early, between the 14th and 21st day of illness. Although this did not bring about a surge of return cases with complications or recurrences, he nonetheless felt that, if there was no pressure on accommodation, a 26 day admission was still preferable to anything shorter.

Active immunisation induced by the subcutaneous injection of gradually increasing doses of haemolytic streptococcal toxin was recommended for susceptible (Dick Test positive) nurses. This, said Dr Benson, 'resulted in the almost complete disappearance of scarlet fever in the nursing staff at the City Hospital over a period of ten years'. He had to admit that reactions, 'unpleasant but not alarming', sometimes followed the course of injections and also conceded that active immunisation 'gave no guarantee of immunity against attacks of haemolytic streptococcal tonsillitis'.[13]

As Dr Benson felt sure that both erysipelas and puerperal fever were also caused by haemolytic streptococci, he recommended the new sulphonamides for both conditions, often combined with blood transfusion when severe anaemia complicated puerperal sepsis. Yet in addition to using these exciting new chemo-therapeutic agents, Dr Benson still adhered to traditional beliefs. In 1938 he wrote:

> I have come to the same conclusions as the late Dr Pospischill, a fever expert of Vienna, who ... told me that he considered fresh air the most important therapeutic agent in the treatment of infectious diseases. The recently extended balconies at the City Hospital afford splendid facilities for fresh air treatment.[14]

The balconies in question were extensions added to the southern end of Pavilion 15 in 1935. Patients were at least partially sheltered from the east

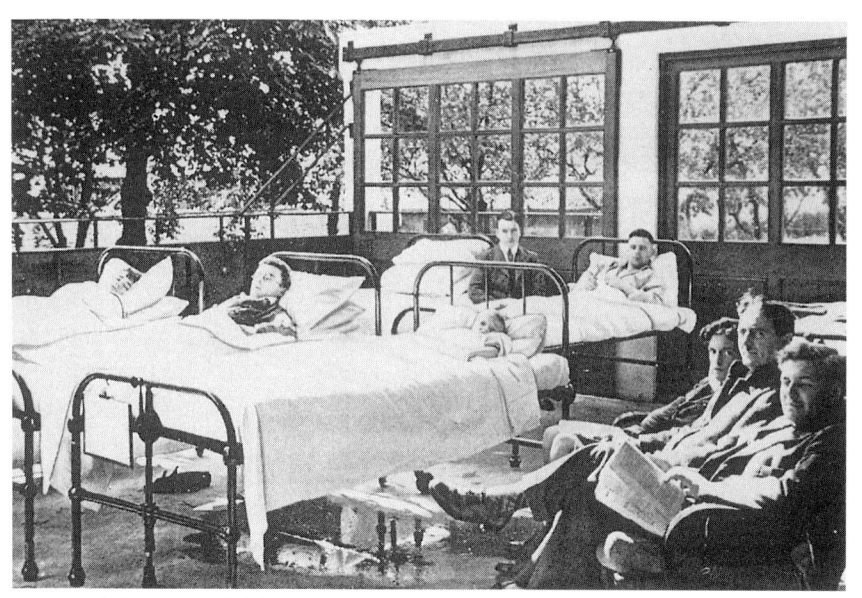

New balcony, probably in Pavilion 15, ca. 1935–36. Note the sliding glazed screens behind the patients. The puddle below the boy's bed is rain water, not incontinent urine! (From Annual Report of the Public Health Department, 1935, p. 31 by courtesy of Edinburgh City Libraries)

and west winds by sliding glazed doors mounted on overhead rollers but the southern aspect remained totally unprotected. Dr Benson reported that:

> The new balconies accommodate 22 and 12 beds respectively in place of the three bed capacity of the previous balconies. Puerperal fever and pneumonia cases respond very favourably to open-air treatment and the patients are highly appreciative of the accommodation provided.[15]

The 1936 Annual Report described further balcony extensions for Pavilions 2 and 17 which were used for patients with septic scarlet fever and those with chest complications after measles and whooping cough.[16]

Other improvements and additions during Dr Benson's time included the conversion of one ward (probably Ward 3) into cubicles. He commented favourably that:

> 138 patients were admitted to the cubicle ward between 6th September – the date of opening – and 31st December (1935). All types of case were handled, including acute measles and chickenpox; no cross infections occurred. The provision of a cubicle ward has simplified administration.[17]

In 1936 this ward took in 143 patients.[18]

A new system of food distribution was introduced in 1935 'by means of special food boxes'. Dr Benson wrote that it had 'given every satisfaction and has done away with the need for reheating food in the ward kitchen'.[19] Nor were patients' comforts neglected. In 1931 an anonymous donor, who was a City Hospital patient's employer, provided wireless installation with loud speakers for four of the wards, and 100 beds were supplied with ear-phones.[20]

In 1925 Dr Benson thanked the MOH, Dr Robertson, for two mercury vapour lamps which were to be used not only for treating acute measles and whooping cough but also 'rickets, glandular tuberculosis, marasmus and debility due to various causes'.[21] Another new item of equipment installed ten years later was a Drinker respirator. Although first used for two patients with diphtheritic paralysis, Dr Benson realised its potential for treating respiratory paralysis due to other causes.[22] Perhaps he was anticipating the poliomyelitis epidemic of the 1940s. By 1936, 21 patients with acute anterior poliomyelitis had already been admitted.

In 1929 Dr Benson drew attention to the steadily increasing number of patients admitted with a provisional diagnosis of puerperal sepsis.[23] From figures of only teens and twenties from 1920 to 1926, there was a sudden influx of patients to 62, 72 and then 153 for the years 1927, 1928 and 1929 respectively. In 1936 there were 194 admissions with suspected puerperal fever and the diagnosis was confirmed in 175 patients. Dr Benson set aside a ward for these patients, many of whom required prolonged and careful nursing, glycerine injections and local irrigations which were time consuming and a burden on staff.[24] In 1923 Dr Benson indicated that the services of a visiting gynaecologist were justified but there is no indication that one was recruited. He also complained that many of the puerperal fever patients, in whom the mortality was particularly high, were referred too late. The death rate in 1925 peaked at 37.5 per cent after which it steadily declined. By 1936 it had fallen to only 9.14 per cent, possibly due to the introduction of the sulphonamide drugs.[25]

Another disease with a dreadful mortality in the pre-antibiotic era was meningococcal infection, then referred to as 'cerebro-spinal fever' or 'cerebro-spinal meningitis' (CSM) The laboratory became important in proving the diagnosis and in differentiating meningococcal from other forms of meningitis. The admission diagnosis of CSM often mistakenly included patients with tuberculous or pneumococcal meningitis, influenza or encephalitis lethargica. Almost all the infants with CSM in the first year of life died, for example 19 of 20 admitted in 1929. That year only 7 of the 49 admissions with CSM of all ages survived, giving an overall death rate of 83.6 per cent.[26] Dr Benson recorded his disappointment with the five different types of polyvalent antimeningococcal sera which he had tried. Although sulphonamides had begun to show potential in the treatment of streptococcal infections, they had not at that stage been employed in CSM.

Dr Benson was well supported by his medical and nursing staff and the Hospital Steward, and he generously acknowledged them in his Annual Reports. Miss Mary Pool, the Matron, continued in office from 1925 to 1943. Sadly Miss McNair, the Assistant Matron, died in 1928 but the cause of death was not recorded in the Report.

In his Report of 1927 [27] Dr Benson proudly produced a table showing that among the nurses, whose numbers ranged between 128 and 161 (mean 149) in the years from 1919 to 1927, the incidence of diphtheria had fallen from 10.34 per cent in 1919 to 0.67 per cent in 1927. The incidence of scarlet fever among the nurses fell from 4.82 per cent to 0.67 over the same years. He prided himself that the routine immunisation procedures were working well and had saved at least £700. He excused the single case of scarlet fever in a nurse in 1928 by explaining that she was highly susceptible and acquired the illness on only her third working day in the hospital. He declined, however, to produce a table of nurses' illnesses in his 1928 Report when he reluctantly had to record, albeit no cases of scarlet fever among the nurses, no less than six cases of diphtheria, three of mumps, two of measles, five of chickenpox and one each of erysipelas and chickenpox.[28] He suggested that four of the nurses who contracted diphtheria may have had false positive Schick reactions and had therefore not been immunised. Fortunately all recovered without sequelae. In 1929, 10 nurses contracted diphtheria. Five were Schick positive and again all survived what were mild attacks.[29]

Dr W. T. Gardiner, the Otologist who treated the ENT complications in streptococcal and diphtheritic patients carried out numerous tonsillectomies, adenoidectomies and mastoidectomies each year, and some paracenteses of ear drums and proof punctures of the para-nasal sinuses. He resigned because of ill health in 1933 and his place was taken in July 1933 by Dr Charles E. Scott, Aural Surgeon. Dr Scott performed no less than 362 tonsillectomies and adenoidectomies and 40 mastoid operations that year on City Hospital patients. The morbidity or mortality from these procedures is not recorded in the Annual Reports.

Mr Frank Jardine, FRCS, was the Consulting Surgeon until 1933 when he was succeeded by Mr C. F. W. Illingworth, FRCS. That year Mr Illingworth carried out operations for appendicitis, intussusception, volvulus, peritonitis, and pelvic abscess in the City Hospital as well as looking after the patients with surgical tuberculosis.

There were still 148 tuberculosis beds in the City Hospital in Dr

Benson's time and 73 of these were set aside for non-pulmonary tuberculosis. In 1932, Dr H. C. Elder, Tuberculosis Officer, was carrying out successful trials of artificial pneumothorax and phrenicectomy to close tuberculous lung cavities. Sometimes these procedures were combined with treatment with the highly toxic antituberculous drug Sanocrysin.

In 1929 90 cases of advanced pulmonary tuberculosis were transferred from Pilton Hospital causing a major strain on the staff at the City Hospital and requiring the temporary employment of additional trained nurses.[30] Unfortunately this influx of tuberculosis patients coincided with a resurgence of diphtheria, 1,535 admissions with suspected diphtheria being received that year mostly in November and December.

Dr Alexander James, the Consultant Physician to the City Hospital, resigned in the autumn of 1930.[31] He had a 'kindly personality' and he often shed light on obscure diagnoses. In retirement he continued to take a keen interest in the hospital.[32]

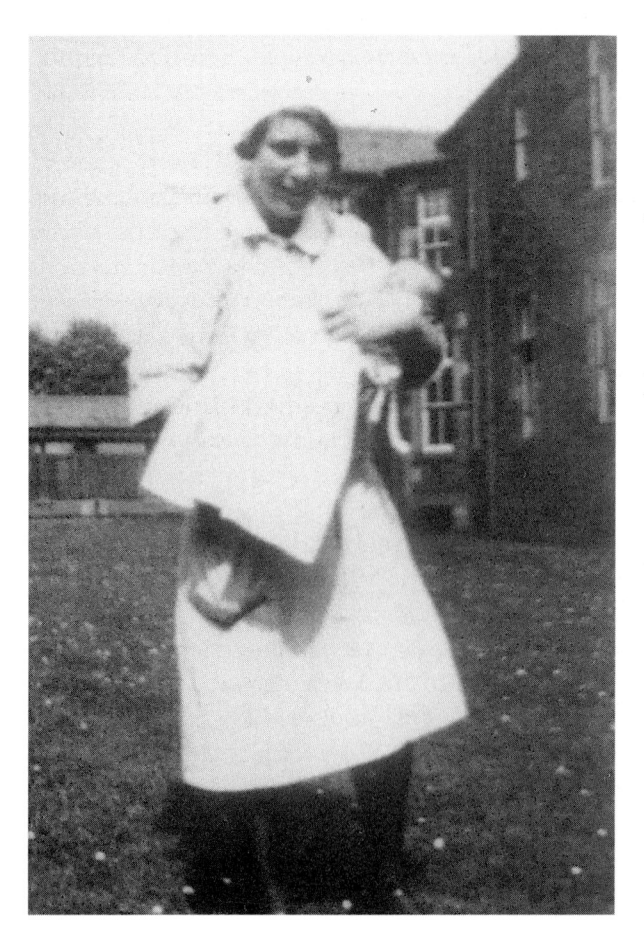

Cerebro-spinal meningitis survivor, 1931 (before sulphonamides and penicillin). Miss J. K. Taylor carries the only baby who survived of the 19 admitted in that outbreak. (By courtesy of Miss J. K. Taylor)

Credit must also be given to Dr Benson's junior medical staff whom he always praised in his Annual Report. Usually the Senior Medical Assistant doubled up as Bacteriologist so combining clinical and laboratory duties. In 1925 Dr Alec Joe, who was to take over from Dr Benson in 1936, covered the interim period between Dr Ker's death and the installation of Dr Benson. Dr G. W. Simpson was Senior Medical Officer and Bacteriologist in 1925 and 1926 when he was responsible for immunising susceptible nurses against scarlet fever and diphtheria. He was followed in 1926 by Dr J. H. D. Lawrie. The Senior Medical Officer in 1927 and 1928 was Dr Douglas and Mr Jimmy Craig was running the laboratory in 1929.

A new senior Medical Assistant, Dr A. L. K. Rankin was appointed in 1929. Dr Benson thought very well of him as 'my right hand man. I cannot speak too highly of his work, clinical, administrative and in the laboratory'.[33] When Dr Rankin left for a post in England in 1934, Dr Benson wrote that his departure meant 'a serious loss for the hospital'.[34] He was replaced by Dr R. C. M. Pearson whose work 'deserves the highest praise'.[35] In the interim between Dr Rankin and Dr Pearson, a Dr Cuthbert had filled the post for four months acting 'with tact and efficiency'.[36]

The medical staff, like the nurses, were exposed to infections in their work although the closer contact of the nursing staff with patients and their sputum and excreta always made them more vulnerable. One nurse died of miliary tuberculosis in 1929, two years after she had entered the hospital service.[37] The Annual Report of 1936[38] still recorded infections in the nurses: five with mumps, four each with scarlet fever and measles, three with phthisis and one each with chickenpox and rubella. But the medical staff too were susceptible. In March that same year the Resident Medical Tuberculosis Officer, Dr J. W. Brydon, died from meningitis following on from streptococcal tonsillitis, otitis media and mastoiditis. Working in a fever hospital was obviously still a risk-prone occupation in the 1930s — irrespective of whether you were a nurse or a doctor.

Two of the stated objectives of the new fever hospital had been to provide teaching — which it was certainly fulfilling — and to carry out research in the laboratory into the aetiology of infection. The laboratory's workload steadily increased. In 1936 10,518 examinations were carried out, most being of throat swabs from scarlet fever and diphtheria patients. Microscopy and the culture of sputum, cerebro-spinal fluid, urine, stool and blood were also performed. As puerperal fever admissions increased, so also did the requirement for uterine cultures. Widal tests were done in cases of suspected enteric fever. In 1932 after the research work of Dr C. E. van Rooyen in Edinburgh, cough plates containing modified

Bordet Gengou medium helped to diagnose patients with whooping cough.

The Hospital Steward appears to have been a lynch pin in the hospital being responsible for the officials in the kitchens, laundry and dispensary. Mr Macdonald held the post from the earliest days at Colinton Mains and retired in 1931 'after 26 years of faithful and unremitting stewardship ...'[39] He was replaced by Mr Stirling, 'a highly efficient successor'.

In Dr Benson's time the ambulance service was improved. In 1930 there were three motor ambulances based at the hospital. Between them they covered 38,843 miles at a cost of 8.1 (old) pence per mile.[40] By 1936 there were four ambulances which were available day and night as the drivers lived in the hospital.

In December 1936 at the age of only 42 Dr Benson resigned his appointment at the City Hospital on account of ill health perhaps as a consequence of rheumatic fever which he had had as a boy. The Annual Report of the PHD for 1936[41] extols his valuable contribution to Edinburgh medicine, to the discipline of infectious diseases, and to the City Hospital. He was regarded as 'a very able lecturer and a sound administrator' whose:

> knowledge of fevers was unsurpassed by any physician in the Kingdom. As a teacher he maintained the best traditions of the Edinburgh School, and during his service at the City Hospital had earned the esteem and high regard of hundreds of Edinburgh undergraduates.[42]

He next became a Medical Officer in the Scottish Health Department from 1936 to 1939. During the Second World War, Dr Benson acted as Company Medical Officer to the Home Guard. He was also a part-time epidemiologist to the Emergency Medical Services of the Department of Health for Scotland and served on the Board of Management of Perthshire, General Hospitals.[43] He made his home in 'Dalnaglar', a large house in Crieff, Perthshire, where he kept a lovely garden. He died in February 1984 at the age of 90 years.

His contribution to the City Hospital was short in terms of years, but he was much more than a caretaker. The hospital remained busy with 3,000 to 4,000 admissions each year with an exceptional peak of 6,033 in 1933. Important structural improvements to the hospital were instituted. He will be best remembered for his brilliance as a teacher who highlighted infectious diseases for the medical undergraduates and postgraduates who were privileged to be taught by him.

PART FIVE

Dr Alec Joe's Superintendentship 1937–60

CHAPTER TWENTY-ONE

1937–41: The Advent of Sulphonamides; Poliomyelitis, Dysentery and Meningitis

When Dr Benson retired in 1936, his natural successor was Dr Alexander Joe whose career up to that time had in many ways been similar to that of Dr Benson. Dr Joe was always known as Alec Joe. He was born in 1894 in Brechin, Angus, where he went to school. Like Dr Benson, his studies in medicine at the University of Edinburgh were interrupted by the First World War. Dr Joe served as a surgeon probationer and won the Distinguished Service Cross for gallantry in the Battle of Jutland. Unfortunately he was captured at sea and spent the rest of the War in German prison camps. After the armistice, he resumed his studies and graduated MB,ChB in 1919, only a year after Dr Benson. He obtained the DPH of Edinburgh and Glasgow in 1923 and the following year graduated MD. His thesis 'Scarlatinal Arthritis: A Clinical and Statistical Study',[1] detailed this rare complication in 49 patients and showed his early interest in infectious diseases. In 1923 he was successful in the examination for the Edinburgh DTM&H. Much later he served as the President of the Scottish Fever Group and in 1942 he was elected FRCPEd.

As a young man his studies under Professor T. J. Mackie in the Department of Bacteriology of the University of Edinburgh gave Dr Joe a firm microbiological foundation for his clinical interest in infection. His colleagues at that time included Professor Sir Stanley Davidson and Dr J. E. McCartney. He next worked as Senior Assistant Medical Officer at the City Hospital where he developed a long-lasting admiration for his chief, Dr C. B. Ker. Dr Joe continued Dr Ker's work of evaluating the Dick Test and he kept records of nephritis in scarlet fever patients. In May 1925 he was appointed Assistant MOH for Edinburgh and Port Medical Officer of Leith.

His first senior appointment, when he was comparatively young, was to succeed the doyen of infectious diseases, Dr E. W. Goodall, as Medical Superintendent of London County Council's North Western Fever Hospital in Hampstead. His research work at that time included air-borne infection, evaluation of Poulton's oxygen tent for the treatment of pulmonary complications of whooping cough, a study on passive immunisation in scarlet fever and puerperal sepsis, an assessment of the standardisation of reagents used for Dick testing and an account of scarlet fever resulting from nasopharyngeal surgery.

Dr Joe, however, yearned to return to Scotland. In 1937 he realised this ambition by being appointed to succeed Dr W. T. Benson as Medical Superintendent of the Edinburgh City Hospital, a post he held for 23 years. He was particularly remembered for his bed-side teaching to undergraduates and DPH course students. He kept up to date with his specialty and was an early contributor to the *Bulletin of Hygiene*. His popular textbook *Acute Infectious Fevers*, first published in 1947, was later translated into Spanish. Articles by Dr Joe appeared in the *Lancet, British Medical Journal, Journal of Hygiene* and elsewhere. Topics included passive immunisation in scarlet fever, the stability of the Schick toxin, scarlet fever after operations on the nasopharynx, the use of placental extracts to prevent measles, and the recently described canicola fever.

Before he retired in 1960, Dr Joe steered the City Hospital through the staff shortages and rationing during and after the Second World War, the smallpox outbreak of 1942 and the epidemic of poliomyelitis in the later 1940s. In 1953 he led the celebrations for the hospital's half centenary.

Shortly after his appointment in 1937, Dr Joe wrote a review of infectious diseases in Edinburgh over the previous 25 years.[2] Since 1913, mainly due to the lower mortality from enteric and scarlet fevers, he showed that for both those diseases, puerperal sepsis, and the other major infections, the death rate had fallen dramatically from 0.89 to 0.26 per 1,000 inhabitants. Fewer patients had the 'septic' form of scarlet fever or the laryngeal form of diphtheria, both previously associated with a high mortality. Although Dr Joe appreciated the improvements in the prevention and treatment of infection, he felt that:

> the predominating factor at work has been the advances made in the housing, nutrition, and general social conditions under which the great mass of the population live.[3]

He could offer no explanation for the fluctuating severity of scarlet fever.

Writing in 1936, Dr Joe was relieved to note that, apart from the nine cases in 1920, there had been no smallpox since 1909. Six years later, however, he was in the thick of Edinburgh's last smallpox outbreak. Typhus too seemed to have disappeared. Yet there were 'new' diseases such as encephalitis lethargica after the First World War, 'infantile paralysis' (poliomyelitis) particularly from 1936 onwards, and bacillary dysentery. Some apparent increases in the rates of infection however, were more artefactual than real. For instance the dramatic rise in the admissions for puerperal fever from 1926 onwards reflected an altered definition of the disease and new criteria for admitting patients to hospital.

Dr Joe reported that scarlet fever and diphtheria had been practically abolished among the nursing staff. He also emphasised important advances in treatment particularly:

> the introduction of scarlet fever antitoxins, the aspiration treatment of laryngeal diphtheria, the treatment of respiratory paralysis in diphtheria and infantile paralysis by the Drinker respirator, the use of Prontosil and related compounds in streptococcal infections including puerperal sepsis, erysipelas, and the complications of scarlet fever, and the more extensive use of intravenous and other methods of injection, such as cisternal and venticular puncture in cerebro-spinal fever.[4]

Structural improvements in the hospital and in particular the provision of more cubicle wards were important innovations. Previously, putting patients with the same disease together in the same ward had seemed sufficient. Dr Joe commented, however, that the interchange of organisms between patients suffering from the same disease, especially scarlet fever, must be stopped and hence the usefulness of the cubicle wards. He was also enthusiastic about the balconies Dr Benson had introduced to increase the fresh air and sunlight for the patients.

Overall Dr Joe wrote – and was quoted by the MOH in the introduction to his 1937 Annual Report – that there had been a change of status of the fever hospital. No longer should it be regarded by public health workers simply as a place for segregating patients with infection. The fever hospital had:

> gained recognition as a centre for the treatment and investigation of infectious disease and for the training of medical and nursing personnel in the special methods applicable.[5]

Dr Joe's team was busy in his first year as Medical Superintendent.[6] A total of 4,663 patients were admitted in 1937, 464 of whom had tuberculosis. The average daily number of beds occupied was 526 with a peak of 745 in December. In the scarlet fever wards several patients acquired measles and chickenpox by cross-infection from scarlet fever patients who were incubating the other infections on admission. It was also an influenza year. At one time 70 adults with influenzal bronchopneumonia were in the hospital whilst the staff themselves were depleted because of the same illness.

Thirty-four nurses completed training and successfully gained State Registration as fever nurses in 1937. All but three proceeded to general training. There were no cases of diphtheria among the nurses that year but this was offset by 21 cases of influenza, 8 of rubella, 3 of chickenpox, 2 of mumps and one each of scarlet fever and erysipelas. Forty two nurses had tonsillitis, practically all due to *Streptococcus pyogenes*.

Of 614 confirmed cases of diphtheria in the wards, 37 died (6.02 per cent). Only three of these deaths were due to asphyxia from airways obstruction, a major change from earlier figures when laryngeal obstruction was the commonest mode of death. Dr Joe wrote that 25 of the 37 diphtheria deaths in 1937 were due to early heart failure. One patient with diphtheritic respiratory paralysis was successfully managed on a Drinker respirator till she breathed normally but then she died of late onset heart failure. Dr Joe was concerned that there were still so many patients with diphtheria which, since the introduction of immunisation, should have been prevented. He also criticised the delay in admitting some diphtheria patients, which prevented the early use of anti-diphtheritic toxin and was responsible for 12 of them dying within 24 hours of admission.

Nine of the 1,432 patients admitted in 1937 with scarlet fever died, a mortality of 0.62 per cent. Today some of these diseases would be classified differently but it is interesting to note why patients with an admission diagnosis of 'scarlet fever' actually died. Three had developed pneumonia; two had appendicitis, and, although promptly operated on, had developed generalised peritonitis; one was admitted with established streptococcal peritonitis; another died of streptococcal septicemia from scarlet fever; one had measles bronchopneumonia together with scarlet fever and the final one was admitted moribund with combined scarlet fever and tuberculous meningitis.

A higher fatality (4.98 per cent) was noted for measles, all 15 deaths in the 301 patients admitted being due to superimposed bronchopneumonia. Dr Joe did not record whether pooled measles immunoglobulin (gammaglobulin) was used routinely or only in severe cases. In collaboration with Professor T. J. Mackie, however, measles serum was being collected from convalescent blood donors, whose response was excellent and 'has enabled us to meet all our hospital demands so far'.

Whooping cough was confirmed in 269 of the 305 patients admitted with this presumptive diagnosis. Forty nine (18.21 per cent) died, of whom 44 were below 2 years of age. Thirty-nine of these deaths were due to bronchopneumonic complications.

Dr Joe used sulphonamides in puerperal sepsis and erysipelas where the mortality was 6.80 and 2.69 per cent respectively. As *Streptococcus pyogenes* was the pathogen confirmed in only 30 per cent of cases of puerperal sepsis, there is little wonder that Dr Joe was not optimistic that the sulphonamides, would cure all the patients. However, he persevered with chemo-therapeutic trials in both diseases whilst pleading for more accuracy in diagnosis and a better classification of severity if meaningful results were to be obtained.[7]

Dr Joe was also keen to employ the new sulphonamide drugs in cerebro-spinal meningitis as serum therapy had proved so disappointing. In 1937 there was nothing to be lost in trying any new form of treatment in an illness where 11 of 16 patients with confirmed meningococcal meningitis died (mortality 68.75 per cent). It was not until 1942, however, that his study of sulphapyridine in meningococcal meningitis was published in the *Edinburgh Medical Journal*.[8]

Among the other diseases, it was heartening to see that all 14 of the patients with enteric fever admitted in 1937 survived. Bacillary dysentery was numerically more important than enteric fever, reflecting its increased prevalence throughout Western Europe. Of 129 patients admitted with bacillary dysentery, flexner dysentery was diagnosed in 30 and sonne in 35. One infant died of flexner dysentery, having being admitted to hospital after several weeks of severe illness. All the others survived and most had a mild, relatively short illness.[9]

The hospital laboratory processed 9,436 specimens in 1936. Most were throat swab cultures for *Corynebacterium diphtheriae* and *Streptococcus pyogenes* and the examination of sputa for tubercle bacilli. Other samples cultured were uterine swabs, cerebro-spinal fluid, stool, urine and blood. The Widal reaction for typhoid fever was carried out on 12 occasions.[10]

Despite their heavy clinical load, Drs Joe, Pearson and A. B. Donald and staff spent 100 hours teaching 333 medical students. Besides 27 doctors attended the two DPH courses held that year.

The fabric of the hospital was not neglected. Balconies were added to Pavilions 14 and 16, raising the number of pavilions with balconies to five. The nurses' home was rewired and redecorated. Worn-out furnishings were replaced in the wards and in the administrative and residential accommodation.[11]

In 1938 Dr Joe noted that admissions to hospital had fallen to 3,685. The reduction in cases of scarlet fever and whooping cough was not compensated for by the usual heavy demand for measles beds. The daily average number of occupied beds was 463 and the greatest number of patients under treatment on any one day was 713.[12]

That autumn, however, 22 patients with poliomyelitis were admitted, of whom seven came from outside Edinburgh. Although Dr Joe hoped this increase of admissions reflected an increased awareness of poliomyelitis, he accepted there might be a true increase in prevalence. Two of the three patients treated with the Drinker respirator recovered. There were only two deaths in all 22 patients (9.09 per cent mortality).

Diphtheria was confirmed in 592 patients admitted with this diagnosis. Thirty-four (5.74 per cent) died, 25 from early heart failure but only three from asphyxia. Of the seven with respiratory paralysis, who were managed on the Drinker respirator, three recovered.

Scarlet fever still accounted for 1,166 admissions, 31.64 per cent of the total in 1938. Only three died (0.26 per cent). This probably reflected three factors: a reduction in the severity of the infection, the use of antitoxin in 215 patients and the treatment of complications such as adenitis and otitis media with suphonamides.

There were 30 deaths from measles in 434 confirmed cases (6.91 per cent mortality), most dying from associated bronchopneumonia. Similarly the seven deaths from whooping cough (11.67 per cent) in 60 patients were all due to bronchopneumonia. Dr Joe emphasised the value of oxygen tents in treating infants with respiratory complications from whooping cough and felt more tents would be needed to cope with future whooping cough epidemics.

Among the non-scarlet fever, streptococcal infections, 14 of the 128 confirmed cases of puerperal fever died (10.94 per cent mortality) and seven of 170 with erysipelas (4.12 per cent). Despite using Proseptinase in alternate patients with erysipelas, Dr Joe noticed no significant difference in mortality but there was a more rapid fall in temperature and cessation of spread of the skin eruption in the group treated with sulphonamide.

The number of patients admitted as suffering from bacillary dysentery nearly doubled in 1938 to 221 compared with 1937. Of these only 101 infections were confirmed in the laboratory, 69 being due to *sonnei* and 32 to *flexneri* organisms. There was only one death.

Although 1938 saw 28 patients with suspected cerebro-spinal meningitis, only 15 proved to be infected with meningococci. Of these 6 died (40 per cent mortality). Yet this horrendous death rate was better than the 68.87 per cent mortality which Dr Joe recorded between 1920 and 1937.[13] Serum treatment was still being given in the first half of 1938 but was then discontinued. Antiserum had been given previously in large doses by the intravenous, intraperitoneal and intramuscular routes as well as by cisternal, ventricular and lumbar puncture but its efficacy was in doubt. Besides, the sulphonamide era had arrived with a bewildering array of drugs from which to choose – Prontosil, sulphanilamide, Proseptinase and Soluseptacide. Dr Joe settled for sulphapyridine. Oral treatment 'and intraspinal injections of soluble compounds'[14] were initially recommended. Intraspinal (presumably intrathecal) injection was, however, discontinued about 1937–38:

> a short experience soon convinced me that the new drugs were dangerous

when given by the last-mentioned route [intraspinal], so that this method was quickly given up.[15]

Those were early days. It has been shown since that severe spinal cord damage results from the alkaline solution in which suphonamide drugs were presented for intrathecal injection.

On 23 July 1942, Dr Joe delivered the Honyman Gillespie Lecture in the Royal Infirmary on 'The Treatment of Cerebrospinal Fever by Sulphapyridine'.[16] He described the results of sulphapyridine therapy in the first 500 consecutive patients. A major outbreak of meningoccal disease had occurred in 1940–41 which sometimes meant that as many as 80 patients were under treatment at the same time. Meningococci were demonstrated in the cerebro-spinal fluid 'in all but a few cases' to whom sulphonamides had been given before admission. In 128 patients meningococci were cultured from the cerebro-spinal fluid. Dr Joe regretted that 'owing to pressure on the medical staff' routine blood cultures were not done.[17] Sulphapyridine was given orally or, if not tolerated, by intramuscular injection.

Although Dr Joe appreciated that the 1920–37 anti-serum treated group of 383 patients (68.7 per cent mortality) was not entirely comparable with the 500 sulphapyridine treated patients in 1939–41, the mortality in the latter group of only 18 per cent must be significant. Despite the toxic complications of the sulphonamides which he carefully documented, he concluded the Honyman Gillespie Lecture by saying:

> There can be no doubt that with the introduction of the sulphonamide drugs we have witnessed remarkable developments in the treatment of infectious diseases. In none has their administration had a more spectacular and convincing success than in cerebro-spinal fever.[18]

For the sake of continuity, the exciting story of chemotherapy in streptococcal and meningococcal infection has been taken on to the early 1940s. Dr Joe's success with sulphapyidine in cerebro-spinal meningitis probably reflects the greater proportion of sulphonamide-sensitive organisms in the 1930s and 1940s than today when sulphonamide-resistant meningococci predominate. Penicillin was still to come.

In September 1939, the Second World War broke out. Dr Joe had to improvise during the privations of the war years and his problems were multiplied in 1942 by the last smallpox outbreak ever to visit the Scottish capital. This is described in the next chapter.

CHAPTER TWENTY-TWO

1939–42: The Second World War and Edinburgh's Last Outbreak of Smallpox

The reorganisation of hospital services to cope with wartime casualties created a shortage of beds for civilians.[1] Both the Western and Eastern General Hospitals were included in the Emergency Hospital Scheme for the reception of the wounded. Even Craiglockhart Institution was made into an emergency hospital and its semi-invalid elderly residents were accommodated in the Northern General Hospital. Bangour Village Hospital likewise was relieved of its function as a mental hospital and, with additional hutted accommodation of 1,400 beds, it became an important casualty hospital.[2] One hundred and thirty male patients were transferred from Gogarburn Institution to Larbert so freeing further beds for the wounded. Because of its unique function to be always ready to receive infectious patients, whether military or civilian, the City Hospital was not asked to make beds available for war casualties.

The MOH, Dr W. G. Clark, stated in his Annual Report for 1939[3] that 31,395 citizens, including 17,811 children, had been evacuated from Edinburgh. Dr Clark commented on how difficult it was to persuade the evacuees to keep clean and of the 'personal abuse and even threats of violence' which medical staff received when attempting to educate parents in the rudiments of hygiene. Most children, however, improved physically and psychologically in the reception areas and 'indeed numbers have definitely announced their intention not to return to the City'.[4]

Although not directly part of the Emergency Hospital Scheme, the City Hospital was doing its bit for the war effort. Overall there were 1,700 more admissions in 1940 compared with the previous year. Dr Joe recorded 4,924 admissions in 1940, of whom 376 had tuberculosis. Of the total number admitted, 663 were members of the armed services. The increased figures were partly explained by 444 patients with rubella and 492 with influenza during 1940, most of whom were among service personnel. Diphtheria cases rose to 671 and measles cases to 465. The outbreak of meningococcal disease in 1940, the most severe in the history of the hospital, resulted in 317 confirmed cases being admitted.

No new major works could be carried out at the hospital during the war. Only essential maintenance was done. Blackout precautions posed problems because of the need to keep the wards well ventilated at night. Patients and staff moved to the subways during air raid alerts but this practice was soon condemned by the Ministry of Home Security which feared that the possibility of fractured gas or steam mains would pose unjustifiable risks. Certain side rooms and wards were therefore rendered blast proof by bricking up windows and by protecting the glass of any unbricked windows with adhesive tape.

Additional clerical workers were required to administer food rationing. Although staff and patients suffered from a lack of variety in food and delays in supply, the nutrition of patients was satisfactorily maintained during the war.

Staff shortages were threatened because of the compulsory registration of certain groups of women but the nursing staff levels were maintained. Of 41 nurses who completed training in 1940, 36 passed the State Examinations as fever nurses. Two proceeded to staff nurse posts in fever hospitals elsewhere and 38 went on to complete their general training. One left to get married. Although the nursing staff numbers kept up, female domestic staff were scarce during the war.

Unlike the First World War, the medical staff numbers were maintained. For the first time since the Great War a lady resident medical officer was employed. In his Annual Report for 1940 Dr Joe singled out Dr A. Whyte, his Senior Medical Assistant, Miss Mary Pool, Matron, and Mr Stirling, Hospital Steward, for their exceptional service during the difficult times. Teaching of medical students continued, 238 receiving over 100 hours of clinical demonstrations on infectious diseases during 1940. A course in hospital administration was also held in 1940 and the DPH course was attended by 15 doctors.

In his Annual Report of 1941 Dr W. G. Clark reported a fall in infectious disease notifications throughout the city.[5] This may have reflected the relatively older population after the evacuees had left. Although 1,070 cases of scarlet fever were notified, the disease was generally mild. Notifications of diphtheria fell from 749 in 1940 to 446 in 1941. None of the 28 people who died that year from diphtheria had been immunised and this fact prompted a major immunisation drive. 52,386 citizens, of whom 18,624 were children under five years of age, were vaccinated against diphtheria in 1941. At some schools acceptance rates touched 92.5 per cent.[6]

By 1941 there were shortages of staff in Edinburgh hospitals particularly of nurses in the tuberculosis wards. After initial salary rises recommended for nurses by the Joint Industrial Council, the Hetherington Committee suggested further increments which it was hoped would improve recruitment. The domestic staff shortage made it difficult to maintain good service in the laundries, kitchens and wards.

It was felt vital to keep up the staffing levels during the war when infections like typhus, secondary to overcrowded, insanitary conditions in the battlefields, could reduce the fighting strength. Dr Clark, therefore, designated the City Hospital to be kept in readiness in case of an epidemic of typhus. Although teams of doctors, nurses, sanitary inspectors, ambulance crews and disinfecting officers were briefed and on standby, they were ultimately not required.

There were even fewer infectious disease notifications in the city as a whole during 1941, and Dr Joe recorded a fall of 1,000 admissions. There were 889 scarlet fever patients, 392 with diphtheria, 272 with whooping cough but still 211 with cerebro-spinal fever. There were more patients with enteric fever (62) and the highest figure to date recorded for poliomyelitis.

All male staff of calling-up age had been replaced by temporary employees, many of whom required training so putting a strain on the remaining permanent staff. Some of the male domestic staff volunteered to stay in the hospital every night in case of emergencies but after a specific Fire Watching Order, the roster shared out the duties with others.

In line with the improved nursing salaries, the City Hospital's junior medical staff had their salaries increased so that they were on an equal footing with doctors working in the Emergency Hospital Scheme. Dr Joe did not state in his report what the increased salary was but pointed out that it ended 'the time-honoured stipend of one guinea per week having continued from the opening of the hospital in 1903 till August 1941'.[7] Presumably the doctors had not previously had to pay for food and lodging. When Dr A. Whyte was called up in November 1941, his place was taken by the lady doctor, Dr Scott Forrest.

The shortage of female domestic staff got worse with a loss of 25 per cent. The situation was aggravated by the unsatisfactory daily workers who replaced them. Rationing continued to impose further administrative problems.

Despite these difficulties, medical education was not neglected: 286 medical students and 15 DPH course postgraduates were taught during 1941. A further course on hospital administration was also held. Two Polish medical students from the Paderewski Medical School[8] at the Western General Hospital visited the City Hospital for instruction in infectious diseases by Polish teachers. Of 29 nurses who completed their training in 1941, 26 became State Registered fever nurses by examination.

By the third year of the war, it seemed as if the City Hospital was settling down despite the shortages of staff and the rationing of food. In 1942, however, Dr Clark in his Annual Report[9] commented on an increase in notifications of infectious disease to 6,959 from 6,260 the previous year. The 2,307 notifications of measles accounted for much of the increase and represented the tip of an iceberg, for the first case in each household under five years of age was the only one required to be notified. There were ten measles deaths. Scarlet fever notifications were close to 2,023, compared with 1,070 in 1941, and there were five deaths. Similarly diphtheria was more prevalent with 480 cases and 31 deaths, but cerebro-spinal fever notifications fell to 84 with a mortality of 16.6 per cent. Dr Joe recorded 885 more admissions than in 1941, most of the increase being due to patients with scarlet fever.

The major anxiety for Dr Clark and Dr Joe in 1942, however, was the resurgence of smallpox.[10] This stimulated a vigorous mass vaccination programme with inevitable complications. In the response to the outbreak, over 360,000 people were vaccinated or revaccinated against smallpox in Edinburgh and the adjacent counties. About 64.3 per cent of the city's population received the vaccine. There were 10 vaccine associated deaths, 8 from post-vaccinial encephalomyelitis. Two children died from generalised vaccinia, one who had dermatitis being accidentally inoculated by a recently vaccinated parent, the other somehow being vaccinated contrary to medical advice. These ten tragic deaths among 360,000 vaccinees or their close contacts must be seen in comparison with the eight deaths among the 36 people who contracted smallpox and the unknown number in the population who might have caught the disease had they not been vaccinated.

In general the citizens of Edinburgh co-operated magnificently by attending vaccination centres. The close contacts of smallpox patients seemed perfectly willing to be isolated in a reception house until pronounced clear of infection. Less close contacts, after revaccination, faithfully attended every day for medical inspection during the post-exposure incubation period which, to be on the safe side, was extended to 18 days. The fear of a widespread epidemic and the natural desire to protect oneself and one's family must have been powerful incentives.

Despite thorough and painstaking detective work in attempting to trace contacts, the authors of both reports on the 1942 outbreak[11] were bewildered as to how smallpox came to Edinburgh and, once established, exactly how it spread.

It is difficult now to appreciate the concern smallpox created in the 1940s. Since the World Health Organisation mounted its successful campaign in the 1960s, smallpox has been totally eradicated, the last naturally occurring case being in Somalia in 1977. Apart from two laboratory acquired cases in England in 1978, there have been no further cases since in the world and, there being no animal reservoir of the disease and no latent form of the virus, we can justifiably relax. This was not the case in 1942.

Smallpox had not been reported in Edinburgh since 1920.[12] The occurrence, therefore, of 36 cases in 1942 alarmed the authorities, because the systems for prevention and containment had not been tested for 22 years. As the 1942 outbreak was the last Edinburgh would ever experience, there follows a brief description of it and in particular the role played by the City Hospital.

The Edinburgh outbreak was not entirely unheralded. In late May 1942 smallpox had been imported off a ship into Glasgow by a seaman who became infected when on shore in Capetown. This resulted in 36 cases being notified in Glasgow between May and July. As in the Edinburgh outbreak there were eight smallpox deaths in Glasgow.

In response to the Glasgow outbreak, the MOH of Edinburgh recommended on 30 June 1942 precautionary vaccination or revaccination for the police, civil defence workers, public utility and transport employees, administrative staff of local authorities and all staff in hospitals and institutions. It was a relief that no cases occurred in Edinburgh during July when Glasgow holidaymakers flocked to the beach at Portobello. Between 21 August and 19 November, however, 29 cases with eight deaths were notified in Fife. Despite careful investigation, no apparent link could be found between the cases in Fife and those in Glasgow.

The Edinburgh outbreak started in the late autumn again without any detectable connection with either Glasgow or Fife. On 28 October a 46 year old man in Ward 13 of the Royal Infirmary, followed on 1 November by a 13 year old boy from the same ward, were transferred to secure isolation in the City Hospital under suspicion of having either chickenpox or smallpox. Two days later the diagnosis of smallpox was confirmed in both. A further seven patients from Ward 13 were diagnosed during November.

Before this, however, on 5 November, two men in the Royal Infirmary Convalescent Home, three miles west of the parent hospital, were discovered to have smallpox. Neither had been treated in nor had any connection with Ward 13. On 5 November a Polish medical student, who had attended neither the Royal Infirmary nor the Convalescent Home, was transferred from a boarding house to the City Hospital, with early smallpox. As he had been out and about in the city throughout the incubation period, it was decided to offer vaccination to the whole population. This became generally available at emergency centres by

8 November. Between 18 November and 13 December 1942, 13 cases of smallpox were notified from the city. Eight of these patients had no discernible association with the Royal Infirmary or Convalescent Home, but five were direct contacts of the other eight cases.

The possibility of 'carrier' or mild cases of smallpox with minimal or no rash was postulated to explain the spread of the disease via 'missed cases'. This seemed unlikely because of the extreme degree of alertness during the outbreak and the intense scrutiny of contacts. It is just possible a mild case of smallpox was misdiagnosed as chickenpox and so disseminated the virus. Fomites were also considered as a possible source of infection, especially among the primary cases that occurred sporadically in the city with no obvious connection with the Royal Infirmary or Convalescent Home.

The prevailing wind came from the south west during the outbreak. No cases were notified in homes or places of work immediately downwind from the City Hospital smallpox hospital, for instance in the Craiglockhart Institution. This was further confirmation of Dr C. B. Ker's postulates nearly 40 years earlier that distant aerial spread of smallpox was exceptionally unlikely.

In Edinburgh 26 males and 10 females were infected. Their ages ranged from a girl of nine months to a retired blacksmith of 79, with a mean age 38.2 years. Many different trades and occupations were represented. Two of the nine unvaccinated patients died. Of the 18 with evidence of only one vaccination, six died. None of the nine who had had prior revaccinations succumbed. In all, five male and three female patients died, four of them being aged 50 years or over. Six of the fatal cases had developed severe haemorrhagic smallpox and the rash in the other two fatal cases was confluent. Fortunately the relatives of the seven who died in the Edinburgh District all agreed to cremation of the deceased.

Close contacts were isolated at Victoria Park House, Newhaven Road, Leith. Formerly a children's home, Victoria Park House had closed in 1939 but was prepared at short notice to receive adult smallpox contacts. By 1942 its former Matron, Miss Bain, had become a ward sister at the City Hospital so was eminently suitable to be in charge of the reception house. It was made as attractive as possible, provided with plentiful food, and appropriately staffed. All the contacts willingly submitted to vaccination or revaccination. The women under observation happily helped with the domestic chores. Between 2 November 1942 and 3 February 1943, 27 people were admitted for observation, usually for 21 days. Three of these people contracted smallpox, the wives of two patients and the infant daughter of another, in the reception house but all had a modified disease, perhaps as a result of their recent immunisation. The reception house also took in four convalescents after recovery from smallpox so that their homes could be further disinfected before reoccupation. The reception house might have been much busier if the Royal Infirmary Convalescent Home had not also doubled up as an observation ward during the outbreak.

The part played by the City Hospital was crucial to the successful termination of the outbreak. Between 28 October and 30 December 1942 when the last patient was admitted, 33 of the 36 smallpox patients were cared for by the City Hospital. A further 23 contacts were under observation in the hospital as suspected cases of smallpox in addition to those in the reception house and the Convalescent Home. All were diagnosed ultimately as suffering from another disease, not smallpox.[13] Six of the eight patients who died passed away at the City Hospital. Of the other two, one patient died in Tranent and another in Cambuslang.[14]

The smallpox hospital at Colinton Mains was rather different from those temporary buildings which were hurriedly finished for the outbreak of February 1904 and which had then accommodated 168 smallpox patients (see Chapter 17). The nucleus of the previous hospital had been the unused wooden structures removed from the Queen's Park after the 1894–95 outbreak. The accommodation used in 1942, however, was probably an amalgam of some of those structures with the addition of buildings from the former Slateford Fever Hospital.

It is likely that Edinburgh and its suburbs had several small fever hospitals which became superfluous after the City Hospital opened in 1903 and more modern ambulances made patient transport easier and quicker. One such was Slateford Fever Hospital described as a 'corrugated iron structure formerly used as an infectious diseases hospital at Slateford by Midlothian County Council'.[15] It was situated between Slateford Road and the Union Canal at the western edge of Meggetland on what is now Alan Park Crescent. It was transferred from Slateford and re-erected at Colinton Mains in 1920 after the city boundaries were extended to include Slateford. The little complex of buildings was nonetheless still shown standing on its original site in a map of 1927.[16] Some of these buildings were used for the nine smallpox patients in 1920 but the whole hospital had remained:

> empty and somewhat neglected until 1939, when it was used as a store for large quantities of bedding, blankets, sheets, towels and other hospital requisites purchased at the outbreak of war.[17]

In July 1942 when smallpox arrived in Glasgow, the Edinburgh Public Health Committee recommended £700 be spent on upgrading the existing buildings at the City Hospital site, providing additional facilities for disinfection and also a mortuary. Although this work had not been completed by November 1942:

> the City Architect mobilized a team of inspectors and clerks of works from his own Department – all skilled tradesmen – who finished the job in a praiseworthy last-minute sprint. The final scrubbing out was done by enthusiastic male workers from the Casualty Services, who took a pride in doing the work quickly and thoroughly, and offered to go back for any similar task.[18]

Such public cooperation was a feature of the wartime spirit.

The Edinburgh Outbreak of Smallpox 1942[19] states that the temporary buildings had 24 beds with quarters for eight nurses. The accommodation added in 1942, besides the mortuary, post-mortem room and a discharge unit, comprised two bedrooms with a bathroom for the male staff.

In addition to the isolation hospital itself, the observation cottages within the grounds of the main hospital were also called into service probably for female patients and suspect cases.[20] Each of these eight separate buildings numbered 9–12 then 23–26 had two, three-bedded, wards and during the outbreak in 1942 'proved their worth'. Even used for female patients (who were less likely to abscond) and suspected cases, the cottages did pose staffing problems, each observation case requiring two nurses, who themselves had to remain in strict isolation.

It is unclear which cottage or cottages were actually used. One of those chosen for female patients is described as only '85 feet away from a fully occupied two-storey diphtheria pavilion'[21] with staff accommodation in a neighbouring cottage. If Pavilion 14 was still the designated diphtheria ward – which would appear unlikely – the observation ward (marked 13 on the original plans and later replaced by the pharmacy) would have been the one used. There is, however, no adjacent cottage for staff. It therefore seems probable that the diphtheria patients were in Pavilion 17 by this time and the two cottages for female smallpox patients and staff respectively would be Cottages 23 and 24 or alternatively the nearby Cottages 25 and 26. Miss J. K. Taylor, who was associated with the Hospital from 1928 to 1969, certainly recalls Cottages 25 and 26 being used for women and children during the outbreak. She also mentions the use of Pavilion 16 for diphtheria and Pavilion 17 for 'Blue Corridor Relief'. Whether Cottages 23 and 24, or 25 and 26 were used, the peripheral situation of these cottages rather than Observation Ward 13 would have been preferable.

At the time of the Glasgow outbreak in June and July 1942, the possibility of smallpox spreading to Edinburgh was anticipated and volunteers were called for from among the City Hospital nurses in case smallpox did come to the capital. The whole nursing staff came forward even though they knew that prolonged restrictions and privations were entailed in nursing smallpox patients. The risk of recently revaccinated nurses contracting the disease itself was of course negligible.

When smallpox arrived in Edinburgh, the two senior ward sisters and the 11 most reliable senior probationers, who were selected, remained on smallpox duty throughout the outbreak. They did not leave the smallpox hospital at any time. Only two reluctantly accepted sick leave, each with a septic finger. These casualties may have resulted from the nursing staff in the isolation hospital doing the domestic chores in addition to their nursing duties. They were, however, assisted by two women from the wartime Casualty Services who had volunteered and were incarcerated with the nurses in the smallpox hospital for the duration of the outbreak. All the washing and cooking had to be done within the isolation compound. Further help came when a retired porter from another hospital volunteered to be gatekeeper, porter and general handyman during the outbreak.

One of the great difficulties in running a smallpox hospital, alluded to by Dr C. B. Ker in the early years of the century and still true in the 1940s, was to maintain adequate medical staff cover whilst strictly adhering to isolation procedures. In 1942, like a *deus ex machina*, help came from a doctor, on home leave in Edinburgh from the Indian Medical Service. He had had experience of managing smallpox and volunteered to serve in the isolation hospital where, in fact, he stayed for 10 weeks providing medical cover at a time when male doctors were especially scarce because of the war.[22]

Food for the smallpox patients and the isolation staff came from the hospital kitchen and was emptied into receptacles placed on tables near the smallpox wards. The crockery and cutlery were kept in the isolation area and washed by the staff so they did not return to the main hospital. The smallpox hospital wash-house was used for the patients' laundry. After a preliminary washing there, it was steeped in a carbolic solution for 12 hours and then uplifted for the main hospital laundry to deal with.[23]

The only discordant voices during the outbreak came from relatives of patients in the main hospital whose visiting arrangements were curtailed. They complained that visiting was only allowed to seriously ill patients and those who had to be accompanied on their discharge home. Some of the wily, long-stay, tuberculous patients who most resented these restrictions:

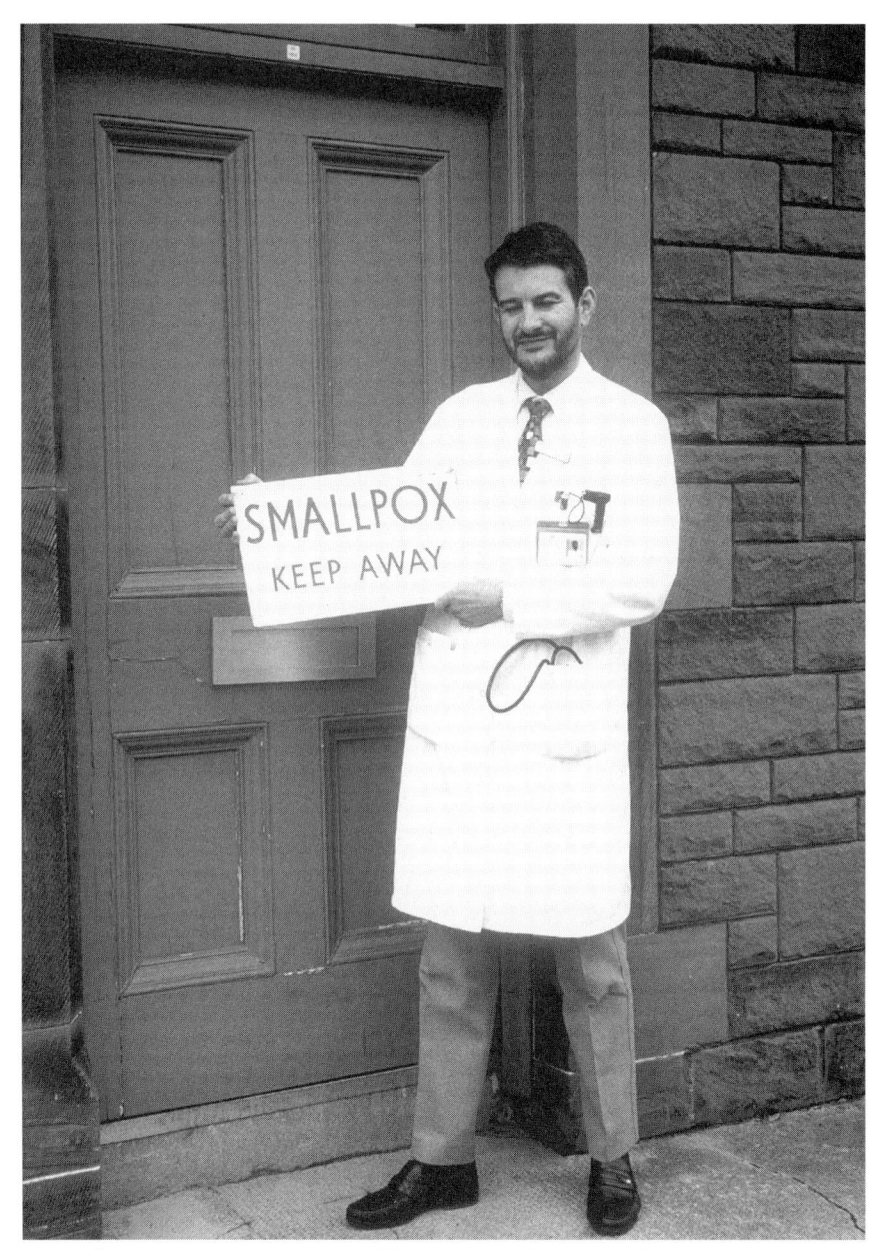

Smallpox warning. Dr P. D. Welsby, ID Consultant, outside Cottage 23 displays the red lettered sign, probably last used in earnest in the 1942 outbreak. (Photo J. A. Gray)

attempted occasionally to contrive their own visiting arrangements at remote parts of the hospital perimeter.[24]

Relatives could take parcels for patients to the Public Health Department in Johnston Terrace, whence they were delivered in bulk to the hospital. The visiting ban was not lifted until 4 January 1943, sixteen days after the last smallpox case was declared non-infectious. The restrictions had been in force for two months and there was general relief when the newspapers announced that visiting could resume.

During this difficult time the morale of the nurses and volunteer helpers in the smallpox hospital remained high. Their only physical recreation was to walk about inside the quarantine area. They could receive but not send letters. Much of their spare time was spent knitting, mending and trying to raise the spirits of their patients which much have dipped whenever there was a death. At Christmas they had a tree festooned with homemade paper decorations. The surviving patients unanimously praised their medical and nursing carers as did the MOH and the citizens of Edinburgh. A lady from the Borders gave £13 for 'the heroic nurses who had saved us from smallpox epidemic in wartime'. Smaller monetary gifts and 'delicacies to eat and books and magazines to read' were also contributed. The gardener at Polton Farm Colony sent beautiful chrysanthemums from his greenhouse to cheer up the patients and nurses. After the outbreak the nurses were rewarded with a 50 per cent addition to salary and a special holiday of either two[25] or four[26] weeks.

Although the part played by the City Hospital was over, the MOH and his team still had much to do. Some homes that had not been fully disinfected still required attention. Compensation had to be paid for clothing and fabrics damaged by formaldehyde. Replacements were given for infected ration books, clothing coupons, national registration identity cards and other valuable printed material that had had to be destroyed. Paper money belonging to the patients and contacts was burned at the Public Health Department in the presence of the MOH who signed certificates requesting banks to supply new notes. Although the sums involved were small, one of the banks sent a representative to witness the incineration.

The smallpox hospital was never used again for its original function and was burned down about 1946 or 1947[27] when it seemed unlikely there would ever be another smallpox outbreak. It was indeed the last time smallpox visited Edinburgh. Contingency plans for smallpox, and later, viral haemorrhagic fevers like Lassa fever, were to contain them initially in Cottage 25. It was last used in 1973 for a Pakistani family under suspicion of smallpox. They were isolated in Cottage 25 for three days after their return from a holiday in their home country. Eventually the suspect child's laboratory tests proved negative for smallpox and the clinical diagnosis of papular urticaria was confirmed.

In 1979 the World Health Organisation declared the global eradication of smallpox.

CHAPTER TWENTY-THREE

1943–47: The End of the War; The Nursing and Domestic Staff; Penicillin; Anxieties about the Coming NHS

The Annual Report of the Public Health Department for 1943 was not published until September 1944, the fifth year of the war. Dr W. G. Clark, the MOH, wrote optimistically. Despite the disruption, rationing and shortages at home, the Allies were making remarkable progress. The D-day landings in Normandy in June 1944, the advances in Italy and, in the Far East, the bombing of Japan and the imminent destruction of the Imperial Japanese Navy in the Battle of the Philippines, all gave hope that the war would be over soon. Dr Clark felt that the war had:

> a toughening effect on the individual and coalescent influence on the community which ... brought out latent powers of resistance. If this communal spirit and purpose were carried into peace-time years, the beneficial effect on the health of the nation would be considerable.[1]

Preparations were made in 1943 for an expected influenza epidemic in Edinburgh but the disease did not affect Scotland as severely as England. Infant mortality was falling partly due to better attendances at ante-natal clinics. Child welfare was also improving with the provision of clinics both for health supervision and the treatment of infants. Twenty-seven nurseries, for children under five years whose mothers were engaged in war work, ensured better care and an opportunity for education on healthier living. Milk, fruit juice and cod liver oil were dispensed in 18 toddlers' playgrounds and nurseries run by the Voluntary Health Workers' Association. Clinics for evacuees were set up at Broomlee Camp and Middleton House. Despite this, 5.2 per cent of children were infested, mainly with lice, although admittedly this proportion was slowly dropping.

Scarlet fever notifications, so high the previous autumn, continued to remain high into 1943 and there was more measles and whooping cough than previously. Fortunately, both the scarlet fever and measles were relatively mild but 19 of the 775 notified cases of whooping cough died. There were fewer notifications and a lower mortality from cerebro-spinal fever. Diphtheria immunisation was being strongly encouraged. Sadly tuberculosis showed an increase especially among young women many of whom were undertaking long hours of war work. A new Government Scheme encouraged infected workers to accept maintenance allowances and leave their work to undergo a course of treatment.

The abbreviated wartime report by the City Hospital's Medical Superintendent[2] recorded 4,432 admissions in 1943 of whom 295 patients were from the armed services. Not surprisingly the 392 admissions with bacillary dysentery were almost three times more than the average over the previous four years. Although 424 confirmed cases of diphtheria were admitted, the hospital death rate from diphtheria of only 3.31 per cent was the lowest since 1931.

The 207 medical undergraduates who attended for clinical instruction received a total of 85 hours teaching. Students from the Paderewski Medical School were also taught at the City Hospital by Polish teachers. On government instructions, DPH courses were abandoned for the duration of the war.

Forty of the 43 nurses who completed training in 1943 passed their State Registration examinations as fever nurses. Of these 33 went on to general training schools, three left to marry, three went into isolation hospitals as staff nurses and one joined the Civil Nursing Reserve. There was a close affiliation with Kirkcaldy Hospital, six of whose seconded nurses passed the State Examination after one year's training and two, seconded from Sanderson Hospital, Galashiels, completed their training in two years and also passed the State Examination. In addition five general trained nurses obtained certificates after one further year's training.

Sadly the Matron, Miss Mary Pool, resigned on health grounds on 15 May 1943. She died in Ireland in March 1944. She was the last remaining member of staff who had worked in the second City Hospital before the move to Colinton Mains in 1903. Except for a period on active service during the First World War and afterwards when she was Matron at the Deaf and Dumb School for a short time, she had been a loyal servant of the Corporation all her working life. Appointed Matron at Colinton Mains in 1925, her:

> whole existence was bound up with the City Hospital and with the improvement of the status of the fever nurse, in the course of the latter spending many long and arduous hours of her scanty leisure.[3]

Miss Pool had continued the tradition of her predecessors by keeping a detailed account of each nurse's progress in the City Hospital Nurses' Register.[4] Her entries begin in Volume VI in neat, upright handwriting compared with the previous sloping, angular calligraphy of Miss Sandford and Miss Thomas. Details are given (usually in red ink) in the Daily

Record Book[5] of the classes attended by the nurses: Anatomy & Physiology, Hygiene, Fever Nursing, Materia Medica and cooking classes. Also entered in red ink are the illnesses suffered by the nursing staff, their sick leave, holidays, any reprimands received and comments on either excellent or unsatisfactory behaviour.

Reasons why nurses left the hospital are recorded. Many only lasted a few months and gave up on account of ill health. Frequently there are comments such as 'A nice girl, quiet and lady like. Left as she was much too susceptible to continue fever nursing' or 'Not strong enough to continue nursing (had Empyema)' or 'Asked to resign because of her condition'. This euphemism for pregnancy is recorded several times as a reason for terminating employment.

Some nurses were criticised for being 'flighty' with porters or male patients. Others came into conflict with ward sisters or the Matron herself 'Left of her own accord. Not at all suitable for training as a nurse. Very impudent manner and resented being corrected' and another 'Left at her own request – a most difficult mischief making girl'. Some were dismissed for being unkind to small patients or for smacking a child, some for dishonesty 'Dismissed for stealing money from nurses and patients' friends' or 'for ordering goods in another nurse's name'. Rules were not to be flouted and one nurse was 'Dismissed for staying out all night without permission [when on night duty] – a girl one could not recommend'. As late as 1930 a third year nurse was 'Dismissed owing to her going to a ward in her scarlet uniform after being forbidden to do so, she was a good nurse also worked well'.

In the 1930s several nurses developed tuberculosis, but whether it was acquired at home or occupationally is not always clear. A few died. In 1934 one entry laconically records of a second year nurse 'A very quiet girl, developed T.B. Warded in Ward 7. Died 2nd June', and another in 1935 'Died influenzal pneumonia 9.4.35 – an exceptionally nice girl (from Isle of Eigg)' and one of several in 1936 'A very nice girl developed T.B. after being 6 months. History of T.B. on Father's side'. Dr H. C. Elder, the Tuberculosis Officer, was called in by Dr Benson to diagnose and treat these unfortunate nurses after admission to Ward 7 at the City Hospital or to the Royal Victoria Hospital. Some of them ultimately made a good recovery.

Similar but even briefer comments appear in the Servants' Record Book.[6] These statements presumably acted as an *aide mémoire* for Matron if she was required to give references later for her domestic workers, many of whom subsequently went into private service. Typical comments were 'could work very well but required constant supervision – Respectable honest girl' or 'Returned on Nov. 19th and was dismissed for not coming back at the right time. Works well under supervision. A little inclined to be noisy but a pleasant willing girl'. On 17 October 1925 one of the servants 'Was sent away for coming in late and through a window – Not a thorough worker though quite willing and anxious'. Dishonesty also occurred. A servant in the laundry whose annual wage in 1927 was £24 'Ran away stole a great many things of value from Miss Brydon also from one of the maids. A very good worker'.

Despite the misdemeanours of a few servants – and nurses – things ran smoothly most of the time. The wards were scrupulously clean. One former nurse[7] in Dr Benson's time recalls the diphtheria wards where a single drop of water on the floor was regarded as a crime by the 'masterful ward maid'. Nurses in the open-air tuberculosis wards all commented on the freezing conditions, for staff as well as patients. One job the nurses all hated was emptying the enamel sputum mugs of the tuberculosis patients.[8] The sputum had to be checked for blood, measured in volume (which was often illegally guessed by eye) and then emptied into a heavy duty paper bag. The mugs were then washed out and sterilised.

The sputum mug routine was regarded as even more unpleasant than the 'slunging' of soiled linen.[9] The practice of dispatching slunged linen from the turrets down the glazed tile chutes into the carbolic tanks outside was discontinued about 1928.[10] In the 1940s, however, linen was still scrubbed on the ward and put in a large carbolic tub before being uplifted for the laundry.[11] Without disposable gloves the nurses' hands and forearms became red and sore despite the liberal use of zinc and castor oil ointment. Sepsis of the fingers and hands was common.

Some aspects of nursing in the 1940s have been vividly recalled by Mrs Jean Day whose career started at Blairgowrie Cottage Hospital in 1942 when aged 17 years. She then began her training at the Edinburgh City Hospital in July 1943. She does not recall Miss Pool, who became ill in 1943 and died in March 1944 but does remember Miss Maggie Broach, the 'elderly but kindly' Assistant Matron who bridged the gap between the retirement of Miss Pool and the appointment of Miss M. I. Adams in November 1944.

From 1944 Miss Adams instituted a new system of nursing education, calling the nurses in training 'student nurses' rather than 'probationers'. Whereas Mrs Day, starting as a probationer in 1943, was thrust straight into the wards on her first day of work, the new student nurses received an introductory course of lectures before going on the wards.

Mrs Day certainly did not have the benefit of any gentle breaking-in period. On her first day she was taken in hand by a nurse who was senior to her self by only one month. They both wore gauze strips wound round the nose and mouth and together they swept the ward floor and afterwards dusted the locker tops. On this particular male tuberculosis ward there was only one domestic and the nurses had to do most of the heavy cleaning, pulling the beds out, rubbing thick polish on the floor then rubbing it off with a 'dummy', a heavy block of wood on top of a thick duster. Patients' lockers were emptied weekly, trundled to the bathroom and scrubbed inside and out. The toilets and bathrooms also had a major weekly clean when the wall tiles were also washed. Flowers were taken out of the wards at night, laid along the corridor and next morning freshened up and returned to the ward.

Mrs Day was bewildered in the male tuberculosis ward to which she was assigned. 'I had never encountered all that coughing and spitting, or rattle of enamel sputum pots.' She hated the daily sputum pot ritual. Some of the patients were on complete bed rest and one or two on 'silence' – possibly suffering with laryngeal tuberculosis. A frightening man with facial lupus lay hidden by a cloth mask. Artificial pneumothorax was carried out on the ward but not other surgical procedures such as phrenic nerve crush or gland dissection. Among the long-stay patients, pressure sores were frequent despite a 4-hourly round with soap and water, methylated spirit rub and talcum powder. Deep sores were managed with ichthyol paste and cod liver oil dressings, which were nauseating for both patients and staff. Two-hourly turning did not yet seem in vogue.

Long before pre-sterilised procedure packs were available, trays and trolleys were set up in the mornings by a nurse assigned to that job. Syringes and needles were boiled, kept immersed under methylated spirit in enamel dishes and finally washed with sterile water before use. Pills for injection were dissolved in a teaspoonful of water heated over a methylated spirit flame. When sputum was difficult to expectorate, it was the responsibility of the nurses, in the absence of physiotherapists, to obtain samples by postural drainage, failing which gastric lavage was used. Smoking was frowned upon. When one senior doctor in the tuberculosis ward asked a patient who had been readmitted if he had stopped smoking and he confessed he had not, the doctor refused to discuss his case with him. His treatment was continued, however, as also for the other patients some of whom, if questioned, would not have been so honest.

For light relief there was a pool table in one of the wards and a piano. A patient called Freddie Cullen, who had previously played in a band, delighted everyone with his piano and accordion music.

Some of the long-term patients were allowed home leave after two consecutive negative sputum cultures. Three negative cultures in a row usually meant they were ready for discharge. There was great joy when a patient was granted home leave or discharge and genuine sympathy for those who relapsed and had to be readmitted. Ambulant patients were allowed to walk round the hospital grounds and 'go to the pines' but sitting in the sunshine was discouraged in case it reactivated the disease.

Aged 19 or 20 Mrs Day had a routine chest X-ray along with her colleagues and was found to have a shadow on one lung. Although asymptomatic she was put on half duty and directed to help the Home Sister. Part of her time off the wards was spent on the hospital's telephone switchboard but occasionally she would briefly relieve nurses on the wards during their meal breaks. Being on the switchboard enabled her to warn the night nurses on each ward when Jennie their 'fearsome Night Sister' was on her rounds. This would 'jolt them out of a sleepy stage, hide the coffee pot and if a young Doctor was sharing the coffee, he could clear out too'. Somehow, even in wartime, they acquired real ground coffee, which they boiled up in a pot and strained through a gauze swab. They were careful not to be caught because eating and drinking on the wards was strictly prohibited.

Mrs Day's tuberculosis was frequently assessed. When she eventually got back to work she was ordered to rest on her half days, and not go to dances or cinemas which were the nurses' favourite entertainments. In time she was declared free of tuberculosis but was disappointed to have been put on half-pay after the first six months of her illness.

Working on the fever wards was similar to the tuberculosis wards except that the patients changed over more frequently and there were fewer sputum pots to empty. Non-essential conversation with patients was discouraged and regarded by the senior staff as 'time-wasting or else as looking for a husband'. Beds were made, remade and tidied incessantly especially before Matron or Dr Joe did a ward round. Tidiness was paramount. With military precision all bed wheels had to face away from the ward doors, as also the wheels of the mobile screens which were in vogue before bed curtains were introduced. Before a visit by Dr Joe or his staff, a linen hand towel, pleated in the shape of a fan, was tastefully arranged behind the taps of a scrupulously clean wash hand basin for the doctors to use. 'There was no animosity in doing this task, just an accepted part of the daily routine'.[12]

Mrs Isobel McFarlane, later a Sister in the whooping cough ward, and her sister Mrs Patricia Hunter, both of whom trained at the City Hospital as Nurses I. and P. McWilliams, also recall the formality of ward rounds. Nurses had to stand with their hands behind their backs. They always knew when Dr Joe was coming as his heels made a clicking sound as he walked along the corridor. He was sometimes accompanied on ward rounds by medical students. On one occasion a male student was ticked off by Dr Joe for addressing Nurse Isobel McWilliams by her first name.[13] Such familiarity was not approved of.

Yet Dr Joe could be generous and understanding. Although very much 'the Chief', he could say to a couple of staff whom he surprised together in the linen cupboard that it was alright 'to visit each other' but they should avoid being caught. After many years of experience he could be dogmatic in his diagnoses. As late as 1954 when a smallpox suspect was admitted off a ship in Leith, Dr Joe flung back the bed clothes and correctly and dramatically pronounced the spots to be chickenpox, so allowing the patient to be transferred from an isolation cottage to a ward. He was always keen to demonstrate the characteristic cough and whoop of a child with pertussis and would wait and listen for a long time with his students until a child obliged. He was rather formal with children, only condescending to waggle a bunch of keys to obtain the babies' attention. Overall the nurses respected him greatly and everyone recognised his diagnostic acumen and administrative ability. Miss J. K. Taylor, later Matron, confirms his lasting devotion to the City Hospital which she shared with him.

Mrs Day recalls many children with dysentery. Flexneri, sonnei and dysenteriae types were admitted into the same ward and treated with sulphaguanidine, a non-absorbable sulphonamide. Batches of patients with dysentery would come in from orphanages, mental homes and, at the end of the war, ex-Prisoners of War. were admitted as well. Despite the unpleasant slunging of dysentery patients' linen by the ungloved nursing staff, any nurse who caught dysentery was reprimanded for not having taken adequate precautions to protect herself.

Visiting patients was not permitted. Relatives could enquire at the hospital about patients and pass over gifts in a set of cubicles specially constructed for the purpose in what later became the Conference Room. The bulletins in the Edinburgh evening newspapers were felt sufficient to keep relatives informed (see Chapter 17). Children settled surprisingly quickly in the wards without their parents but were probably very unsettled on their return home. Letters from patients were taken for disinfection before posting. Clothing was bundled up, taken into a windowless cell and fumigated. Mrs Day recalls taking clothes there, lighting a small lamp under a container with six formaldehyde tablets, and then, before the fumes began, making a dash for the door and finally locking it securely behind her.

Mrs Day unfortunately contracted diphtheria after her tuberculosis. She had been staffing in the male diphtheria Ward 14 and, after developing a sore throat for a few days, was diagnosed as suffering from faucal diphtheria. Apparently she had not been Schick tested that year and it was presumed her immunity was low. She was admitted to the cubicle Ward 3 where all sick staff were cared for 'like private patients'. After intramuscular antitoxin, she was told to do nothing for herself, presumably to safeguard her from myocarditis. Rather than be fed, however, she was allowed to lie on her side and eat her meals herself. One of the hospital porters sent her a bunch of red roses with a card saying: 'May the fragrance of Dr Joe's roses speed your recovery'. Dr Joe's eyesight was poor but she was terrified he would recognise his garden blooms when he came on his ward rounds. Fortunately he did not enquire where they had come from. She got better after seven weeks in hospital followed by a month's sick leave.

Nursing laryngeal diphtheria patients in the steam room of Ward 14 and caring for their tracheotomies was another task the nurses found taxing but also interesting. The inner tracheostomy tube was cleaned, apparently very efficiently, with a feather dipped in sodium bicarbonate solution. Strictly only Schick negative nurses were assigned to this duty and Mrs Day's immunity should have been checked beforehand. She may have derived her own illness from 'specialing' a tracheostomised diphtheria patient.

On night duty Mrs Day looked after an adult male patient paralysed by poliomyelitis who was nursed in the Drinker cabinet respirator. Many of the nurses were intimidated by this unwieldy apparatus whilst sympathising with the unfortunate patient within.

By contrast, scarlet fever nursing was a soft option. The ritual evening bathing of children with scarlet fever was supposed to speed up desquamation, although it was of very doubtful benefit. All nurses had to have a Dick test before working on the scarlet fever wards. Pink uniforms were worn although, by Mrs Day's time in the 1940s, scarlet fever nurses were only segregated from their colleagues in the dining room by a wooden barrier rather than a glass partition as formerly. Nonetheless they still used a separate entrance to the dining room.

Although Mr Morham had designed the nurses' home, the recreation hall and other facilities along the most modern lines in the 1890s, the nurses in the 1940s regarded them as old fashioned. Mrs Day recalls that the home was austere and the only recreational aspect of its recreation hall was 'one elderly, crackly wireless set'. There were, however, occasional staff concerts held there. One nurse in particular, who had trained as a violinist with the D'Oyly Carte Opera Company, gave a fine performance. Junior doctors and nurses poked fun at their seniors in hospital reviews which were well received, suggesting that there was a more relaxed attitude than before. One post-war dance was held during Mrs Day's time but, as she was on night duty, she could not attend.

She recalls the large ground floor sitting room of the nurses' home and two sick rooms for nurses not ill enough to be warded. Staff nurses had their sitting room on the first floor, ward sisters theirs above this, whilst Matron's flat occupied the top floor of the east wing. Discipline also extended into the nurses' home. The bedrooms were bleak and nurses were forbidden too many personal fripperies on their one and only chest of drawers. Untidy or improperly made beds were liable to be stripped by the Home Sister and had to be remade when the nurses came off duty. Bathrooms were 'old fashioned cubicles' and pranksters would sometimes throw cold water over the top of the partition onto some unfortunate nurse enjoying a hot bath on the other side.

Windows on the ground floor of the nurses' home were nailed in such a way that they could only be slightly opened. Although an obvious fire hazard, this was supposed to deter intruders rather than keep errant nurses in. Mrs Hunter and Mrs McFarlane [14] remember that the nurses on the ground floor managed unobtrusively to remove the nails from windows in their bedrooms and in the sitting room to allow revellers to creep back into the home after 10 p.m.; others had access to a secret ladder leading up to a first floor window from outside. Once a month a pass to 11 p.m., or exceptionally to 1 a.m., was permitted or else a single night's sleeping out was allowed.

Professional etiquette in the 1940s forbade nurses from going out with doctors, porters or ambulance men. It was even considered improper and over-familiar to say 'Good morning!' to a porter in the corridors. Yet, unlike 1905, practical joking was taken in good part. A bewildered probationer, unaware that a 'long stand' referred to a tall type of drip stand, was sent to the nursing office for a quite differently interpreted long stand. Similarly, in her first week of nursing, Mrs Hunter was sent to another ward by a senior colleague to fetch a pair of Fallopian tubes.

At the end of three years' training there was a tough oral examination in addition to the written and clinical tests. In the practical exam nurses could be asked to lay out trays for any procedure from a simple enema to a blood transfusion. The ongoing assessment books, which evaluated a nurse's progress throughout her training, were also scrutinised.[15] The State Examination Certificate as a Registered Fever Nurse would then be awarded to successful candidates.

In 1944 Dr W. G. Clark, the MOH, reported fewer notifications of infectious disease in the city.[16] Even so, there were 1,222 cases of scarlet fever and 1,124 of measles. Only the first child aged less than 5 years with measles in a family was notified so the actual incidence was much higher. Both illnesses had become milder, only three deaths occurring from scarlet fever and none from measles. There were 306 cases of diphtheria, the lowest incidence since 1899, and 12 deaths, again the lowest reported mortality ever. Perhaps as a result of the war, there were 766 notifications of bacillary dysentery.

Dr Clark paid tribute to the five hospitals most concerned with providing facilities for the wounded under the Emergency Medical Service (EMS) Scheme. These were the Western General with accommodation especially for Poles, the Eastern General, the Southern General (Craiglockhart Hydropathic) with beds for Norwegian service men, Gogarburn and, finally, Bangour which accommodated by far the greatest number of service personnel. Each of the hospitals had a quota of German and Italian prisoners of war who 'added to the international character of the strangers within our gates'.[17]

Although City Hospital had no EMS commitment as such, 425 service patients were among the 4,461 patients admitted during 1944.[18] The average number of beds occupied per day was 434 with a peak of 536 at the end of December and a trough of 355 at the end of August. Much of the end-of-year increase was due to bacillary dysentery with 949 admissions of whom 597 were bateriologically confirmed. Dr Joe commented 'that the ultimate responsibility in the case of this disease must literally be put in the hands of the individual citizen, and that much higher standards of personal hygiene must be inculcated'.[19] Mortality for diphtheria patients in hospital was falling and that for cerebro-spinal fever at 5.71 per cent 'has reached what ten years ago would have been regarded as a fantastically low level'. Meningococcal meningitis was still treated with sulphonamides but, as Dr Joe pointed out:

> The most important event of the year from the medical stand point was the release of penicillin for civilian use in infectious hospitals. Much careful work will be necessary before a balanced verdict on the value of this remedy can be presented.[20]

On 1 November 1944, Miss M. I. Adams, formerly Matron of the Isolation Hospital in Norwich, took up her appointment as Matron of the City Hospital in succession to Miss Pool who had died in March 1944. Like her worthy predecessors, Miss Adams held office for a very long time, relinquishing her post in September 1965 after nearly 21 years as Matron.

Wartime restrictions continued during Miss Adams' first two years in office. Although the adoption of the Hetherington Report by the Joint Industrial Tribunal had improved the salaries and conditions of service of domestic staff, few were recruited and shortages persisted. Fortunately, enough nurses were available but Dr Joe and Miss Adams found difficulty in obtaining ward sisters willing to work with tuberculous patients.

Rationing continued for several years after the war. Along with the Nursing Register, the Record of Rationed Butcher Meat Purchased is preserved. Weekly returns were made and submitted every two months to the Ministry of Food then temporarily housed in the College of Art, Lauriston Place. They included the number of patients, particularly service men and women for whom a special allowance was given, the cost of meat and the amounts sanctioned by the Ministry of Food. All this wartime form filling required extra clerical staff and greater expense.

During and immediately after the war, patients' food was nourishing, reasonably plentiful but monotonous. For children in the whooping cough ward during the war years, breakfast consisted of porridge, bread and jam and milk. Mid-morning orange juice and a biscuit were given, followed by lunch of soup, mince, potatoes and cabbage with semolina as a sweet. Supper was simply bread and jam and milk again. Supplements of a teaspoonful of malt and 'Parrish's Syrup' were also given daily in those vitamin conscious times.[21]

Identity cards were issued to nurses during the war. These 3 in × 4 in pieces of brown cardboard carrying the nurse's name were embossed

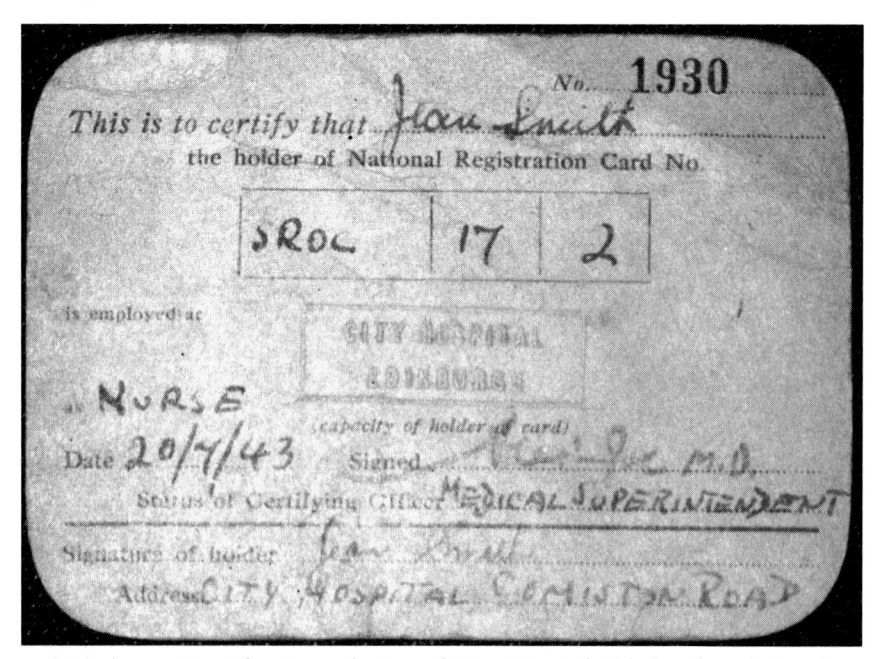

Nurse's war time identity card stamped City Hospital, Edinburgh and signed by Dr Alec Joe, 20.7.1943. (By courtesy of Mrs Jean Day, née Smith)

with City Hospital letter stamp and signed by Dr Joe. They were supposed to be worn on duty perhaps as proof of identity for the staff who were nursing service personnel. Mrs Day records they were mainly used to wave at the entrance to cinemas and the *Palais de Dance* so allowing the nurses to jump the queue and be admitted at forces' prices. She cannot remember having to show her identity card at any other time.

At the end of the war Mrs Day recalls scrubbing out the side wards which had been sandbagged against blast in the event of an air raid. As it happened there were few raids over Edinburgh. Enemy aircraft had circled the city in October 1939 during an attack on the Forth but no bombs were dropped on the city itself.[22] Subsequent raids were light and spasmodic with the dropping of incendiary rather than high explosive bombs. The expected civilian bombing casualties therefore did not arrive. However, the beds that had been set aside in other hospitals, for civilians and for military casualties before the D-day landings, were put to good use. They helped to reduce the waiting lists of voluntary hospitals in other parts of the country and allowed key civilians working in munitions factories or in industry to get back to work promptly.

Education continued during 1944. Dr Joe and his staff taught 234 medical undergraduates and Paderewski Medical School students attended clinics at the City Hospital with Polish teachers. A two-week introductory course for newly enrolled nurses was successfully introduced by Miss Adams. Of the 39 nurses who completed three years fever training in 1944, 34 passed the State Examinations. Together with nurses from Kirkcaldy and Galashiels, a total of 36 proceeded to general training. Five nurses already generally trained gained the Fever Certificate after only one year at the City Hospital.

Dr Joe's Report for 1944 acknowledged the assistance of Dr Scott Forrest who helped to prepare the Annual Report, and Miss Broach who had acted as Matron until Miss Adams took over. Mr Stirling, the Steward, also received honourable mention. His administrative skills had been tried to the utmost during the staff shortages and rationing imposed by the war. At Christmas 1944, the Lord Provost, Rt Hon. Sir John Falconer and the MOH visited the Hospital. Accompanied by Drs Clark and Joe and Miss Adams, the Lord Provost was photographed on the steps of the general offices showing his chain of office to a group of smiling nurses.[23]

The end of 1944 ushered in a severe outbreak of measles, which peaked in January 1945 when 1,784 cases were notified (the first in each household below the age of 5 years). Altogether 2,920 such cases were notified in 1945 and there were 16 deaths. Of 494 notifications of whooping cough, there were 17 deaths, but only one of the 1,029 patients with scarlet fever died. Among 362 cases of diphtheria, there were 13 deaths. Bacillary dysentery, with 752 notified cases, was numerically second only to scarlet fever. Dr Clark dealt with 193 contacts of smallpox from ships, but happily no cases occurred in Edinburgh.[24]

1945 was a light year for the City Hospital, with only 3,890 admissions. Of these 302 had tuberculosis, mostly advanced, and 80 of them died. That year, by comparison, the Royal Victoria Hospital admitted only 132 rather less severe cases. The lot of tuberculosis patients at the City Hospital was brightened by concert parties and visits from choirs. An occupational therapy enthusiast encouraged handicraft and other kinds of diversional therapy. A library scheme also operated for long-stay patients although books sent to the infectious diseases hospital could not be returned.[25]

Dr Joe commented that 342 of the City Hospital admissions were of service patients in this, the last year of the war. He was concerned by the numbers with dysentery and the 20 per cent increase in diphtheria

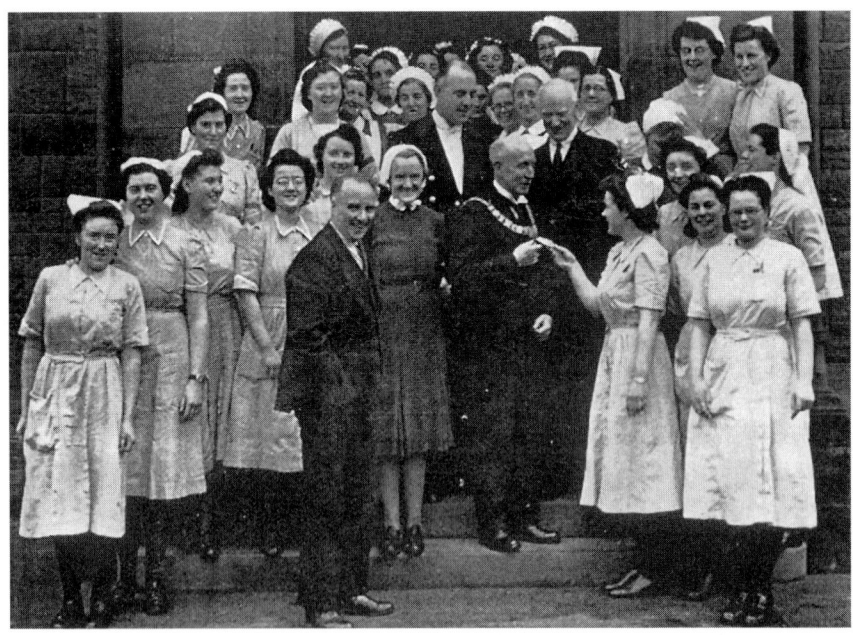

Christmas visit of Lord Provost, 1944. Nurses in front of the general offices admire Sir John Falconer's chain of office. Left to right: Dr Alec Joe, with hands characteristically in his pockets, Miss M. I. Adams, Matron. Behind Sir John, is the MOH, Dr W. G. Clark, wearing a dark tie. From Annual Report of the Public Health Department, 1944, p. 33. (By courtesy of Edinburgh City Libraries)

patients. Hygiene was obviously being neglected – hence the dysentery problem – and he recorded in one children's ward that 60 per cent of those of school age had head lice.[26] Well into the 1960s on top of the admission sheet for each paediatric patient there were two boxes to be ticked, one for 'Head clean' and the other 'Body clean'. Tooth combs and antipediculosis shampoos were used to remove the nits' eggs and the 'mechanised dandruff', as the active lice were termed.

Removal of blackout precautions restored proper ventilation in the wards. Fire watching ceased. Food was plenteous but the variety poor and frequent milk puddings became monotonous. Recruiting domestic staff and nurses remained difficult. Two hundred and twenty-one medical students attended for infectious diseases teaching and Polish students from the Paderewski School were accommodated again.

Miss Adams appointed an Assistant Sister Tutor. Forty nine nurses completed their three years training but only 35 passed their State Examination. Affiliations with Kirkcaldy and Galashiels continued. In 1945 the end of the war in Europe was marked by the resumption of the nurses' Annual Garden Party and Prize Giving with Reunion. This time the Lady Provost graced the occasion and presented the prizes.

In 1946, Dr Clark reported the lowest ever number of scarlet fever and diphtheria notifications.[27] Of 172 cases of diphtheria, 10 died. The drive for more complete diphtheria immunisation continued. Demobilisation after the war was associated with housing shortages. Food remained poor. Although the birth rate inevitably rose, so too did infantile mortality but the overall death rate for all age groups in the city fell.

Dr Joe reported 2,991 admissions in 1946 of which 285 were for tuberculosis. There were 125 service patients spread over all the wards. Diphtheria admissions fell to 188, the lowest in the hospital's records. Whooping cough mortality fell to 3.75 per cent and that for measles to 0.41 per cent.

Dr Joe saw to the replacement of old equipment and had the buildings repaired and painted inside and out. Despite the employment, especially in the TB wards, of male orderlies, recently demobbed from the RAMC, there remained shortages in nursing and domestic staff. In mid-September only 115 of a possible 156 nurses were on duty. Many were on special leave because of family illness. Two hundred and eighteen medical students received instruction and the Polish students were again made welcome. The DPH courses, in abeyance during the war, were resumed in the spring and summer terms.

Nursing education continued and the introductory training period for new entrants was increased from two to three weeks. Of 35 nurses completing the three year training in 1946, 31 passed the State Examination as fever nurses. Kirkcaldy and Galashiels sent nurses for fever training as before. Thirty-one nurses left for general training and nine left to be married. At the nurses' Prize Giving and Reunion on 26 June, the presentation of the C. B. Ker Memorial Medal was resuscitated after a lapse of about 20 years. It was won by Nurse A. Adams for the best record of practical and theoretical work. The prizes were presented by Dr C. C. Easterbrook, formerly Medical Superintendent at the Crichton Royal Mental Hospital, Dumfries. Appropriately enough he had been a Resident in the second City Hospital in 1894 and had been a close friend of the late Dr Ker. He recalled that at the request of Miss Sandford, the then Lady Superintendent of Nurses, he had given a course of lectures to the nursing staff, the first in the history of the hospital. Lectures were delivered at 7.30 a.m., the most suitable time for both day and night staff.

At the end of Dr Joe's Report for 1946[28] he recorded, courteously as ever, his appreciation of the work done by the Matron, Steward, heads of departments, and ward sisters. He would miss the support of Dr Scott Forrest who was leaving to undertake postgraduate studies. She was replaced by Dr A. Whyte who returned from war service to resume his appointment as Senior Assistant. When he accepted another post in December 1946, he was to be succeeded by Dr Margaret Main.

Although the National Health Service (NHS) was still two years away when he wrote his Annual Report of 1946, Dr Clark, the MOH, gave it only a cautious welcome. His own Public Health Department would be reduced to staffing and equipping health centres, providing maternity, child welfare and midwifery services, health visiting, home nursing and after-care of the sick. His major task would remain the prevention of ill health. Sadly, from the infectious diseases angle, this would mean his separation from the fever hospital which would be run by a Regional Hospital Board, and so disrupt the total management of infection by the local authority. He agreed, however, that the means test for contribution to care in municipal hospitals should disappear, that medical directors of hospitals should have greater freedom to place patients in hospitals suitable for their needs, and that the grouping of hospitals on a regional basis would help to provide institutional care for the chronic sick in an ageing population. Was Dr Clark anticipating devolution when he wrote in 1946:

> A point in favour of the new service, is that it takes cognisance of purely Scottish needs and it is likely to be directed by Scotsmen with an intimate knowledge of Scottish problems.[29]

The population of Edinburgh rose from 459,430 in 1946 to 485,664 in

1947 due to the continuing demobilisation of service personnel after the war.[30] The city's birth rate rose and death rate fell. Epidemic infections were not yet conquered but trends pointed to some control now taking place. Over 10,000 children received primary or maintenance diphtheria immunisation in 1947. Only 50 cases of diphtheria were notified with two deaths. Measles, for which there would be no immunisation for several decades, still caused 1,403 notifications (of the first child less than 5 years in the family). Whooping cough figures showed a rise to 790 cases and there were 20 deaths. At the turn of the century, 320 beds had been allocated in the third City Hospital for scarlet fever. In 1947 there were only 310 *notifications* of scarlet fever in Edinburgh with no deaths for the second year running. Only 72 cases of puerperal sepsis were recorded and, thanks to sulphonamides and penicillin, no deaths resulted. Compared with the previous year, 1947 saw the notifications of infectious diseases fally by 795 to 4,203 and the City Hospital admitted only 2,796 patients of whom 224 had pulmonary tuberculosis.

Yet if the classical fevers were genuinely in decline, some newer infections were prominent. In 1947 Dr W. G. Clark reported 172 cases of poliomyelitis from the Lothians and Borders requiring the use of seven 'iron lungs' (mainly Drinker-type cabinet respirators), five of which were loaned from other hospitals.[31] The 151 Edinburgh cases showed a typical seasonal preponderance increasing in the late summer and autumn.

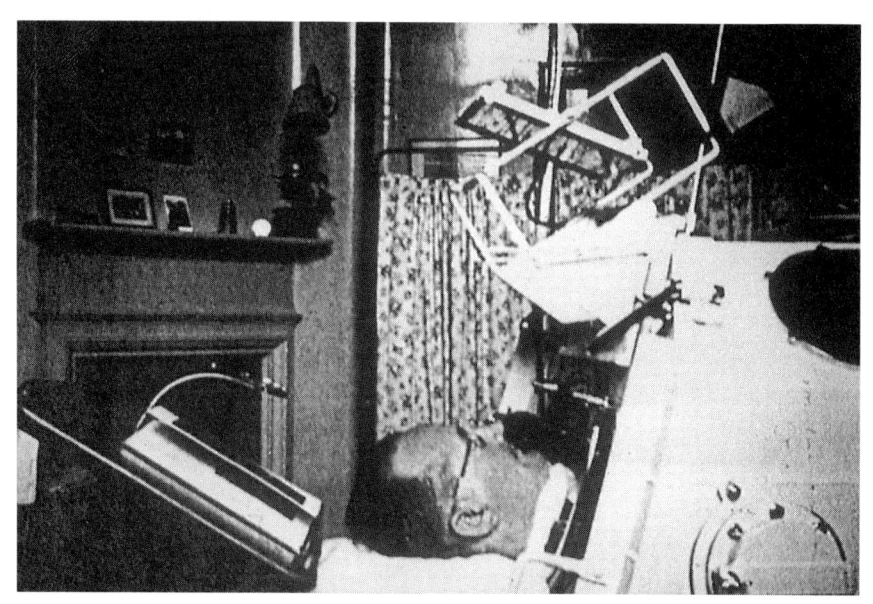

Poliomyelitis patient with respiratory paralysis in a Drinker cabinet respirator (iron lung) ca. 1947. (By courtesy of Miss J. K. Taylor)

Most affected were children between 5 and 15 years of age (38 per cent) and next those under 5 (36 per cent). Seven of the 19 deaths were in children under 5 years. General practitioners received a circular in mid-August covering the clinical features and offering consultations where the diagnosis was uncertain.

In 1947 Dr Joe's team admitted all of the 172 patients notified with poliomyelitis from the city and neighbouring countries. The hospital mortality was 12.20 per cent and many survivors were permanently crippled. The staff were severely stretched and often six of the seven cabinet respirators for treating respiratory paralysis were in use simultaneously. Four physiotherapists joined the establishment temporarily and the services of an orthopaedic surgeon and a neurologist were called upon. Dr Joe had correctly predicted in 1938 that 'in coming years this disease will make a regular contribution to our hospital admissions'. When he alluded to this forecast again in 1947[32] he was of course unaware that the Salk and later Sabin poliomyelitis vaccines would virtually eliminate the disease within the next decade.

Although there were only 44 patients with bacillary dysentery and six with enteric fever admitted in 1947, Dr Joe pointed out that 79 infants and children were admitted with gastroenteritis. The overall mortality rate of 16.45 per cent was even higher than that for cerebrospinal fever and poliomyelitis. Managing gastoenteritis was labour intensive and the average length of admission was 30 days. Ideally Dr Joe would have wished a unit with single-cot cubicles but, until that could be arranged, he set aside a ward purely for the treatment of infantile gastroenteritis. This may have been Ward 2A.[33]

The shortage of full-time nurses was partly compensated for by the employment of non-resident part-time nurses. Although some attended regularly, others did not and the staff wastage was high. As the part-timers were reluctant to nurse tuberculosis patients, an extra burden was placed on the full-time nurses. In 1947, 38 nurses completed training and 29 became State Registered Fever Nurses. Affiliation with Kirkcaldy Hospital and the County Hospital, Haddington, continued but there were no nurses from Galashiels. On 25 June 1947 at the Annual Prize Giving and Reunion the C. B. Ker Memorial Medal was presented by Dr John Ritchie, formerly a City Hospital Resident and later MOH for Dumfries, who spoke eloquently on the early days of the hospital.

In April 1947, the Catering Officer reorganised and increased the kitchen staff appointing male cooks and a male kitchen superintendent. Electric trolleys were introduced to deliver food quickly to the wards. In 1947 also an occupational therapist was appointed to provide diversional therapy such as toymaking, woodwork, rug making and embroidery.

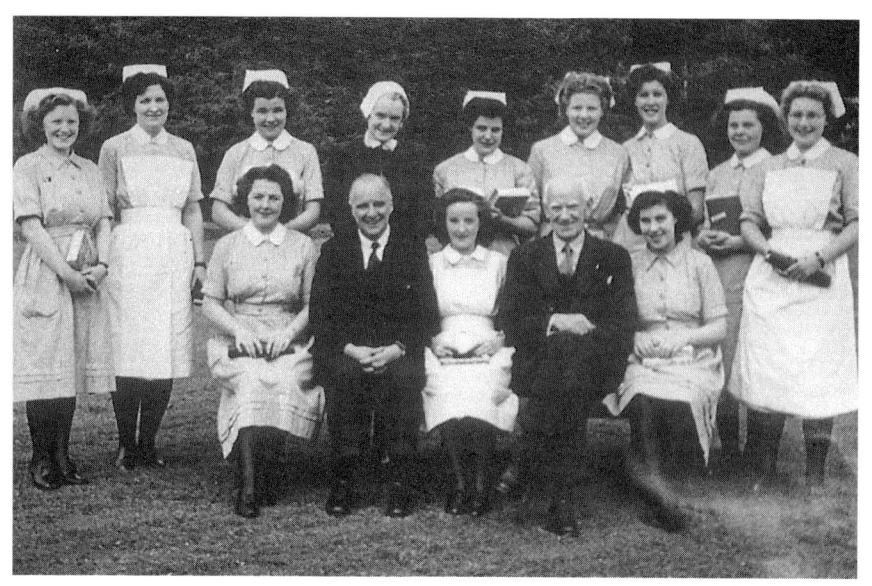

Nurses' Prize Giving, 1947 or 1948. Dr Alec Joe is at the left centre with Miss M. I. Adams, Matron, behind him. Dr W. G. Clark, MOH, is sitting at right centre. (By courtesy of Miss J. K. Taylor)

Library services for the patients also became available. Sadly Dr Joe could report no progress in 1947 with upgrading of the laboratory owing to difficulty with labour and materials.

The Medical Superintendent's Report for 1947 ended on a nostalgic note. With the National Health Service coming in the next year, it was the last offical Report he would make to the Medical Officer of Health. Dr Joe wrote:

> whatever may be the new arrangement for its management, it [the hospital] will require to work hand in glove with the medical officer of health in the future as in the past, and there is not likely to be the slightest disturbance in the close mutual collaboration which has always existed.[34]

Dr Joe thanked the Corporation and its Public Health Committee for their 'lively and almost paternal interest' over the years. He also thanked his Matron, Miss Adams, for her endeavours with nursing recruitment and Dr Margaret Main, his Senior Assistant, who had coped with the poliomyelitis outbreak in September 1947 when Dr Joe had been on annual leave.

At the end of 1947 no one really knew how the new National Health Service would work out. It signified major changes in the care of the sick and the prevention of disease. For the City Hospital it meant administrative separation from its parent body the City of Edinburgh Corporation which had nurtured it for nearly seventy years. Nonetheless it was essential that the links between the Public Health Department and the hospital should be maintained even though from 5 July 1948 the hospital would be administered by the South Eastern Regional Hospital Board (Scotland).

CHAPTER TWENTY-FOUR

The Early Years of the NHS; The Bacteriology Laboratory; Thoracic Surgery Unit; and the Half Centenary Celebrations

Despite his forebodings about the introduction of the National Health Service, Dr W. G. Clark, the MOH, wrote in his Annual Report for 1948 that in Edinburgh the actual transition took place smoothly and with no disturbance to hospital routine or to the local authority's remaining services.[1] Experienced administrative staff were shared between the Public Health Department and the new hospital boards of management. Indeed, during the first few months of the NHS some of the Corporation's officers helped the new boards on an agency basis.

Dr Clark reported that the city's infant mortality rate for 1948 had fallen dramatically from 49 to 34 per thousand births. Sadly there was a slight rise in the still-birth rate at 29 per thousand and 15 mothers died in childbirth compared with 12 in 1947. The death rate in the population from all causes was 12.2 per thousand, the lowest in the city's history. Only one of these deaths was from diphtheria (in an unimmunised child) among only 14 cases of diphtheria notified. This reflected the success of the immunisation campaigns.

Statistics for tuberculous were less satisfactory[2] and, although there were fewer deaths, the number of notifications increased from 1945 to 1948, probably as a result of the war. Dr Clark found it disturbing that the nursing shortage meant that there were insufficient staffed hospital beds in which to isolate tuberculous patients. More and more people were going voluntarily to the Mass Radiography Unit for chest x-rays and the number attending the city's dispensaries had doubled over the preceding eight years suggesting a greater public awareness and concern about tuberculosis. Dr Clark mentioned that a controlled trial of BCG vaccine would shortly take place. This had been thwarted many years earlier because of Sir Robert Philip's animosity with Calmette (see Chapter 19). Its introduction was delayed further by the outbreak of the Second World War in 1939. Notifications of non-pulmonary tuberculosis were steady in 1948 and there were fewer deaths from this form of the disease. Dr Clark hoped to increase the availability of tubercle-free milk and so improve these statistics even further.³

At the beginning of the NHS the seven Edinburgh hospitals previously administered by the Public Health Department came under the control of the South Eastern Regional Hospital Board (Scotland). These were the City Hospital, the Royal Victoria Hospital, the Eastern, Western and Northern General Hospitals, Bangour Hospital and Gogarburn Certified Institution. Overall these hospitals represented about 4,500 beds of which the City Hospital had 557. Below the Regional Hospital Boards were Boards of Management often taking charge of a group of hospitals. Thus the City Hospital now came directly under the Royal Victoria and Associated Hospitals Board of Management together with four other hospitals, the Royal Victoria Hospital, Southfield Sanatorium and the smaller hospitals at Loanhead and Newtonloan.

Agency services were provided for some time after the start of the NHS from previous authorities such as the Edinburgh Corporation, Midlothian County Council and the Tuberculosis Trust.⁴ There were, however, delays in providing Regional Advisers. Besides:

> Another major difficulty has been that the considerable financial independence which it was hoped would be granted to the Boards of Management has not been realised, and the time spent in preparing a 'case' for the Regional Health Board and the delay in getting approval has seriously impeded progress on many urgent projects, and the appointment of urgently required additional staff".⁵

Such sentiments remain familiar in the NHS today.

Dr Joe chose the inception of the NHS to write a synopsis of the history of the hospital entitled *Edinburgh City Hospital: A Noteworthy Enterprise of Fifty Years Ago*⁶ and he quoted extensively from the work of Bailie James Pollard.⁷ In his own report on the City Hospital Dr Joe wrote that 1948 was 'probably the most momentous year in the history of the City Hospital ...'⁸ on account of the arrival of the NHS and the changes in administrative control from local authority to health board.

Yet the functions of the hospital were not altered in any way. In fact Dr Joe's greatest concern in 1948 was the fall in the number of nurses in training from 114 to 84. Every effort was made to recruit more. It was hoped that the recently introduced Whitley Council Regulations for improved salaries and conditions of service would also help. To encourage prospective nurses to enter training in infectious diseases and tuberculosis, the three-year training period was cut to two, but even this failed to improve recruitment. Only thirty nurses completed training in 1948 of whom 26 passed the State Examination as fever nurses.

Kirkcaldy, Galashiels and Haddington continued to send nurses for fever training and, without the 11 extra nurses they provided, the City Hospital could barely have functioned. Twenty-two nurses went on to general training elsewhere and two left to become married. Nurse Jean Ewing was presented with the C. B. Ker Memorial Medal for 1948 by the MOH. This gesture of solidarity between the hospital and the Public Health Department confirmed that the connections so valuable before the NHS were still being fostered.

The nursing shortage occasionally made Dr Joe reluctant to admit patients with less serious forms of illness. Not every mild case could be accommodated. Fortunately in 1948 admissions fell to 2,651, of which 229 were tuberculous, and there were no major epidemics.[9] Scarlet fever accounted for most admissions (874 with 744 confirmed) followed by measles with 329 confirmed cases. Of 308 bacillary dysentery referrals only 182 were bacteriologically confirmed, 176 being due to *Shigella sonnei*. None died. Sadly there were 18 deaths among the 94 patients with unspecified forms of gastroenteritis (19.15 per cent mortality) who were accommodated in the new gastroenteritis ward.[10] Only 18 of the 187 suspected cases of diphtheria were confirmed and only one died. There were 30 confirmed cases of poliomyelitis with two deaths.

Fifteen confirmed cases of cerebro-spinal fever were admitted. Thanks to sulphonamides and penicillin, only one patient died. These drugs were also valuable in treating the otitis media and bronchopneumonia complicating measles. It was in fact a great time to try out each new antibacterial agent as it was discovered. Polymyxin, 'one of the more recent antibiotics', was used but without spectacular success in some of the 92 patients with confirmed whooping cough who were admitted during 1948.[11]

There were 191 tuberculosis beds at Colinton Mains in 1948. Ever since the National Health Insurance Act of 1911, 48 of these beds for male tuberculous patients had been situated in 'temporary structures', Wards 28 and 28A within the former Poor Law Institution at Craiglockhart. In 1911 they were taken over by the local authority and staffed by City Hospital doctors and nurses.

> For a variety of reasons the original wards continued in general use until the end of 1948, when additional accommodation was found for the patients in Ward 7 of the City Hospital. This belated change marked a great improvement in the ward facilities and amenities which was much appreciated by patients and staff alike.[12]

During 1948 Professor T. J. Mackie, the second holder of the University's Chair of Bacteriology, supervised the upgrading of the City Hospital's laboratory. This was put in the capable hands of Dr Archie T. Wallace who was to provide devoted service for many years. During 1948 the laboratory examined 6,260 specimens (which included 44 from autopsies).[13] Mr Jimmy Craig had been recruited as the City Hospital's Laboratory Assistant some time after the First World War.[14] He had possibly previously done laboratory work in one of the armed services. He coped single handed with a heavy workload for many years, supported by Edinburgh University Department of Bacteriology whilst under the nominal supervision of only one senior clinician. He collaborated with joint projects run by the university on aspects of scarlet fever and diphtheria so was associated both with Professor T. J. Mackie, Dr J. E. McCartney, and Dr Helen Wright of the university department and with Dr A. L. K. Rankin of the City Hospital. Jimmy Craig became responsible for all the scientific work of the laboratory until 1945 when, sadly, he developed tuberculosis and died shortly afterwards in Southfield Sanatorium.

During Dr W. T. Benson's Superintendentship, a part-time porter at the City Hospital, Mr William Webber, became friendly with Jimmy Craig and, with Dr Benson's permission, worked with him in the laboratory whilst continuing his portering duties. Mr Webber later rose to be the City Hospital Bacteriology Laboratory's Chief Medical Laboratory Scientific Officer. He gained the Fellowship of the Institute of Medical Laboratory Scientific Officers with a thesis on the sensitivity of tubercle bacilli to para-amino salicylic acid (PAS)[15] His cheerful smile, luxuriant wavy white hair, enthusiasm for organisation, and his keen participation in the Salvation Army will long be remembered.

Dr Archie Wallace (MB, ChB, Edinburgh, 1931) acquired the DPH in 1936. After general practice in Dingwall, he was Assistant Bacteriologist to the Royal Infirmary of Edinburgh and up to 1940 was Junior Tuberculosis Officer to the Edinburgh Public Health Department. During the war he served in the RAMC in Africa and Italy. After the war he became Lecturer and soon after Senior Lecturer in the University Department of Bacteriology. In 1948 was appointed as Bacteriologist to the City Hospital where he served faithfully until he retired in 1974.

Dr Wallace was awarded his MD degree in 1959 and was elected FRCPEd in 1979. He was meticulous, painstaking and totally devoted to his work. His expertise in the laboratory diagnosis of tuberculosis and in the sensitivity testing of tubercle bacilli to new chemo-therapeutic drugs, made him invaluable to Professor John Crofton's team with which he collaborated in the now famous studies of the 1950s. On leaving the City Hospital he worked for four years as Bacteriologist to the Libyan Tuberculosis Service.[16] Few who met Archie Wallace or who had the

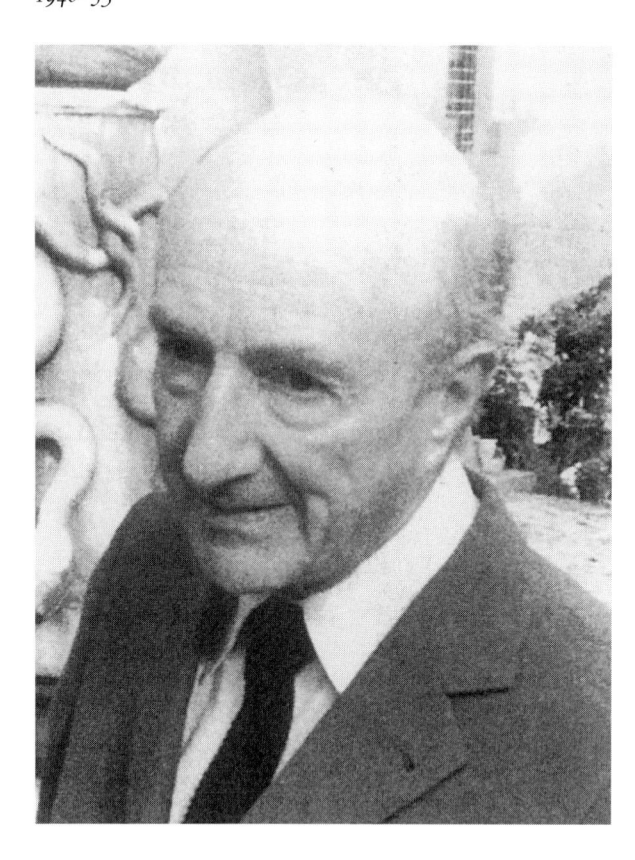

Dr Archie T. Wallace, Consultant Bacteriologist and expert in the laboratory diagnosis of tuberculosis. (By courtesy of Mr Charles J. Smith)

privilege of working with him could forget his modesty and almost saintly dedication to his work. He died in 1992 having spent his later years at Nunraw Abbey.

By the end of 1948 about half the hospital was equipped with cables to take alternating electric current.[17] and this allowed Dr D. H. Cummack to use the newly installed x-ray equipment in Cottage 13. Unfortunately even then it could not be fully utilised because of the staffing difficulties. Dr Cummack from the Western General Hospital (see Chapter 29) gave generously of his time to set up the City Hospital's X-ray Department.

Among the medical staff, Dr Margaret Main, who had coped so well during the poliomyelitis outbreak of 1947, resigned in July 1948. She was replaced as Senior Assistant Medical Officer by Dr George Sangster who became one of the City Hospital's much loved and respected physicians.

Dr Sangster had qualified MB, ChB, from the University of Aberdeen in 1937. Before the outbreak of war he became interested in the part played by certain strains of *Escherichia coli* in infantile gastroenteritis. This formed the basis of his thesis for the MD which was awarded in 1949.

His studies were interrupted, however, by the war and, like Drs Benson and Joe before him, he was commissioned Surgeon Lieutenant in the Royal Navy; he saw active service in the Dieppe Raid of August 1942. He later wrote papers on canicola fever, paratyphoid fever, mycoplasma infection, viral and bacterial meningitis as well as infantile gastroenteritis. He was later appointed Consultant Physician in Infectious Diseases, having previously held the title of Assistant Physician. In 1971, he was awarded the MRCPEd.

Short, prematurely bald and standing with his feet at 'a quarter to three', Dr Sangster was affectionately known as 'Wee George'. Although a reluctant lecturer, he was a patient and dedicated teacher at the bedside. Decades of nurses, medical students and doctors (including your author) benefited from the uncanny clinical and diagnostic skills he imparted, laced with a delightful, dry, couthy humour. His favourite phrases became part of the folklore of the Infectious Diseases Unit. A scraggy, malnourished, dehydrated infant would be commended to the paediatric Ward Sister as a 'wee bairn needing some intravenous mince and tatties'. He liked nothing more than to be in the wards especially when there was a difficult diagnostic problem. All too often he would confound everyone by proposing, correctly, some obscure diagnosis which not even the 'experts' had contemplated.

Dr Sangster loved to tinker with mechanical or electrical gadgets especially when any new monitoring equipment arrived on the ward. Before the tiny clinical laboratory across the corridor from Ward 15 was closed under Health and Safety at Work regulations, Dr Sangster would be in his element with the microscope examining blood films for malarial parasites or for the atypical monocytes of glandular fever. He loved to count white blood cells in cerebro-spinal fluid and search for meningococci, pneumococci and *Haemophilus influenzae*. He was so keen to view the 'enemy' as he termed the bacteria that he would often snatch specimens from tardy resident doctors and process them himself.

Dr Sangster served for many years as Honorary Secretary of the Hospital's Medical Staff Committee and Honorary Secretary of the Society for the Study of Infectious Disease. He also organised several highly successful Scottish-Scandinavian Conferences on Infectious Diseases.

In 1980, his last year as a Consultant, he was plagued by ill health but he rarely, if ever, allowed himself to be off sick. Typical of the man, he delayed what was to be a curative nephrectomy until a few days after he retired. His health restored, he tended his beloved garden and took his wife on holiday abroad. It seemed unjust that he should die of a cerebral tumour only months after retirement. He is still sadly missed.

In Dr Sangster's second year at the City Hospital, Dr W. G. Clark's Annual Report for 1949 [18] commented on 'another good year' with lots of warm sunshine, a lengthening of the span of life, falling rates for maternal and infant mortality, fewer notifications of scarlet fever and diphtheria and a 10 per cent reduction in deaths from tuberculosis despite the notification of 661 new cases.[19] Measles and scarlet fever appeared to be getting milder with only one death from measles (in 1,392 cases) and, for the fourth year running, none from scarlet fever (in 1,183 cases). Sadly six of the 760 patients notified with whooping cough died. Other major notifications were for dysentery (277), influenzal pneumonia (111) and poliomyelitis (27).

Under the new NHS regulations, certain boundaries were removed and 171 of the 2,713 admissions to the City Hospital in 1949 came from outside Edinburgh.[20] The numbers were augmented further by the closure of several small county fever hospitals. There were 161 cases of tuberculosis admitted. Of 930 suspected cases of scarlet fever the diagnosis was confirmed in 845. Although a milder disease than before, this was the largest number of scarlet fever admissions since 1944. Only seven cases of diphtheria were admitted, with no deaths. Cases of puerperal sepsis fell to 21, an all time low.

The greatest number of patients in the hospital on any one day in 1949 was 433 and the lowest 322 which was as well because of the continuing shortage of nurses. Kirkcaldy, Galashiels and Haddington were still providing nurses but this was the last year of the affiliation with these hospitals. Altogether 30 nurses completed training and 26 of them passed the State Examination to become Registered Fever Nurses. On 22 June 1949 Lady Fraser of the Nursing Committee of the South-Eastern Regional Hospital Board (Scotland) gave an address and presented the nurses' prizes. The C. B. Ker Memorial Medal was won by Nurse Alice Binning with Nurse Margaret Murdoch her runner-up.[21] In 1949 six sections comprising 261 medical students received a total of 90 hours of instruction. The DPH and other courses for postgraduate doctors and general practitioners also continued.

The X-ray Department was fully functional by 1 February 1949. During the year, 2,034 X-rays were carried out on tuberculous patients, 500 on fever patients and 400 on members of staff. In the teaching block at the north east of the hospital site, a spare room was fully equipped for the Bacteriology Laboratory, which opened in July 1949. Further enlargement and an animal house were envisaged as later developments.

In his Annual Report for 1950,[22] Dr W. G. Clark commented on the rise in notifications of infectious disease to 7,209, which was 2,153 more than in 1949 and the highest since 1945. Part of this increase was real because of an epidemic of measles in the spring and summer and part because the previously voluntary notification of whooping cough had became compulsory in 1950. There were then 1,768 cases of whooping cough of which 74 per cent were in children under five years of age. Three died. There was also an increase of dysentery with 551 notifications, the highest for six years. Sixty-nine cases of poliomyelitis were reported with six deaths, the greatest number since the epidemic of 1947. For the fifth year in succession there were no fatal cases of scarlet fever and for the second year in succession no diphtheria fatalities. The death rate for tuberculosis fell to 48 per 100,000 of the population, the lowest ever recorded for the city.[23] BCG vaccine was being used from March 1950 to protect tuberculosis contacts.[24]

In the spring of 1950 in response to a serious outbreak of smallpox in Glasgow, the Edinburgh Public Health Office carried out 1,386 vaccinations. 15,000 doses of lymph were distributed for use by hospitals and general practitioners. Eighteen contacts from SS *Chitral* which had imported the smallpox to Glasgow were kept under surveillance. Two who developed suspicious rashes were admitted to the City Hospital, but fortunately neither turned out to have smallpox.[25]

The increase in notifications of infection in 1950 was reflected in the admission figures for the City Hospital.[26] Including 152 cases of tuberculosis, the total annual admissions rose to 3,412, 699 more than in 1949. Of these, 649 came from catchment areas outside the city under the new NHS arrangements. Twenty-five service personnel were admitted. The daily average bed occupancy, including tuberculous patients, was 389 and the greatest number on any day was 445 (in February) and the lowest 342 (two days before Christmas).

Of 1,081 confirmed cases of scarlet fever admitted in 1950 there were no deaths. Dr Joe now attributed this as much to penicillin as to the diminution in the severity of the disease. Despite reducing the hospital stay from 28 to 21 days for patients with scarlet fever, there were few re-admissions. Only two cases among 115 suspects admitted had proven diphtheria and neither patient died. Similarly there were no deaths among 269 patients with a confirmed diagnosis of measles. As with scarlet fever, penicillin may have helped to reduce the mortality in measles when used for the bacterial complications such as otitis media and bronchopneumonia. Only nine of the 22 suspected cases of puerperal sepsis were confirmed and none died. Dr Joe called it 'a disappearing condition'. Of 89 confirmed cases of poliomyelitis, 57 were from Edinburgh and 32 from outside the city. The mortality was 6.74 per cent.

Nurse recruitment remained difficult in 1950, especially for the tuberculosis wards. Eighteen of the 22 nurses who achieved State Registration proceeded to general training elsewhere. Courses were held for the first time by the British Tuberculosis Association and five of the City Hospital Nurses passed the examination. At the nurses' Prize Giving and Reunion on 28 June, the Lady Provost presented the C. B. Ker Memorial Medal to Nurse Margaret Pringle. The runner-up was Nurse Agnes Balfour.[27]

Instruction of medical undergraduates continued with 90 hours of teaching provided for 235 students. Postgraduate courses were held for the DPH students and an advanced course in medicine for general practitioners.[28]

In 1951 Dr W. G. Clark reported that the notifications of infectious diseases in the city had fallen by 166 to 7,043 and, for the first time, no case of diphtheria was notified.[29] Measles and whooping cough together made up 4,394 of these notifications. Scarlet fever figures were reduced by more than half of those in 1950 to 451 cases. The number of poliomyelitis victims in the city dropped from 69 in 1950 to 41 in 1951. An outbreak of dysentery peaking in February and March accounted for 996 notifications.

The City Hospital admitted fewer patients in 1951 (2,802 compared with 3,412 in 1950) and 173 of these had tuberculosis.[30] The average bed occupancy was 340 patients. Eighty-six patients died, 38 from tuberculosis and 48 from fevers. There were no deaths from diphtheria (no confirmed cases), scarlet fever, measles, puerperal sepsis, enteric fever, erysipelas, rubella and mumps. Most surprisingly too, there were no deaths among the 22 confirmed cases of cerebro-spinal fever admitted, presumably because of the prompt use of penicillin. The fatality in the 177 confirmed whooping cough cases was 4.52 per cent. Four of the 58 confirmed cases of poliomyelitis died (mortality of 6.9 per cent). An emergency electric generator was installed in Ward 14 to supply the cabinet respirators in the event of a power cut.[31]

Although only two of the 478 confirmed dysentery patients admitted in 1951 died, the large number of dysentery patients and the prolonged admission they required, was affecting hospital staffing.[32] Dysentery patients tended to be asymptomatic in 7 to 10 days but often occupied a hospital bed for several weeks till clear of infection on bacteriological grounds. Both oral sulphonamides and streptomycin were tried on patients with bacillary dysentery with little apparent effect. Chloromycetin (chloramphenicol) and sulphonamides were given to babies with gastroenteritis and Dr Joe reported that both seemed to be beneficial.[33] Neither is advised today.

Nursing recruitment picked up slightly with 30 more nurses in training or in part-time employment than in 1950. There were still shortages on night duty and at weekends and the reliance on part-timers weakened the system and increased the risk of cross-infection.³⁴ Twenty-three nurses became State Registered Fever Nurses and two passed the examination for the Certificate of the British Tuberculosis Association. On 11 July 1951, Mrs Blair, Chair of the Nursing Committee of the Health Board, presented Nurse Janet Learmonth with the C. B. Ker Memorial Medal. Her runner-up was Nurse Janet Anderson.³⁵ Sadly nosocomial infections still affected the nurses, three being absent for long periods with pulmonary tuberculosis, and one each with pericarditis, pleurisy and 'rheumatism' (presumably acute rheumatic fever).

In October 1951, after the internal reconstruction of the adjacent joiner's shop, a major extension to the laboratory allowed it to handle more tuberculosis samples.³⁶ In all the laboratory processed 20,447 specimens from the City Hospital and 1,752 from the Royal Victoria Hospital.³⁷ The X-ray Department took 4,409 X-rays of which 2,486 were of tubercular patients. The physiotherapy department carried out 5,584 treatments on 156 patients, mainly concerned with poliomyelitis and tuberculosis victims.³⁸

As a 'result of the disappearance of the extra-mural school' only 188 medical students attended for the usual 90 hours of instruction in clinical infectious diseases. Eight postgraduates came on the DPH course whilst others attended the advanced course in medicine. The Professor of Tuberculosis, now Professor John Crofton, also used the tuberculosis wards for undergraduate teaching.

Between 1948 and 1951 considerable modernisation was carried out at the hospital.³⁹ Old equipment was replaced, stainless steel sinks installed and beds fitted with vi-spring mattresses. Improved bedside lockers and overbed tables were introduced. The slunges were modernised. Specialised medical and X-ray equipment was installed. It was hoped a new boiler house and laundry would be up and running by 1952.

With the imminent introduction of thoracic surgery, the new operating theatre in Cottage 11 ⁴⁰ was almost complete and also the upgrading of Wards 6 and 6A in which the surgical patients would be accommodated. Ward 12, another former observation cottage to the south east of Ward 7, was being converted into a recreation centre for tuberculous patients.⁴¹ Each of the tuberculosis wards was adopted by one of the Edinburgh churches so that there were regular visits by parishioners and the clergy.

A Group Catering Officer was appointed in 1951 with principal duties at the City Hospital. Better food and more interesting menus for patients and staff were soon introduced but low pay for the cooks was a deterrent to recruitment. New kitchen equipment, however, was provided and more electrically heated trolleys for delivering food to the wards.⁴²

The Scottish Branch of the Red Cross started running a trolley shop service with comforts for the patients. A committee was formed to run patients' concert parties and other entertainments.[43] Film shows were given for long-term patients during the winter. Television was still in its infancy but by 1952 the Infantile Paralysis Fellowship had generously supplied television sets for poliomyelitis patients.

By 1952 the Annual Report of the Public Health Department no longer contained a report on the City Hospital. Dr Clark, the MOH, bemoaned the loss of control of the infectious diseases and tuberculosis hospitals and the mass miniature-radiography service which were now the responsibility of the Regional Hospital Board. He did, however, comment on the good will and communications still existing between the different administrations.[44] In 1952 there were no deaths in Edinburgh from diphtheria, scarlet fever, typhoid, poliomyelitis, or whooping cough. Apart from tuberculosis, the incidence of notifiable infection was low. Scarlet fever now appeared a relatively mild illness. Of the 752 notified cases, 304 patients were nursed at home.[45]

The City Hospital admitted 3,050 patients in 1952, 244 of whom had tuberculosis.[46] Fever patients from outside the city numbered 466 and 32 came from the armed services. The average daily bed occupancy was 384 with a peak of 431 in November and a trough of 323 in early

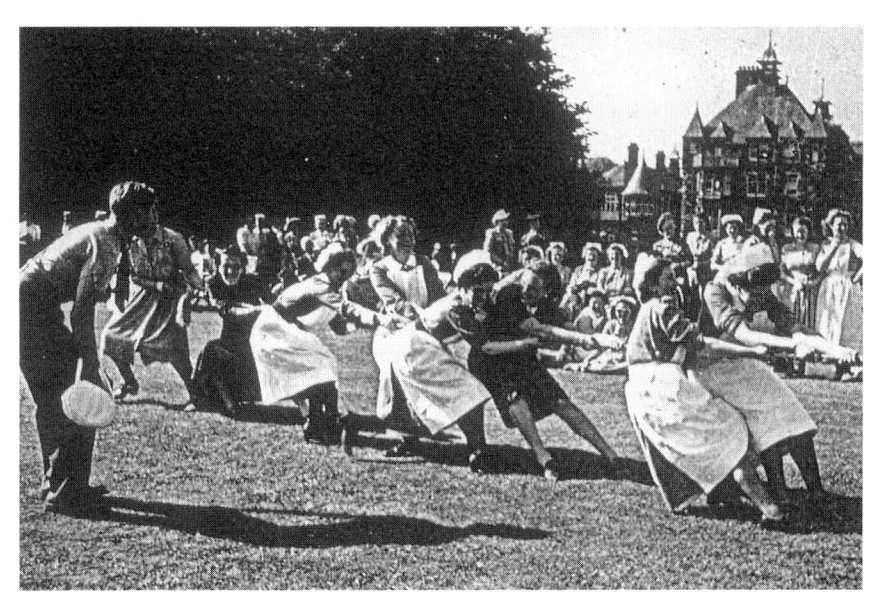

Senior sisters' tug o' war (against the doctors) ca. 1950s. The south west wing of the nurses' home is in the top right of the picture. (By courtesy of Miss J. K. Taylor)

January. Of the 68 deaths, 19 were from tuberculosis. The greatest number of confirmed cases of any disease was scarlet fever with 699 patients, followed by 419 with measles, 139 with chickenpox, 123 with rubella, 115 with infantile gastroenteritis and 112 with pneumonia. Many of the 186 suspected pneumonia cases were referred by Bed Bureau. Their mortality was 12.5 per cent. There were 30 confirmed cases of poliomyelitis from 64 suspected cases and a mortality of 6.67 per cent. Despite Dr Clark claiming no whooping cough deaths in 1952, Dr Joe did record one death out of the 74 confirmed patients admitted to the City Hospital,[47] but this patient may have been admitted from outside the city.

On 19 April 1952 a major new development began with opening of the thoracic theatre for the treatment of patients with surgically amenable pulmonary tuberculosis. By the end of the year Mr Andrew Logan and his team had carried out 152 major operations. This new theatre together with 43 beds in the reconstructed Pavilion 6 formed the Thoracic Surgical Unit. Wards 6 and 6A were divided into smaller rooms each containing between 2 and 5 beds and in Ward 19, previously empty, staffing was found in January 1952 for an additional 10 tuberculous patients. By the end of the year, Ward 19 housed 28 patients.[48]

Before the Thoracic Surgery Unit opened, City Hospital patients requiring operative treatment were transferred either to the Eastern General Hospital or the Royal Infirmary.[49] From 1952, however, there was a regular list of non-cardiac thoracic surgery cases at the City Hospital. Later cardiac surgery services were opened up by Mr Wade, Mr McCormack and Mr Walbaum who, with Mr Logan, formed an impressive team at the forefront of technical advances in their specialty.

Mr Andrew Logan, popularly known as 'Charlie Logan', graduated MA at the University of St Andrews in 1926 and then MB, ChB in 1929. Soon after he became a FRCSEd and FRCSEng. In 1964 he was elected FRCPEd. He served in the RAMC achieving the rank of Lieutenant Colonel and, in addition to being Consultant in Thoracic Surgery to the Regional Hospital Board, he was Consultant to the Army in Scotland, and Reader in Thoracic Surgery at the University of Edinburgh. A meticulous surgeon, he operated on patients with mitral stenosis, in which he became a leading expert, and on patients with oesophageal cancer besides carrying out more routine thoracic surgical procedures. He is a tall man, very much a 'Chief', and a disciplinarian with a wicked sense of humour. He acknowledges that he reputedly told a junior whom he was reprimanding 'It's not all your fault. I must take some blame for having appointed you!' Mr Logan retired from the City Hospital in 1972 but continued to operate in South Africa thereafter.

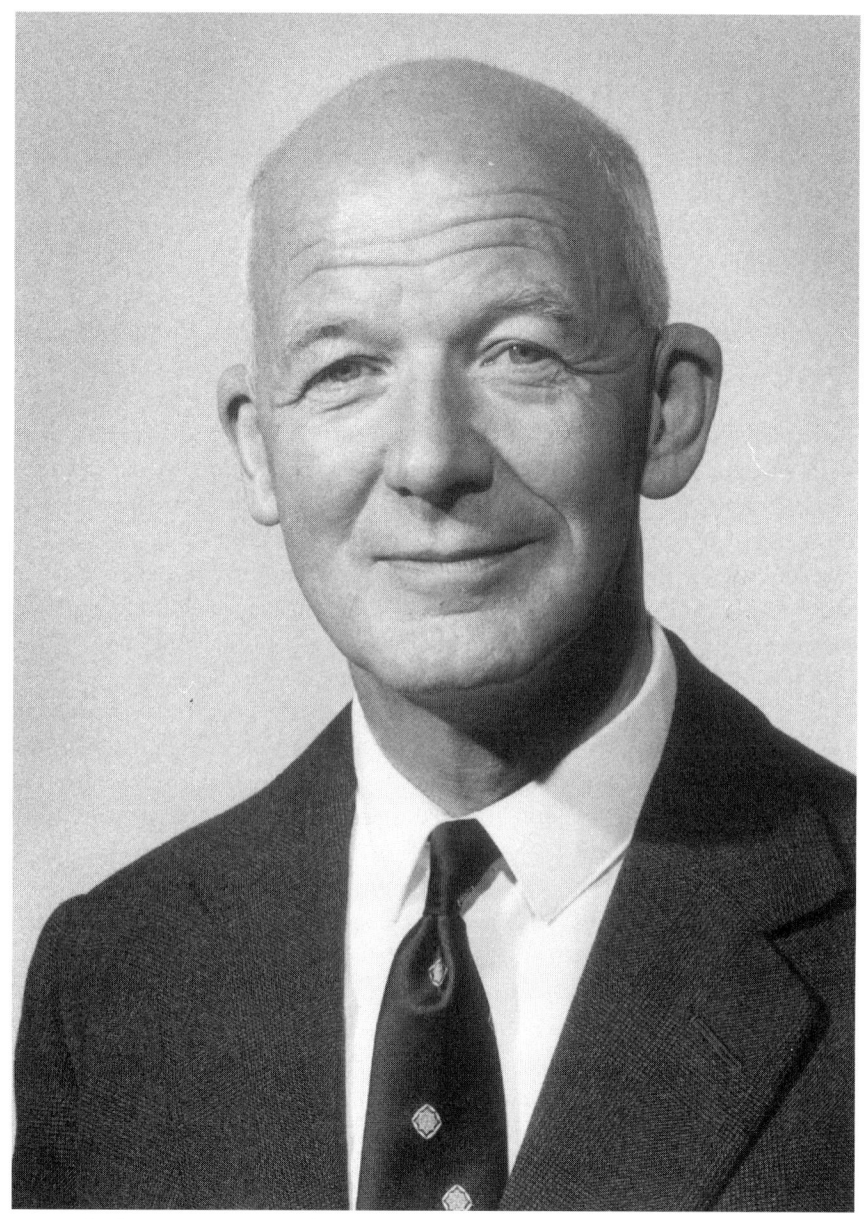

Mr Andrew Logan, Consultant Cardio-Thoracic Surgeon, about 1970. (By courtesy of Mr Andrew Logan. Photo: John K. Wilkie, by kind permission of Mrs Wilkie)

Mr R. J. M. McCormack, known as 'Bobbie McCormack', was another experienced member of the team. He was a flamboyant man in mood and dress, often sporting a pink spotted bow tie at a time when most medical men were still conservative in their attire. This marked him out as the controversial and colourful character that he was. By his own admission, he was often nervous before major surgery, but nonetheless he achieved highly successful results. He had graduated MB, ChB (Edinburgh) with honours in 1944 and later became FRCSE, FRCSEng, and FRCPEd. He had served in the RAMC overseas and, like Mr Logan, worked in both the Eastern General Hospital and Royal Infirmary before coming to the City Hospital.

In 1964 after visiting centres in the USA Mr McCormack requested funds for the introduction of cardiac bypass surgery.[50] This application would have been strongly supported after the highly experienced Dr Archie C. Milne, who came to the hospital in 1953, was made Consultant with administrative responsibility for anaesthetic services at the City Hospital in 1965.[51] Unfortunately in 1967 it was decided that only those cardiac patients who did not require bypass surgery would be operated on at the City Hospital, those who did being referred to the Royal Infirmary.[52] Mr McCormack served the City Hospital well on the Board of Management of the Royal Victoria and Associated Hospitals and, in succession to Dr N. W. Horne, he became Chairman of the City Hospital's Medical Staff Committee. He also initiated the idea of Friends of the City Hospital starting with a young volunteers group.[53]

Mr Philip Walbaum who became an experienced cardio-thoracic surgical Consultant to the South-Eastern Regional Hospital Board (Scotland), had, like Mr McCormack, graduated MB, ChB with honours in Edinburgh in 1944. He became a FRCSEd in 1948. Like some of his eminent predecessors at the City Hospital he had served as Surgeon Lieutenant, but this time in the RNVR.

Another thoracic surgeon with lists at the City Hospital was Mr J. D. Wade. He was a Cambridge graduate, MA and MB, BChir in 1939, and later FRCSEng and FRCSEd. He had been a Clinical and Research Fellow in Massachusetts General Hospital and was noted for his experimental work on high blood pressure. Like his colleagues Mr Logan, Mr McCormack and Mr Walbaum he also carried out cardiac surgery. Together they provided excellent service to patients in Edinburgh over many years.

At the request of the Regional Hospital Board 214 tonsillectomies were carried out at the City Hospital in 1951–52 in a bid to reduce the waiting list for ENT operations at the Royal Hospital for Sick Children.[54]

In addition, 10 scarlet fever patients of the City Hospital had tonsils and adenoids removed during convalescence.[55] This activity by the ENT surgeons signalled the start of their long association with the City Hospital where they were to take over Pavilions 2, 3 and 4 in 1965.

Nursing recruitment remained a problem in 1952. Although the total number of nurses rose by eight, and trained part-time nurses were increased from 24 to 42, there were only 60 student nurses in training at the end of 1952 compared with 70 in 1951.[56] The thoracic surgical theatre, the surgical tuberculosis beds in Pavilion 6 and the opening of Ward 19 for additional patients with respiratory tuberculosis, all increased the demand for nurses. This was especially so in the tuberculosis wards. Sadly not even:

> the combined effort made by the City Hospital Committee and the Presbytery, when a number of medical men and nurses spoke at church services, had little apparent effect in inducing suitable candidates to come forward.[57]

Nonetheless, 22 nurses completed training and passed the General Nursing Council's trial examination for admission to the fever part of the Register. Two general trained nurses were also admitted to the Fever Register and six obtained the Certificate of the British Tuberculosis Association. In all, 16 nurses went on to general training. At the nurses' Prize Giving and Reunion on 9 July 1952, Lady Mathers presented the C. B. Ker Memorial Medal to Student Nurse Denis Hand, the first male nurse to receive the award. Student Nurse C. MacKay was the runner-up.[58]

Although 1952 should have been a 'blank year' for the instruction of medical undergraduates because of the extension of the course from five to six years, 52 students attended for various reasons and received 30 hours of clinical teaching. Besides, 19 DPH students were taught at the City Hospital, and the Professor of Tuberculosis continued his teaching rounds in the tuberculosis wards.[59]

In 1952 the laboratory performed tests on 33,559 samples, the X-ray Department carried out 5,331 investigations and the physiotherapists gave 15,528 treatments to 228 patients.[60]

In the Annual Report of the Public Health Department for 1953, Dr H. E. Seiler, who succeeded Dr W. G. Clark as MOH, reported 6,647 notifications of infectious disease, an increase of 396 from 1952.[61] Part of this was due to the greater prevalence of bacillary dysentery which reflected the pattern throughout Scotland. Most cases were due to *Shigella sonnei* although there was an increase in *Shigella flexneri* cases too. There were 61 reports of poliomyelitis, most late on in the season. There was a big drop in the number of measles cases but a huge increase in whooping cough with 2,048 notifications, compared with only 782 in 1952; 258 were admitted to hospital and four died.[62] Of the 619, mainly mild, cases of scarlet fever, 236 were treated at home.[63] Dr Seiler commented on one of the five patients notified with typhoid fever, a service man from the Suez Canal Zone. He had been flown back to the UK where he developed overt typhoid fever, emphasising the rapidity with which infection could now spread by air travel.[64]

The City Hospital admitted 3,862 patients in 1953 (361 with tuberculosis), the highest annual admission figure since 1945.[65] The number admitted from outside the city boundary was 603 partly reflecting an increase in patients from West Lothian after the closure of Tippethill Hospital for infectious patients.[66] The average daily bed occupancy was 409 with a peak of 479 in late November and a trough of 362 in late August. Of the 74 deaths, 36 were in tuberculous patients and 38 in fever patients. One six year old, unimmunised girl died of diphtheria, having been admitted late on the fourth day of her symptoms. She was the only confirmed case of diphtheria in 1953, suggesting that the uptake of diphtheria vaccination was now high enough to keep a satisfactory herd immunity.[67]

Although Dr Joe[68] showed that 62 confirmed cases of poliomyelitis were admitted in 1953 with a mortality of 3.23 per cent, he recorded that in all, 85 cases were notified.[69] The outbreak began with a single case in June and slowly built up to a peak of 28 cases in October and 25 in November then fell to 8 cases in December. Overall there were slightly more than in 1952[70] suggesting incomplete immunisation in the community against poliomyelitis compared with diphtheria.

There were more part-time and full-time trained nurses in 1953 but still only 255 nurses altogether, the same as in 1952. Many were on short-term contracts and only 62 in training. Twenty-one completed their fever nurse programme and obtained State Registration before going on to general medical and surgical training elsewhere. Nine received the British Tuberculosis Association Certificate. On 7 July 1953 at the nurses' Prize Giving and Reunion, Lt Col A. D. Stewart, former Chairman of the Board, presented the prizes and delivered a highly original address 'describing and commenting on some outstanding scenes and experiences in his own life'.[71] On 16 September a study day, mainly concentrating on tuberculosis, was attended by 60 nurses from several hospitals, including the City Hospital.

Now in their fifth rather than their fouth year of training, because of the lengthening of the curriculum, 148 medical students attended the City Hospital and received the usual 90 hours of instruction. They were again divided into six sections. Thirteen postgraduates attended the DPH course. A refresher course was held for general practitioners and an Advanced Course in Internal Medicine for prospective hospital doctors.[72]

The work of the laboratory increased dramatically, 47,610 examinations being made in 1953. This largely comprised diagnostic tests for dysentery, salmonellosis and tuberculosis.[73] Sensitivity testing on tubercle bacilli for streptomycin, isoniazid and para-aminosalicylic acid formed an important part of Professor Crofton's onslaught on tuberculosis and increased the laboratory's workload.

The X-ray Department was also busy in 1953. X-rays on tuberculous patients, fever patients and staff came to total of 6,837 examinations. The workload of the physiotherapy department also increased with 19,155 treatments carried out on 363 patients of whom 266 had tuberculosis. In the surgical theatres, 240 major and 341 minor operations were performed and 784 minor procedures.[74]

There were delays in the conversion and equipping of the boiler house and laundry. It had been difficult to keep up sufficient steam pressure when changing from the old to the new laundry system so completion of Stage I would take until September 1954. The nurses' home needed complete modernisation as did the interior of the former servants' home. Shortage of married accommodation came about because the thoracic surgical registrar was obliged to be resident in the hospital at all times.[75]

Dr Joe was not someone who could allow an important anniversary to pass unnoticed. On 13 May 1953, exactly 50 years after the royal opening of the hospital by King Edward VII, Dr Joe arranged a Jubilee Thanksgiving Commemoration Service. It was held in the recreation hall of the nurses' home. Among those attending were Lord Provost James Miller and Lady Miller, Lord Mathers, Chairman of the Regional Hospital Board and Lady Mathers, Bailie Mossman, Chairman of the Board of Management and a large congregation including many who had been present at the Royal Opening Ceremony in 1903.[76]

The service was conducted by Rev. George D. Monro, MA, Church of Scotland Chaplain, and the Order of Service was typewritten on a single pink sheet.[77] With the Pentlands clearly visible through the large bay windows of the recreation hall, the service began appropriately with the singing of the metric version of Psalm 121 'I to the hills will lift mine eyes, from whence shall come mine aid …'. There were three hymns, two prayers, including the Lord's Prayer and a rendering of Beethoven's anthem 'Creation's Hymn'. The first of the two scripture readings was taken, from the Old Testament, Isaiah 61, v. 1–3, and the second from the New Testament, the Gospel according to St Mark 1,

v. 29–42 describing Christ's casting out of devils and the cleansing of the leper.

The focal point of the service was Dr Joe's address.[78] He first described the 1903 royal opening in detail, not even sparing his audience the account in *The Scotsman* of the lack of refreshments for spectators (see Chapter 16). Dr Joe then told the story of the development of the second City Hospital on the old Infirmary site and the final decision to build at Colinton Mains Farm, the strong influence of Dr C. B. Ker in the first 25 years and the increasing reputation the hospital gained under his guidance. Despite the enormous advances in the prevention and management of infections in the first half of the twentieth century, Dr Joe argued strongly for the retention of the fever hospital. There had been after all between 24 July and 3 December 1947 in Denmark 2,722 poliomyelitis patients admitted to the fever hospital in Copenhagen and as many as 70 victims at a time had required assisted ventilation. Dr Joe propounded:

> Only those who are satisfied that that cannot happen here are in a position to discount the necessity of the fever hospital ... Let us pause therefore and ponder well before we discard the fever hospital and what remains of its trained staff.

The subsequent problems of viral hepatitis, staphylococcal endocarditis and HIV infection from the 1970s onwards have gone a long way to justify his prophecy of 1953.

Dr Joe said he would have liked to have described all the advances of the last 50 years and compared and contrasted the infections at the turn of the century with the present situation and the modern wonder drugs available to treat them. He would have wished:

> to think back on the off duty pursuits of the staff in the early years when life began at Morningside Station at the horse tram terminus and compare with the present when the bus runs almost to our own door, and even the sisters possess their own private motor transport; or to wax nostalgic for the days when only fields intervened between the hospital and the Pentland slopes. Some day a chronicler may appear among us to relate all these things as well as the solid achievement in our special work.

In conclusion Dr Joe requested the congregation's 'earnest good wishes for the hospital as it goes forward to what lies ahead in the next fifty years'.

CHAPTER TWENTY-FIVE

1954–60: Changing Patterns of Disease

In his Annual Report for 1954, the MOH, Dr H. E. Seiler praised the good relations which had developed in connection with the prevention of tuberculosis because of the meetings held by Professor J. W. Crofton with other consultants in the city.[1] Dr Seiler also reported that, by mid-November 1954, 595 children had participated in a study requested by the Department of Health and supported by the Advisory Committee on Medical Research in Scotland. This 'Triple Antigen Investigation' was designed to assess the relative immunity conferred against whooping cough by a combined diphtheria, whooping cough and tetanus vaccine compared with whooping cough vaccine separately followed by a combined diphtheria and tetanus preparation. If successful, the triple antigen (which was later adopted and is now given at the same time as vaccines against poliomyelitis and *Haemophilus influenzae* type B) would reduce the number of injections needed. It was hoped that this would make primary immunisation procedures more acceptable and improve uptake.

There were 403 fewer notifications (6,244) in 1954 compared with 1953, fewer scarlet fever cases and no diphtheria cases, but a slight increase in the number of measles cases.[2] Of the 44 notified cases of poliomyelitis, all but three were probably acquired in the city. The 1,046 bacillary dysentery notifications were the highest ever. The figure could have been boosted by both improved diagnosis and references to the disease in the press, which encouraged more patients to seek medical advice. Most patients were only mildly unwell, but a few were seriously ill.[3] Whereas there had been 72 deaths from whooping cough in 1903, there were only 7 deaths in all from this disease between 1952 and 1954.[4] Compared with 1930 when there were 1,278 notifications of scarlet fever, with eight deaths, 1954 saw only 416 notifications and no mortality.[5] Dr Seiler commented on the incidence of *Salmonella typhimurium* food poisoning associated with office parties serving egg sandwiches. Imported Chinese liquid egg preparations were also implicated.[6]

The City Hospital admitted 3,763 patients in 1954, 427 with tuberculosis,[7] compared with 3,862 in 1953, representing a decrease of 99 admissions. Two thirds of the fever admissions came from the city itself rather than from outlying catchment areas. The daily average bed

CITY HOSPITAL   EDINBURGH 1954

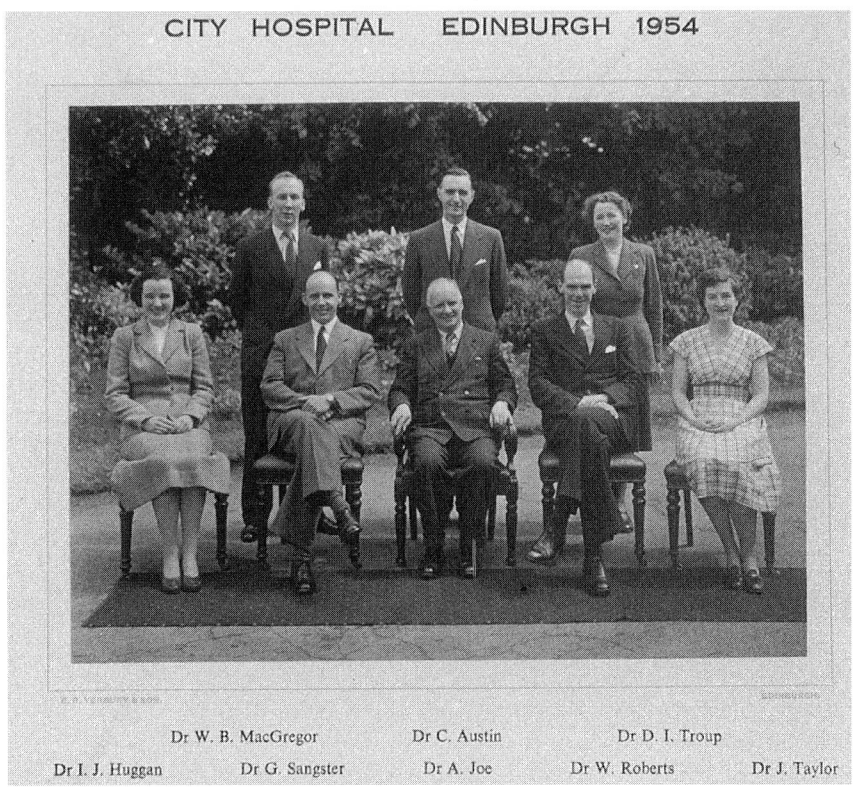

Dr W. B. MacGregor   Dr C. Austin   Dr D. I. Troup
Dr I. J. Huggan   Dr G. Sangster   Dr A. Joe   Dr W. Roberts   Dr J. Taylor

Dr Alec Joe, Dr George Sangster and medical staff, 1954 (Photo: E. R. Yerbury & Sons, Edinburgh, by kind permission)

occupancy was 409 compared with 408 in 1953. Of the 77 deaths, 33 were attributed to tuberculosis. The admissions for suspected scarlet fever rose to 857 patients, the highest since 1950, but only 771 of these were confirmed in hospital. There were 663 confirmed cases of bacillary dysentery and 150 of infantile gastroenteritis. Patients with gastroenteritis, together with the 88 confirmed cases of poliomyelitis and 63 patients with pneumonia, were far more labour intensive for the nurses than the numerically superior cases of scarlet fever. There were three deaths each from poliomyelitis and infantile gastroenteritis giving a respective mortality of 3.41 and 2.0 per cent. The other important illnesses in 1954 were measles and whooping cough with 368 and 162 patients respectively.

Dr Archie Wallace kept busy in the laboratory as the Royal Victoria Dispensary was also sending sputum samples for analysis and sensitivity testing of tubercle bacilli. Dr Wallace reported an increase of 13,000 examinations above the 1953 figure, bringing the total number to 60,615. The X-ray Department reported 8,036 examinations, of which 6,622 were for tuberculosis. The physiotherapists carried out 23,605 treatments and the surgical theatres carried out 311 major operations and 1,626 minor operations and procedures.[8]

Although the nursing complement rose to 267 in 1954, this was still unsatisfactory as many were untrained or part-time members of staff.[9] However, 24 student nurses completed their training and 18 passed the General Nursing Council's examination for inclusion in the fever part of the Register. Twenty-one went on to general training. Nine nurses were awarded the British Tuberculosis Association's Certificate. At the annual Prize Giving and Reunion, Lady Miller presented Student Nurse Anne Fairley with the C. B. Ker Memorial Medal. Her runner-up was Student Nurse Agnes Kirkwood.

Medical students were as usual divided into six sections; 162 students received 90 hours of clinical instruction. Twenty-three postgraduates attended the DPH course, and the refresher course for general practitioners continued.[10]

The fabric of the hospital was also improved in 1953. Pavilion 15 was reopened after reconstruction of the sanitary annexes and the formation of wooden partitions dividing most of it into one and two-bedded cubicles. New bed curtains increased privacy for patients and reduced work for the nurses moving mobile screens.

The laundry services and linen supply were reorganised with a view to central pooling of all linen issues and also in an attempt to reduce losses. Stage I of the laundry renovation took even longer than expected but it was hoped the new group system would be functioning on a modified scale by March or April 1955.[11]

Dr H. E. Seiler, the MOH, recorded only 4,179 notifications of infection in 1955, a dramatic drop with 2,065 fewer cases than in 1954.[12] Although there was less whooping cough and scarlet fever, there were still 1,034 cases of bacillary dysentery and 40 of poliomyelitis. Amongst 'new' diseases he reported a child with Weil's Disease and five piggery workers with canicola fever, another spirochaetal zoonosis. There were 1,053 cases of measles, counting only the first child in the household under the age of five years.[13] Passive protection with gamma globulin for infants at risk of measles was now available from the Health Department.

Dr Joe also recorded a dramatic fall in admissions to the City Hospital, there being 3,039 in 1955 compared with 3,763 in 1954 even though the number with tuberculosis rose to 453.[14] The average daily bed occupancy fell to 346. Of the 79 deaths, 51 were among fever patients and 28 among tuberculosis patients. For the first time in the history of the hospital there were no whooping cough deaths among the 66 confirmed cases admitted. Diarrhoeal illness accounted for most admissions with 555 confirmed cases of bacillary dysentery (357 *Shigella sonnei*, 197 *Shigella flexneri*, and one *Shigella newcastle*), 15 confirmed cases of enteric fever, 59 confirmed cases of salmonellosis (45 with *Salmonella typhimurium*) and, finally, 125 infants with gastroenteritis. This gave a grand total of 754 patients with bacteriologically confirmed diarrhoeal illness compared with only 362 cases of scarlet fever and 216 with measles.[15] The proportion of patients with these diagnoses was changing radically.

Of 136 admissions with suspected poliomyelitis only 55 were confirmed; two died. The Edinburgh Branch of the Infantile Paralysis Fellowship lent the hospital an elongated bath, based on the American Hubbard design, for use by adult patients with paralytic poliomyelitis.[16] This allowed the patient to 'swim' a few strokes whilst supported from a harness attached to a pulley suspended from rails in the ceiling. These ceiling rails could still be seen in a side room of Ward 16 until the 1990s although the tank beneath had long since gone.

Reconstruction work was completed in both Wards 7 and 7A, the patients moving in during November 1955. They seemed to appreciate the division of the two large open wards into three smaller more intimate ones.[17] The laundry pooling system was extended to cover more than half the items. Redecoration of the nurses' home was proceeding but there were no funds for better central heating, hot water supply and basins.

Another development in September 1955 was the introduction of the shop and Sub-Post Office controlled by the City Hospital Welfare Association. During their first two months they both proved to be welcome additions for the staff and patients.[18]

The number of nurses dropped from 167 in 1954 to 152 in 1955. The universal lack of recruitment to fever hospitals would soon lead to a shortage of senior trained fever nurses as well as probationers. Seventeen City Hospital nurses completed training and 15 passed the General Nursing Council's examination in fever training. Eleven went on to general training. Seven City Hospital nurses received the British Tuberculosis Association Certificate that year. On 7 July 1955, at the nurses' Prize-Giving and Reunion, Miss H. O. Robinson, OBE, Nursing Officer to the Department of Health for Scotland, presented the C. B. Ker Memorial Medal to Student Nurse Diana Thomson. Student Nurse Margaret Black was runner-up.[19]

The 142 medical students received the usual 90 hours of clinical instruction in infectious diseases. Eight postgraduates attended the DPH courses.[20]

Because of the fall in admissions in 1955, Dr Archie Wallace carried out only 53,807 examinations in the laboratory, 6,808 fewer than in 1954. The X-ray Department issued 7,565 reports and the thoracic surgeons recorded 291 major operations and 947 minor operations or procedures. The physiotherapists carried out 19,309 treatments on 495 patients.[21]

Following the fall of notifications of infection in 1955, the next year saw an epidemic of measles in the first six months and of whooping cough later in 1956.[22] Compared with 999 notifications of measles (first in the household under the age of 5 years) in 1955 there were 2,542 such notifications in 1956 with three deaths. Similarly, following the 624 cases of whooping cough in 1955, the MOH reported 1,731 cases in 1956, probably reflecting the natural fluctuation in incidence of whooping cough. There were 1,024 notifications of bacillary dysentery mostly among children although one elderly man with dysentery died. Of the 39 reports of poliomyelitis all but two were from Edinburgh itself. Fortunately 21 were non-paralytic.[23]

The City Hospital admitted 2,741 fever patients and 503 tuberculous patients in 1956,[24] an increase overall of 205 patients on the previous year. The average number of admissions between 1951–55 inclusive was 3,303. The daily bed occupancy was 335 with a maximum of 401 in early July and a minimum of 256 at the end of December 1956. There were 72 deaths in 1956, 43 fever patients and 29 with tuberculosis. The most commonly confirmed diagnoses were bacillary dysentery (493), measles (411), scarlet fever (246), whooping cough (215), chickenpox (127), and infantile gastroenteritis (109). As confirmed in Dr Seiler's Report for 1956,[25] poliomyelitis cases seemed less severe and Dr Joe only needed to use a respirator for one patient. The swimming tank used by paralysed patients was moved into the bigger side room of Ward 16.

Nursing staff numbers dropped further to a total of 114, 38 less than in 1955 and 53 less than in 1954. Most losses were among untrained, full-time staff. It seemed likely that the fever part of the General Nursing Council's Register would shortly close. In 1956 only 11 nurses completed training and passed the Fever Certificate examination. Two were given the Certificate of the British Tuberculosis Association. On 11 July 1956, Student Nurse Elner J.J. Pettitt was presented with the C.B. Ker Memorial Medal by Miss R.H. Pecker, OBE, RGN, who had been Registrar for the General Nursing Council (GNC) in Scotland for many years.[26]

The 140 medical students received the usual 90 hours of clinical instruction. Seventeen postgraduates attended the DPH course.[27]

The laboratory carried out 58,578 examinations, including 65 autopsies.

The X-ray Department performed 8,979 examinations, of which 7,430 were on tuberculous patients. The physiotherapists carried out 20,180 treatments on 542 patients and again most of these (283) were patients with tuberculosis. In the surgical theatres 307 major operations were carried out and 635 minor operations or procedures.[28] The demands for X-rays, physiotherapy and thoracic surgery reflect the intense activity generated by Professor John Crofton's crusade against tuberculosis.

On the fever side of the hospital, Dr Joe generously acknowledged the support that he received from Dr George Sangster, his Assistant Senior Medical Officer, and Miss M. I. Adams, the Matron, who retired at the end of September 1956 after nearly 21 years in office. Miss J. K. Taylor, the Assistant Matron, was promoted to Matron and held the post for the next four years.

By August 1956 the new laundry was sufficiently complete for work to be transferred from temporary premises. When Southfield Sanatorium moved its laundry to the City Hospital, all the hospitals in the Group were sending laundry to the central site. Negotiations were in progress to take laundry also from Rosslynlee Mental Hospital. Maintenance on rhone pipes continued with work completed on four ward blocks. Redecoration in the nurses' home was nearly finished but funds were still insufficient for services to be improved. The shop and Sub-Post Office reported a good first financial year.[29]

In 1957 Dr H. E. Seiler reported that the first limited supplies of poliomyelitis vaccine had been received in May the previous year. Immunisation was restricted to children born in the month of March in the years 1947–54[30] and 1,682 of them were vaccinated. By 1957 supplies of vaccine had increased and all children born between 1947 and 1954 were offered vaccination. To encourage uptake there was wide press coverage and letters were sent to the parents of school children. By late 1957 even the cohort of children born in 1955–56 could be covered. This vaccine was the less acceptable Salk killed vaccine given by three injections rather than the Sabin oral 'sugar-lump' live vaccine which succeeded it. Dr Seiler reported only seven cases of poliomyelitis from the city of Edinburgh in 1957,[31] but this probably reflected a non-epidemic year for poliomyelitis, rather than an early effect of vaccination.

Altogether in 1957 there were 5,395 notifications of infectious disease (including 468 with tuberculosis) compared with a total of 7,386 in 1956. There were fewer notifications of measles and whooping cough and both the illnesses were less severe. Dr Seiler commented, however, on the worrying increase in food poisoning although notifications of bacillary dysentery showed a fall. Infectious hepatitis (mostly what would now be called type A) was an important cause of morbidity in schools but, as the disease was not at that time notifiable, no figures are available.[32] Both this and the continuing problems of gastroenteritis prompted a campaign to improve school hygiene.

The other major disease of 1957 was influenza type A. It began in early September and reached a peak over the next two months; 60 per cent of school children were affected but adults were the most ill and 58 deaths were recorded.[33] The impact of influenza admissions to the City Hospital in 1957 was to hasten the change of function of some of the tuberculosis wards to the care of non-tuberculous chest diseases. Overall there were 2,970 admissions to the City Hospital in 1957 and 186 of these had non-tuberculous respiratory illnesses and 435 medical or surgical tuberculosis. There were, therefore, many fewer fever patients in 1957 (2,275 compared with 2,741 in 1956).[34]

The 74 admissions so far unaccounted for in the figures for 1957 represent the elderly patients taken into Pavilion 19, the function of which had changed to become the first Geriatric Medicine Unit in the City Hospital. Special mechanical hoists were installed for lifting the elderly patients.[35] The 36 nominal beds were opened in February 1957. Elderly patients in this unit accounted for 20 of the 102 deaths in the hospital in 1957.

The most frequent diagnoses among fever patients in 1957 were bacillary dysentery (330), measles (216), infantile gastroenteritis (147), whooping cough (140), scarlet fever (133, the lowest figure for 30 years), rubella (124), and pneumonia (108). There were no confirmed cases of diphtheria and no deaths among the patients with measles, whooping cough, scarlet fever, erysipelas, enteric and puerperal fever. There was one death among the 26 patients with cerebro-spinal fever and one among the nine with poliomyelitis. Although active immunisation against poliomyelitis was available that year, it may have been too early for it to be totally effective. Among 'newer' diseases, 58 cases of aseptic meningitis were admitted, the outbreak starting with three nurses from a children's home. All made a complete recovery. Although no virus was isolated, Dr Joe suspected an ECHO viral infection.[36]

Nurse staffing levels fell by eleven among the full-time untrained staff. Twelve nurses completed training and gained the GNC certificate as fever nurses. Two passed the examination of the British Tuberculosis Association. At the Garden Fete, which replaced the nurses' Prize Giving and Reunion, the sum of £257 was raised for the Benevolent Fund for Nurses and for staff amenities. The C. B. Ker Memorial Medal was not presented, perhaps because of the alterations in the pattern of nurse education. A combined training programme with the Royal Infirmary was sanctioned by the GNC. Candidates would train at the City Hospital up to their preliminary examination then transfer to the Royal Infirmary to complete their training for the general part of the Register. Besides, student nurses were to start in the Preliminary Training School at Carlton House, Carlton Terrace, under the auspices of the Southern Hospital Board of Management. Despite advertisements, recruitment of senior nursing staff to the City Hospital was so difficult that no one applied for the post of Sister Tutor. Some of the staffing gaps at training level were to be filled by seconding eight nurses from the Western General Hospital and three from Leith Hospital. Even then the nursing complement remained worryingly low.

Medical student training continued as before with 155 attending in 1957. Twenty-one postgraduates came on the DPH course. The laboratory processed 60,380 specimens the X-ray Department took 7,530 plates (5,563 on tuberculous patients). The physiotherapy department recorded 12,370 treatments on 357 patients. The surgeons carried out 179 major operations and 316 minor operations and procedures.[37]

Apart from the conversion of Wards 19 and 19A for use by elderly patients, it was hoped that some of the tuberculosis wards could be upgraded but there were insufficient funds to proceed. Wards 18 and 18A were to be converted over the winter. At least two thirds of the hospital were now powered by alternating current rather than by direct current. About half of the hospital's rhones and lightning conductors had been overhauled. Road resurfacing, last done in 1948, was hampered by underfunding, only £2,000 of the necessary £8,200 being allocated.[38]

By 1957 the City Hospital laundry took washing from all the hospitals in the group, also from Rosslynlee, Longmore and Liberton Hospitals and more recently from the Northen General Hospital as well. The weekly throughput was about 25,000 articles. An allocation of £14,500 for new machinery would push up the throughput to 40,000–50,000 articles weekly and, when the final equipment was installed between November 1957 and January 1958, a throughput of 50,000–60,000 items per week was expected.[39] Centralisation of laundry services was obviously economic, but it did cause major concern in the 1960s and 1970s when ageing equipment required repair or replacement.

In his Annual Report for 1958,[40] Dr Seiler recorded a drop in the notifications of infectious diseases to 4,899 compared with 5,395 in 1957. Much of the infection was due to measles (1,753) and dysentery (1,041) and the number of scarlet fever notifications had gone up by 129 to 277. Two outbreaks of salmonella food poisoning totalling 62 cases were tracked down to infected milk and South African frozen egg products respectively. There had also been a smallpox scare when a lascar seaman disembarking from the liner *Circassia* in Liverpool was reported to have the disease. This served as a reminder to encourage maximum uptake of smallpox vaccination in the city.

The city's health programme in 1958 concentrated on the highly successful mass X-ray campaign which included 308,747 citizens, 84.4 per cent of the population over the age of 14 years. During the campaign 424 cases of tuberculosis were discovered, mostly in men aged over 60.[41] Much of the planning and coordination of the campaign, a combined effort between Professor John Crofton's team at the City Hospital and City's Public Health Department, was carried out by Dr (later Professor) James Williamson and Mr Alec Welstead, the highly efficient Group Secretary to the Edinburgh Royal Victoria and Associated Hospitals Board of Management since 1952.

The Annual Report of the City Hospital for 1958,[42] recorded 3,977 admissions. The average annual number of admissions had been 3,709 (1943–47), 2,928 (1948–52) and 3,324 (1953–57); so Dr Joe could argue that beds for infectious diseases were still essential. Of those admitted in 1958, 2,662 were fever patients, 417 had tuberculosis (medical or surgical) and 42 were geriatric. During the reconstruction of the ENT Department at the Eastern General Hospital 234 beds had been lent by the City Hospital – and may, incidentally, have boosted the annual admission figures. Of the 161 patients who died in 1958, 42 were fever patients, 26 were tuberculous and 68 were non-tuberculous respiratory disease patients; 25 died in the geriatric wards.

Most of the fever patients in 1958 were suffering from bacillary dysentery (396), measles (357), scarlet fever (222) and infantile gastroenteritis (208).[43] Antibacterials were then popular in the management of bacillary dysentery, most of which was due to *Shigella sonnei*. Of the 354 patients treated with oral streptomycin, 343 (96 per cent) were bacteriologically cleared with one course. Other oral drugs including neomycin, chlorhydroxyquinolone and tetracycline were tried, but oral streptomycin proved the most satisfactory.[44] Doubtless the chest doctors, adhering strictly to the triple therapy which included injectable streptomycin for treating tuberculosis, must have been alarmed by their colleagues on the infectious diseases wards using oral streptomycin on its own. The risk of spreading resistance to tubercle bacilli was ever-present.

Antibiotics do not appear to have been employed at that time in the management of infantile gastroenteritis. The causative organism was found in 75 of the 208 patients. Of these, 29 had *E. coli* stereotype 026, 25 had type 0111, 19 had type 055 and there was one patient each with types 0119 and 0128.[45] The now notorious *E. coli* 0157 was not among the isolates in 1958. Dr Sangster, who had written his MD thesis for Aberdeen University on infantile gastroenteritis, did most of this research.

In 1958 the nursing staff numbered 266 in all, boosted by 61 nurses from the Western General Hospital and 15 from Leith Hospital. There were 27 nurses in training for fevers. Only one of three nurses who sat the British Tuberculosis Association examination was successful.[46] Eleven nurses passed the fever component of the GNC examination and eight of these proceeded to general training.[47] Such was the continuing understaffing, however, that the Report went on to state:

> Any future developments in the function of the hospital will depend on a successful solution of the nursing problem, and all thinking in such developments must take the provision of an effective nursing service as its starting point.[48]

During 1958 160 medical undergraduates were taught and 15 postgraduates attended the DPH course. The laboratory's workload increased to 73,694 examinations in 1958. The X-ray Department carried out 8,014 examinations, 6,881 of which were for tuberculosis. The physiotherapists treated 688 patients delivering a total of 17,028 treatments. There were 291 major operations and 817 minor procedures carried out in the surgical theatres.[49]

Improvements to the fabric of the hospital continued in 1958. At the cost of £22,000 Pavilion 16 was to be renovated to accommodate 34 patients mostly in single cubicles between the two wards. A further £2,000 was granted for the upkeep of the roads, but the money arrived late in the year when the weather was bad so progress was slow. Further work was done on the rhones and down spouts some being described as 'paper thin'.[50] They were after all about 55 years old.

The hospital laundry was excelling itself and further developments in 1958 allowed it to process 65,000 articles weekly. Despite early teething troubles, by the end of September, 1958, the cost per item fell from 3.1d to 2.5d and it was hoped that even this could be improved upon.[51]

A much needed improvement in the hospital's telephone system was envisaged by the General Purposes Committee of the Board of Management at its meeting on 6 October 1958.[52] It proposed two switchboards with 75 extensions and five outside lines at an estimated cost of £130 to instal and £278 per annum to run.

A meeting of the Board of Management on 20 August 1958[53] discussed a demand by the Edinburgh Corporation to close the hospital's west gate. The Corporation was then building the new secondary school at Firrhill and wished the west gate closed. They asked the hospital authorities to fund part of the cost of the roadway along the old field from Oxgangs Road North. In the interests of patients, staff and ambulances, the Board of Management resolved strongly to resist this pressure. A year later the Corporation had agreed to form a pedestrian footpath bordering the frontage of the school on the west access roadway to the hospital. Vehicles were to use a new roadway to be laid along the west perimeter fence of the school from Oxgangs Road North.[54]

The Annual Report of the Public Health Department for 1959[55] showed 986 fewer notifications of infectious disease compared with 1958. Excluding 331 cases of tuberculosis, Dr Seiler reported 3,582 infections. Measles (1,257), dysentery (731) and an increased number of whooping cough cases (600) formed the bulk of these notifications. No poliomyelitis was reported and, for the third year running, no notification of diphtheria. Surprisingly there were still 255 notifications of scarlet fever. Perhaps in response to the recently introduced Food Hygiene (Scotland) Regulations there was a decline in the number of food poisoning incidents.

Exciting changes were taking place at the City Hospital.[56] In May and June 1959, the Tuberculosis and Respiratory Diseases Unit under Professor Crofton moved to the City Hospital from Southfield Hospital which thereafter was to house geriatric patients. The Southfield Hospital Research Laboratory moved into Ward 4 at the City Hospital and continued working on respiratory pathogens including mycoplasma and viruses. Alteration of accommodation, purchase and transfer of equipment together cost £1,500. Funding from the Wellcome Trust would later make Ward 4A into a prestigious research laboratory continuing the work on respiratory pathogens. Later it would also fulfil a similar research and service role as the Regional Virus Laboratory. Work on the conversion was scheduled to start early in 1960.

The new X-ray Department, medical out-patients department and the offices for the Professorial Unit would be housed in the former servants' home (New Medical Block) which had almost become obsolete with the run down in resident domestic staff.[57] The site of the X-ray Department, formerly in the upgraded observation Cottage 13, would be converted into a new pharmacy. It would be adjacent to a new Steward's main store which would be moved across the roadway from its original site north of the kitchens. Funds were allocated for this work which was to start by 31 March 1960.

On the infectious diseases corridor, work had been completed on the new cubicles in Pavilion 16. It was opened on 10 November 1959 by Lady Mathers, wife of the Chairman of the Regional Hospital Board, with various official guests attending.[58]

The City Hospital laundry was processing between 58,000 and 72,000 articles weekly at 2.5d per item. Considerable expenditure was made on repairs and maintenance. The hospital roads cost £2,000. It was hoped that an annual allocation would be given to prevent the state of disrepair that had needed so much correction in 1956. A further £2,000 was spent on repairs to all the rhones except those in the former servants' home, Ward 3 and the animal house. Despite the neglect over 60 years, very little rot was found in these buildings. In the mortuary, however, £1,000 worth of repairs was needed to combat quite serious dry rot.[59]

In anticipation of his retirement the next year, Dr Joe announced that he wished to terminate the lease on the Medical Superintendent's house, having decided to buy a new home in the vicinity.[60] He was the last Superintendent to live in the house, which later became the offices of the Board of Management.

In his Annual Report for 1960[61] Dr Seiler commented on the increase in notifications of infection to 5,303 (4,994 excluding tuberculosis). Much of this was due to more measles and whooping cough. Scarlet fever notifications numbered 243 and erysipelas 51, both showing small reductions on the 1959 figures. Only one case of poliomyelitis was notified and again no diphtheria recorded. Bacillary dysentery, however, continued to be prevalent with 643 notifications, all but 13 of which were due to *Shigella sonnei*.

In March 1960 Dr Alec Joe, Medical Superintendent of the hospital and general physician in the infectious diseases wards retired after 23 years of service to the hospital. His Superintendentship was taken over by a consultant in chest medicine, Dr N. W. Horne who changed the title to Physician Superintendent. Dr Joe's clinical duties in infectious diseases became the responsibility of a new Consultant, Dr J. McC. Murdoch.

Dr Joe did not live long to enjoy his well-earned retirement. He died suddenly on 25 November 1962 leaving a widow and a daughter. Few clinicians had more experience of the transition from the infectious diseases so prevalent when he took up his appointment in 1937 to the relative calm of 1960. In 1937 his team had managed 614 patients with diphtheria of whom 37 died and 1,432 with scarlet fever of whom 9 died. In 1960 there had not been a single confirmed case of diphtheria admitted to the City Hospital for the previous seven years and the number of notifications of scarlet fever in the whole of Edinburgh had fallen to 243.

Dr Joe had carried out research with the newly introduced sulphonamides and later penicillin noticing their dramatic effect on patients with scarlet fever, erysipelas and meningococcal meningitis. He had coordinated the in-patient care for the victims of the last outbreak of smallpox in Edinburgh in 1942. With increasing difficulty due to the lack of nursing staff, he coped with the problems affecting the hospital during the Second World War and the subsequent outbreaks of poliomyelitis, dysentery and infantile gastroenteritis, all diseases requiring intensive nursing care.

Dr Joe always championed the status of the fever hospital and was reluctant to give up any ward accommodation for administrative purposes. As late as March 1959 he objected to the double side room in Ward 17A being used by the Superintendent Engineer as an office. He pointed out that, of the eight cottages available for emergency accommodation, five had already been utilised by the administration, two being used temporarily as offices by the Board of Management.[62]

Dr Joe will perhaps be best remembered for his love of the hospital he served, his teaching ability and the mutual affection that he and his staff had for one another. He:

> always enjoyed what he called a 'cerebral holiday' at a hospital party or with a few cronies at Simpsons in the Strand or the old University Club in Edinburgh.[63]

After he retired:

> The way in which his old seniors and residents at the 'City' never failed to keep in touch with their old chief was an earnest [mark] of the respect in which they held him.[64]

The author of an addendum to his obituary in 1962, who was possibly Professor Robert Cruickshank, wrote:

> He was of a vintage of fevers men of whom few others are now left, and many hundreds of his students and staff will cherish fond memories of him as teacher and colleague.[65]

PART SIX

Dr N. W. Horne's Superintendentship 1960–74, Two Decades of Change, 1974–94, and the Closure

CHAPTER TWENTY-SIX

1960–74: The Building Boom Years; Infectious Diseases, Pyelonephritis, and Tropical Medicine

Changes in Administration

On 14 July 1959, Dr D. M. Alston and Mr Alec G. Welstead, respectively the Chairman and the Group Secretary and Treasurer of the Board of Management of the Edinburgh Royal Victoria and Associated Hospitals, met with representatives of the Regional Hospital Board, the University of Edinburgh, the Public Health Authority and their own Board of Management to discuss the future of the City Hospital. Dr Joe was due to retire in December 1959 but in fact did not leave until the end of March 1960 as he was granted a three month extension of service until his successor arrived.[1] There was general agreement that the remit of the infectious diseases wards should be widened to include all aspects of infection such as the problem at that time of hospital staphylococci. The holder of the new consultant post in infection was to be responsible for administering his own wards but should not necessarily be the medical administrator of the whole hospital.

At the meeting of the Board of Management on 21 October 1959[2] it was resolved that one of the chest physicians, whilst retaining most of his clinical work, should take over the medical administration of the hospital. He should, however, be relieved of the lay aspects of administration either by the appointment of a Hospital Secretary or by strengthening the staff of the Group Secretary and Treasurer so that his team could take over that work. In making this appointment of Physician Superintendent, the Board was to take into consideration the recommendations of the City Hospital's consultants. The Board expected some difficulty in delineating the exact responsibilities of the Physician Superintendent and the Hospital Secretary, but insisted that a distinction must be drawn.

Despite some dissent, the Board decided to write to each of the consultants at the City Hospital asking them to recommend a Physician Superintendent.[3] At the same time the Board asked Drs Alston and Seiler to represent its views on the committee appointing the new Consultant Physician for the infectious diseases wards. By 16 December 1959, the

Board heard that the infectious diseases consultant post had been offered to Dr James McCash Murdoch who would take up his duties on 1 April 1960.[4]

On 20 January 1960, the Board agreed that the new Physician Superintendent should administer the whole hospital, including the infectious diseases wards.[5] By 16 March 1960, a fortnight before Dr Joe was to leave, the Board announced that the medical administration of the whole hospital would be under the care of the chest consultant, Dr Norman W. Horne, who would become the new Physician Superintendent.[6]

The Board of Management decided to move its offices from Cottages 23 and 24 into the spacious surroundings of the recently vacated house of the Medical Superintendent at the west of the hospital's main gate. Unfortunately, because of the blocking of a ventilation space in the house early in the century,[7] some dry rot had invaded. Until this was rectified, the Board's Offices could not move from Cottages 23 and 24. This in turn delayed the transfer of Dr Murdoch's original offices from the side rooms of Ward 17 into Cottage 23, but the moves were eventually all completed satisfactorily.

The Building Boom

The period of Dr Horne's Superintendentship (1960–74) ushered in an era of intense building activity for the hospital. Most of the buff coloured brick buildings were erected during this time and some old buildings were refurbished and put to new uses. Over the course of a few years the hospital was to have the Wellcome Research Trust Virus Laboratory constructed in Pavilion 4, and a New Medical Block formed out of the original servants' home and containing the X-ray Department, an outpatient clinic, a small respiratory physiology laboratory, chemistry laboratory, medical offices and a centralised medical records room. A pyelonephitis unit was established in Pavilion 14. The Board's offices were expanded within the former Medical Superintendent's house. Pavilions 8 and 15 were refurbished, the latter with cubicles for infectious diseases patients. The City Hospital laundry took over washing from the Western General Hospital and, after enlargement and updating, could cope with a throughput of 80,000 items weekly. Much needed repairs and improvements were made to the hospital roads, exterior lighting, covered ways and underground ducts.[8]

In 1963 the Tropical Medicine Unit moved from the Eastern General Hospital to the City Hospital which was to be its home for the next nine years. With fewer nurses and domestics living in the hospital and with the alteration in use of the former servants' home, more changing room accommodation was needed. A new brick building was therefore constructed east of the main gate and south of the former porter's lodge. It opened in 1964 as the much welcomed non-resident staff changing block.

In 1965 the in-patient facilities for the Ear, Nose and Throat Department opened in Pavilions 2, 3 and 4 which had been completely remodelled to provide three operating theatres and 93 beds. Apart from some beds and cots in the Royal Hospital for Sick Children, the City Hospital then provided for the bulk of ENT surgery in Edinburgh.

The new medical residency on the tennis court of the former Medical Superintendent's home was almost complete in 1965 but not occupied until 1966. Its 36 study bedrooms accommodated the living-in medical students and the junior doctors. A new brick-built pharmacy, pharmacy store and general stores building was in use by 1967 on the site of Cottage 13 which had temporarily housed the X-ray Department before its move to the New Medical Block. The space occupied by the former Steward's store and dispensary to the south of the original administrative offices was later used for the hospital shop, Sub-Post Office and a part-time branch of the Bank of Scotland. The remainder of the central site block (the former kitchens and dining rooms) became accommodation for the departments of physiotherapy and occupational therapy. A much needed 150-seat lecture theatre was also created. By 1971, the new kitchens and communal dining room to the west of Pavilion 2 had come into use. Instead of the doctors eating separately, all staff would eventually take meals together in the large, open-plan dining room.

By 1974, much of Pavilions 18 and 19 had been upgraded for the proposed Burns and Plastic Surgery Unit which was to have come to the City Hospital but which eventually never did. With modifications, Pavilions 18 and 19 were developed further and opened in 1976 as the new Care of the Elderly Unit. The Geriatric Day Centre in Ward 22 opened the following year.

Much of the impetus for the refurbishment of old premises and the building of new ones came from go-ahead leadership in the Board of Management. Its Chairman was a Loanhead general practitioner, Dr Douglas M. Alston, and later Mr C. J. Phillips of Phillips, Knox & Arthur, Quantity Surveyors. They had the enthusiastic support of Dr Horne, the new Physician Superintendent, Mr Alec Welstead, the Group Secretary and Treasurer, and Mr Geoffrey Redmond, the City Hospital Secretary.

There were, however, many frustrations along the way, for budgets were as tight as they are now. If adequate funds were not forthcoming from the Regional Hospital Board in time, the Board of Management had to down-scale previously agreed projects or see building schedules falling behind in their dates of completion. Mr Welstead had a particular flair, however, for utilising any money still available at the end of each financial year. He always had a series of schemes and projects instantly ready and costed to which spare cash could be devoted.[9] In this way many small, and some large, developments were funded. There was immense pride in the hospital with so much new building. Morale was high and it looked as if the hospital's future was secure.

Dr N. W. Horne

The City Hospital owes much to Dr Norman Horne, Physician Superintendent from 1960 until 1974. A quiet, unassuming man with charming manners, it would be unjust to pass too quickly over the major contributions he made both as the medical administrator of the City Hospital and as a fine clinician whose opinion was widely sought. He was born in Aberdeen and moved to London and then back to Edinburgh, where he attended George Watson's Boys' College. His early and long-lasting interest in sport was realised at school where for two seasons he opened the batting for the First Eleven cricket team. He entered medical training at the University of Edinburgh at the age of 17 and graduated MB, ChB in 1940. Resident posts followed in the Royal Infirmary with Professor W. T. Ritchie and Professor (later Sir) Derrick M Dunlop.

Dr Horne had only been married for three months when the Royal Air Force Volunteer Reserve (RAFVR) posted him overseas for three years and he served in many parts of the world. On his return to the UK, Professor Dunlop recommended him to Professor Charles Cameron, the second Professor of Tuberculosis, who appointed him Assistant Physician to Southfield Hospital in 1948. He had passed the MRCPEd. examination in 1947 and was elected a Fellow in 1954. From 1950 to 1954 he was Medical Superintendent at Southfield Hospital. He was appointed in 1953 as a NHS Consultant Physician in Respiratory Diseases and Tuberculosis at the City Hospital having charge of beds in Wards 4, 5 and 18. He was also first a University Lecturer and then a Senior Lecturer in Respiratory Medicine and Tuberculosis.

Dr Horne wrote extensively on respiratory diseases and tuberculosis. He was much involved in Sir John Crofton's trials of new antituberculosis drugs in the 1950s. His popular *Modern Drug Treatment of Tuberculosis*, co-authored by Dr J. D. (Ian) Ross (Health Horizon 1958), was a non-profit-making, practical handbook for doctors working in the developing world. The seventh edition appeared in 1990 under Dr Horne's name alone, after the death of Dr Ross. *Clinical Tuberculosis* (Macmillan 1992) under the joint authorship of Sir John Crofton, Dr Horne and Dr Fred Miller was also directed at those working in developing countries. Earlier

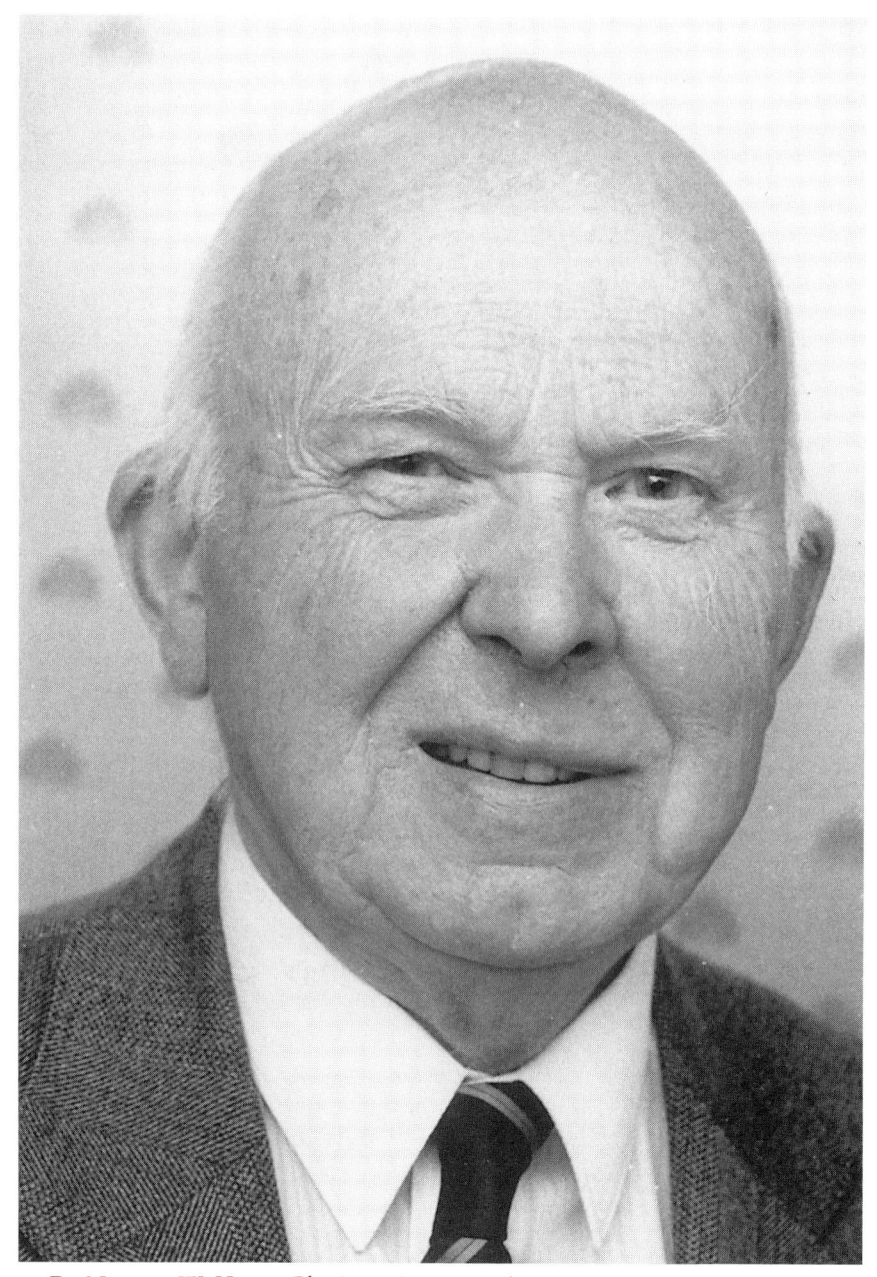

Dr Norman W. Horne, Physician Superintendent 1960–74 and Consultant Chest Physician. (By courtesy of Dr N. W. Horne)

Dr Horne had contributed the chapter on Respiratory Diseases in Davidson's *Principles and Practice of Medicine* (Churchill Livingstone). Recently he wrote on 'Tuberculosis and other Mycobacterial Diseases' for the twentieth edition of Manson's *Tropical Diseases* (W. B. Saunders 1996) and has co-authored a chapter on 'Renal Tuberculosis' for the next edition of the *Oxford Textbook of Medicine* (Oxford University Press).

Dr Horne has been President of the British Thoracic Association and was President of the European Region of the International Union against Tuberculosis and Lung Disease from 1982 to 1988. In 1982 he was appointed Chairman of the Chest Heart and Stroke Association of Scotland. In 1966 he took a year away from being Physician Superintendent when he was invited to be Visiting Professor of Medicine at the University of Baroda, north India.

Dr Horne is always punctual and his written and spoken work is meticulously rehearsed and prepared. He was a popular physician, teacher and lecturer. He is also a keen churchman and a former gardener and remains devoted to sports news. One highlight of his days at the City Hospital was the annual cricket match played in the hospital grounds between his own medical team and a non-medical side of paramedical and administrative staff captained by Mr Alec Welstead. Dr Horne was a competent wicket-keeper, and Mr Welstead a keen batsman. Dr Horne ruefully recalls the painful black-eye he sustained on the cricket pitch when a young Australian doctor, whom he is too loyal to name, proved to be an unexpectedly vicious bowler. All was forgiven later in the enjoyment of the traditional post-match strawberry tea.

In 1974, Dr Horne's post of Physician Superintendent ceased with the reorganisation of the NHS in Scotland. He remained active, clinically as well as administratively, being the Chairman of the newly formed South Lothian Division of Medicine from 1974 to 1981. He finally retired in 1982.

Mr Alec Welstead

Mr Welstead, like Dr Horne, originally hailed from Aberdeenshire. He is a tall, lean man with much charm and a great sense of humour. His uncanny ability to direct funds to the City Hospital that would otherwise have been lost at the end of each financial year made him very popular. He was a meticulous minute writer and sat in as Group Secretary and Treasurer not only on the meetings of the Board of Management but on the General Purposes Committee, Medical and Allied Services Committee and the Finance Committee of the Group. Thanks to his careful documentation of the proceedings of these committees, much information remains available today.

Mr Welstead can recall many amusing and strange anecdotes about the hospital. When he first arrived, he was bemused by the underground ducts and walkways below the corridors. He was informed by a young house doctor that it was possible to walk through them from almost any point in the hospital, including the old residency, and end up in the nurses' home. Mr Welstead tactfully avoided asking to what purpose this knowledge could be put. (See Chapter 15.)

On another occasion Mr Welstead received word that several nights previously a group of nurses, returning late to the nurses' home and hoping to sneak in undetected by the Home Sister, had met two men in the dark struggling away from the hospital with what appeared to be a heavily laden children's cot. When the nurses eventually owned up to this strange encounter, they were unfortunately too late to help the police with their enquiries. Seemingly earlier that evening the hospital shop had been burgled and the thieves had found the abandoned cot an ideal vehicle for spiriting away the safe and cartons of cigarettes that they had appropriated.[10]

Dr J. McC. Murdoch

When Dr Horne became Physician Superintendent in April 1960, he had already been a consultant at the City Hospital for seven years. At the same time the new Physician in infectious diseases (ID) began his 23 year consultant career at the hospital taking over Pavilions 14–17 which became known as the ID Corridor. James McCash Murdoch, often referred to as 'McCash' or 'Big Jimmy', regarded himself as one of 'Falkirk's bairns' and had indeed worked at one time in Falkirk and District Royal Infirmary. His medical training was at Anderson's College Medical School, Glasgow, where the standard of teaching was very high and attracted many Americans.[11] James Murdoch's life-long links with the USA may therefore have originated when he was a student at Anderson's College. He qualified LRCP, LRCSEd, LRFPSGlas with the conjoint examination in 1944. He passed the MRCP examination in 1950 and was later elected FRCPEd and FRCPGlas.

During his military service, some of which was spent in India, he drove the Viceroy's car and he promised himself that one day he too would own a Rolls Royce. In time he most certainly did – a succession of them. As a Senior Registrar he worked at the National Hospital for Nervous Diseases, Queen Square, London, then in Edinburgh Royal Infirmary he came under the influence of Professor Sir Derrick Dunlop and Professor Sir Stanley Davidson.

In 1960 Dr Murdoch was appointed to succeed Dr Joe in the ID wards at the Edinburgh City Hospital, in a post that he was to hold

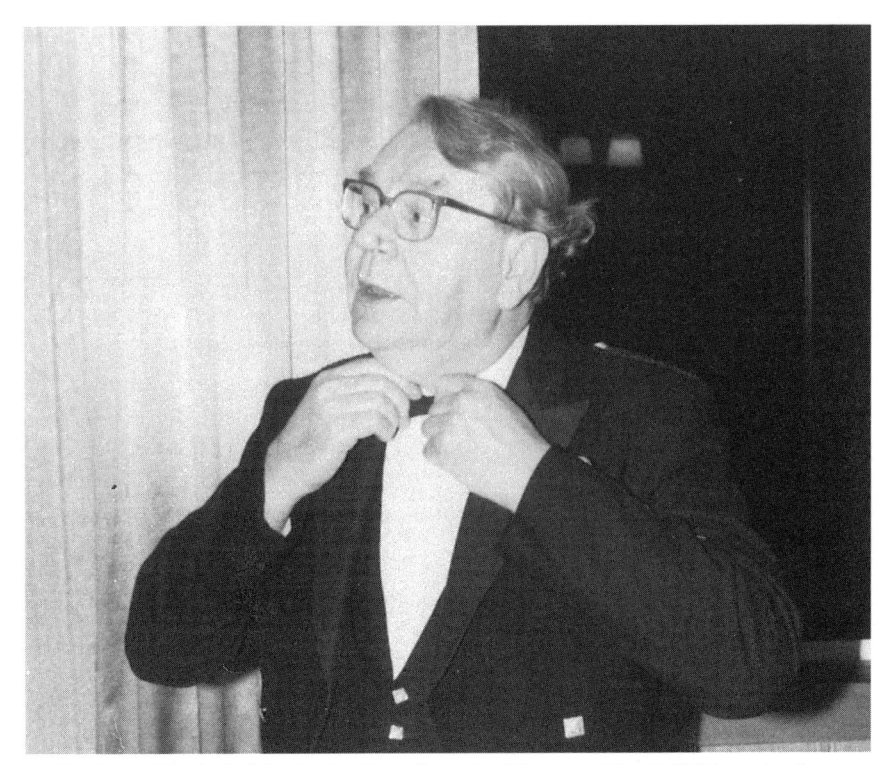

Dr James McCash Murdoch, Consultant in Charge of the RIDU, 1960–83 adjusting his Highland Dress bow tie. (By courtesy of Mrs Irene Murdoch)

until he retired aged 60 in 1983. He quickly made his mark not only in the hospital, but also far beyond as a researcher and a memorable, flamboyant, lecturer and bed-side teacher.

The Pyelonephritis Unit and Infectious Diseases

Dr Murdoch's interests lay in the natural history of urinary tract infection in women and in the chemotherapy of all types of infection. There were few antibiotics that he had not written a research paper about. He maintained a strong link with the therapeutics industry, often being among the first to conduct clinical trials on newly developed antimicrobial agents. Aminoglycosides, nitrofurantoin, cycloserine, the new penicillins and cephalosporins, lincosamines and quinolones were among those he studied. His *bête noire* was the sulphonamide group of drugs, and woe betide any unwary student who chose a sulphonamide for one of Dr Murdoch's patients.

By contrast, his favourite preparation for treating uncomplicated coliform urinary infections was cycloserine, an agent seldom used for that indication by anyone who had not been taught by Dr Murdoch. When he had been working with tuberculous patients he had noticed that the third or fourth line antituberculous drug cycloserine was also effective in low, relatively non-toxic doses in eradicating *Escherichia coli* urinary infections. He was to conduct many trials with cycloserine in the Pyelonephritis Unit he set up in Pavilion 14 of the City Hospital soon after his appointment. Funding came largely from the Scottish Hospitals Endowment Research Trust.

The Pyelonephritis Unit aimed to study the natural history of urinary tract infection in female patients and the risk of later developing hypertension and renal failure. Five or six years previously Dr Edward H. Kass in the USA had quantified urinary infection and coined the term 'significant bacteriuria'. This led to an avalanche of research in urinary infection all over the Western world. In keeping with contemporaneous researchers, Dr Murdoch showed that morbidity and mortality was low in adult females except where the urinary tract was obstructed or when repeated reflux of infected bladder urine in childhood had already caused irreparable kidney damage.

Pari passu with this study, Dr Murdoch used many antibiotics including intravenous kanamycin and cephalosporins for patients with bloodstream infections. For the less serious or chronic urinary infections he employed both short- and long-term courses of oral antimicrobials, often including cycloserine. Edinburgh general practitioners were quick to see the advantage of the Pyelonephritis Clinic for their patients with chronic urinary infections whom they thankfully referred in large numbers. These women were regularly followed up, some of them for decades. Many became reluctant to give up long-term antibacterial treatment which also prevented unpleasant post-coital cystitis and urethritis. It was sometimes a battle to discharge from the clinic women who had been indoctrinated with the idea that without long-term antibiotic prophylaxis they were doomed to die an early death from kidney failure or the complications of high blood pressure. The follow-up clinics in Ward 14 on Tuesday and Wednesday mornings, therefore, were always well attended.

Dr Murdoch enlisted the help of Mr W. Selby Tulloch and later Mr J. E. Newsam, urological surgeons, from the Western General Hospital. A combined medical and surgical approach was used for patients with obstructive uropathy or other surgically correctable causes of resistant infection. On Tuesday afternoons the urological list carried out in the thoracic theatre included nephrectomies and pyelolithotomies. The tiny operating theatre in Ward 14A, formerly designed for tracheostomies when the ward catered for patients with diphtheria, was next used for cystoscopies and retrograde pyelography. It was upgraded at a cost of

£600.[12] A massive ante-deluvian X-ray machine was installed, probably a relic from the days when Cottage 13 had been the hospital's X-ray Department. Despite this cumbersome and potentially dangerous equipment, the Consultant Radiologist, Dr W. Norman Thomson, and his devoted radiographers could produce surprisingly high quality films, which were developed in the adjacent dark room, and so were instantly available for the surgeons to see.

James Murdoch's work was recognised internationally. To use his own words he quickly 'jetted into orbit' attending and addressing conferences all over the world. During the 1960s and 1970s the Minutes of the Edinburgh Royal Victoria and Associated Hospitals Board of Management and its Medical and Allied Services Committee record his frequent requests for study leave. By the end of 1966 he was well known in medical centres and universities in the USA, notably New York, Boston and Florida. He had visited Australia twice as well as New Zealand, Germany, Switzerland and several Scandinavian countries. At the Board of Management meeting on 18 January 1967,[13] at the request of Dr Alston, the Chairman, Dr Murdoch, gave a summary of his recent lecture tours in New Zealand and Australia (September 1966), Ethiopia and India (September–October 1966) and Gainsville where he was the visiting scientist at the University of Florida (November–December 1966). In July 1967 he was to address the 46th South African Medical Congress in Durban.[14]

It is often asked of men such as James Murdoch 'Who looks after your patients when you are away so much?' to which he would give the apocryphal reply 'Just the same doctors as when I'm there!' He had the good fortune to be ably supported on the clinical side by the conscientious Dr George Sangster and the high calibre junior staff whom he had recruited. Among them in the early days were James Syme, later a Consultant Paediatrician in Edinburgh, Alastair Geddes, later Professor of Infectious Diseases in Birmingham, Colin Spiers, later Clinical Research Physician with Eli Lilly, Herbert Pullen, later Consultant in Infectious Diseases in Leeds, the late William (Bill) Ford, later Professor of Experimental Pathology in Manchester and Sydney Selwyn, later Professor of Medical Microbiology at Westminster and Charing Cross Hospitals. Many of these eminent men owe their introduction into the world of medical publications to Dr Murdoch's enthusiastic encouragement. The Unit produced many scientific papers and was often represented at international meetings.

Dr Murdoch was a big, impressive man in every respect, a fine raconteur, a bon viveur, full of *bonhomie*, and with his wife Irene, a genial and generous host. He knew his Robert Burns well and his large, kilted presence was in demand at medical society and golf club dinners where he recited the works of the Bard.

In June 1960 Dr Murdoch had charge of 220 infectious diseases beds, over one third of the total of 612 beds in the hospital at that time.[15] He soon asked for and obtained funding for a third house physician[16] and an additional senior house officer,[17] claiming that the work generated by the Pyelonephritis Unit and clinical teaching justified this increase in staffing. In 1963 he succeeded in obtaining a Senior Registrar who took part in a rotation scheme with the other major hospitals, and Dr A. M. Geddes was the first appointed. In February 1965, Dr Sangster assumed full clinical responsibility for Wards 15 and 16 following the recommendation of the Review Committee which graded him as of Consultant status from July 1963. There were then by 1965 two Consultants, a rotating Senior Registrar, two Senior House Officers and three House Physicians in the Infectious Diseases Unit.

The next request for Senior House Officer staffing for the Infectious Diseases Unit was triggered by the prolonged outbreak of paratyphoid type B which continued from December 1962 until December 1963 peaking to 44 admissions in January 1963. Altogether 141 patients were taken in, requiring ten additional nurses in a newly opened ward. The ratio of 62.5 nurses to 100 patients was below the acceptable minimum and highlighted the shortage of nursing as well as medical staff.[18] Up to 89 patients at any one time were under treatment for paratyphoid. In those days patients were kept in hospital until pronounced non-infectious after six consecutive negative stool cultures.

Viral Hepatitis

Beginning in January 1967, patients suffering from 'infective jaundice' regularly appeared in the hospital's admission figures. As there were few investigations in those days it is difficult in retrospect to know what kind of hepatitis these patients had. Many probably had type A, the common, orally acquired and usually mild hepatitis whose prevalence has decreased since the development of an effective vaccine. Some, however, must have had type B hepatitis, then known as syringe transmitted or serum hepatitis, which caused the tragic Edinburgh outbreak of 1969–70.

This outbreak led to several deaths among dialysis patients in a renal unit as well as killing two surgeons related to that department and a Medical Laboratory Scientific Officer who was accidentally inoculated with infected blood. In May 1970, the Physician Superintendent Dr Horne spoke to the Board of Management about this outbreak of what would probably now be termed a virulent variety of hepatitis non-A, non-B.[19] The Regional Hospital Board had set up an advisory panel and the staff of the Infectious Diseases Unit were praised for their responsible attitude when exposed to considerable danger themselves. There was then no form of active immunisation against viral hepatitis nor did gloves and aprons always protect staff attending these very ill patients.

Miss Margaret Kerr, a stalwart ex-Royal Naval Nursing Sister, was in charge of Ward 16A where most of the ill patients with hepatitis were nursed. She bravely led a devoted team of nurses who coped in inadequate accommodation with this distressing and politically sensitive outbreak. In 1973 Sister Kerr was justly recognised for her services during this difficult time by being awarded the MBE.

Media interest in the hepatitis outbreak was intense. A reporter to a Scottish daily newspaper who was caught gaining access to ward 16A by misrepresentation, was soundly criticised and an apology was later received.[20] Americans visiting the UK would telephone the unit from London to ask if it was safe to attend the Edinburgh International Festival in view of the outbreak of 'yellow jaundice' affecting the city.

Dr Hugh A. Raeburn, Senior Administrator Medical Officer, and Miss Brayton, Regional Nursing Officer of the Regional Hospital Board, boosted nursing staff morale by visiting the unit during the outbreak. They promised upgrading of hepatitis accommodation in Ward 16A. This began a fortnight later[21] and was rapidly completed.

In addition to the improved accommodation this hepatitis incident brought about, the introduction of the sterile syringe service for the hospital had previously been accelerated because of the risks perceived in transmitting hepatitis viruses. Early in 1962 the Board of Management felt that a sterile syringe service would be safer and reduce costs by saving staff time. It would cost about £2,500 per annum.[22] The Regional Hospital Board was at first reluctant to implement the sterile syringe system despite the anomaly of seconding nurses from the Royal Infirmary or Western General Hospital who were already familiar with the system in their own hospitals. When these nurses came to learn about control of infection at the City Hospital they were amazed to find no sterile supply service. The Board of Management then threatened to hold the Regional Hospital Board responsible for any cases of syringe transmitted jaundice that could have been avoided by the introduction of a sterile supply.[23] Moreover they would consider reporting the Regional Hospital Board to the press if that happened.[24] This had the desired effect. Although the Regional Board could not fund a sterile syringe supply for all the wards at once, they agreed to give priority to the Infectious Diseases Unit.[25] By July 1962 the full system was in place either with sterilised or disposable items.[26]

The infectious diseases wards had remained busy since Dr Murdoch took up his appointment in 1960. Admissions averaged about 200 every

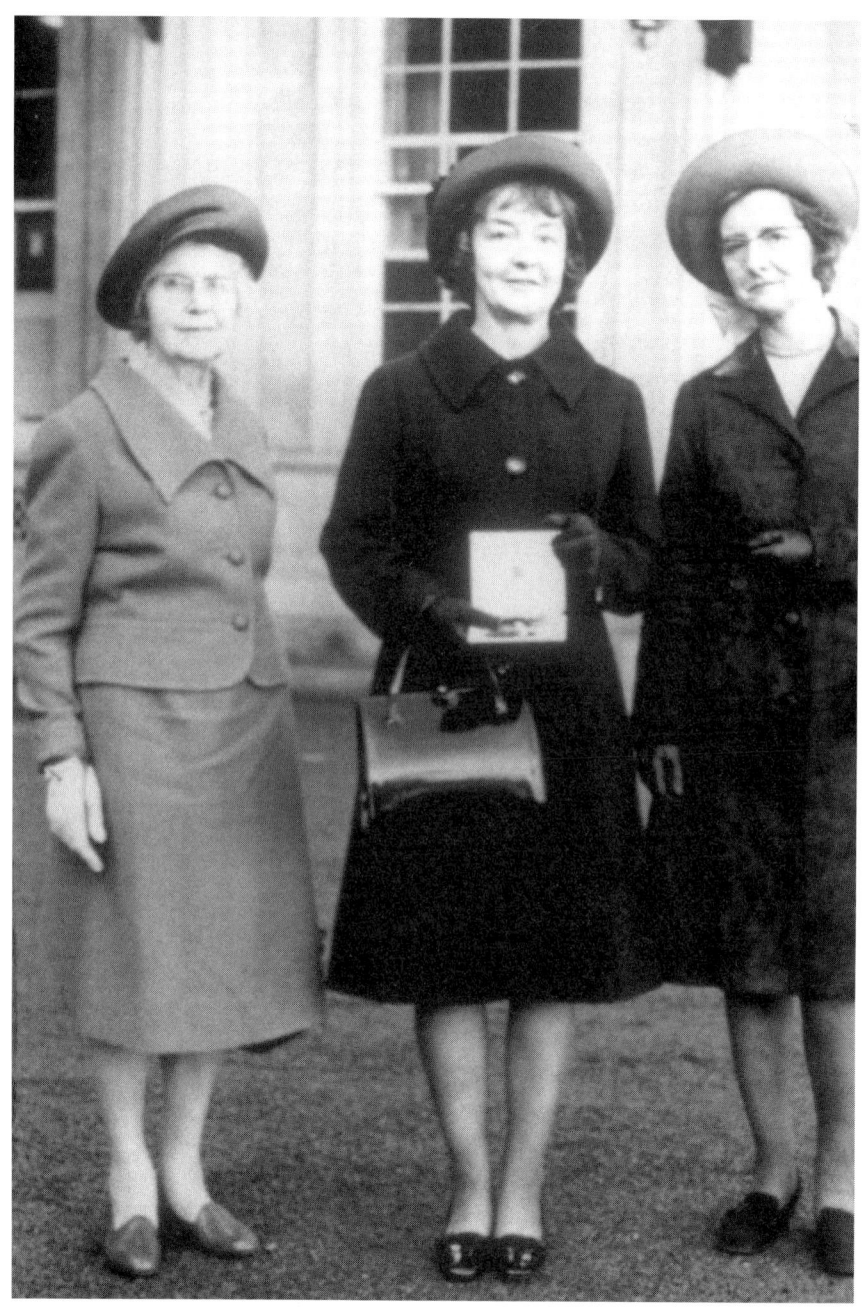

Sister Margaret Kerr, with her mother and sister, shows her MBE at Buckingham Palace, 1973. (By courtesy of Miss Margaret Kerr)

month of whom between 20 and 100 were women taken into the Pyelonephritis Unit for investigation of urinary infections. After much pleading Dr Murdoch secured funding for a third Consultant to the unit and in September 1969 I took up the new post. After qualifying in Edinburgh in 1959 and working in an Arab hospital in Aden during service with the Medical Branch of the RAF, I passed the MRCPEd. examination in 1965. Then followed positions including Research Registrar with Dr Murdoch, Registrar and Senior Registrar posts in Bristol and London and finally my Consultant appointment at the City Hospital. The hepatitis outbreak of 1969–70 was therefore my 'baptism of fire'. After serving on several committees in the Royal College of Physicians, I was elected FRCPEd. in 1974. In 1989–90 I was President of the British Society for the Study of Infection. With various colleagues I have been co-author of articles on infection, the three editions of *Antibacterial Drugs Today* (Adis Health Science Press) and the ongoing *Colour Guides in Infectious Diseases* (Churchill Livingstone). I retired in 1995 to continue as Principal Medical Officer at the Scottish Widows' Fund for two further years and to find time to write this book.

The Tropical Diseases Unit

Another department joined the City Hospital in 1963. An overall shortage of geriatric accommodation had occurred and it was decided to move some beds from Southfield Hospital to the Eastern General Hospital. To make room, the Tropical Diseases Unit moved from the Eastern General Hospital to Ward 20 in the City Hospital.[27] The original budget for upgrading Ward 20 to receive the tropical patients was whittled down from £9,500 to £3,000 which meant that heating, plumbing and electrical services could not be renewed. Dr Frederick J Wright, Consultant in Tropical Medicine, reluctantly had to agree to a very modified upgrading.[28] The memorial library, which was about to be installed at the Eastern General Hospital by the Ex-Far East Prisoners of War (Ex-FEPOW) Association, was set up later at the City Hospital.[29]

Dr Wright had qualified through the University of Cambridge and the London Hospital in 1932. He gained his MD and DTM&H in 1935 and was later elected FRCP (Lond & Ed). He was a Consultant to the Ministry of Overseas Development and a medical specialist to the Government of Kenya. He wrote several books and chapters in multi-author texts and papers on brucellosis and tropically acquired illnesses. Quiet spoken and a devout Christian, he worked closely with missionary organisations.

The Tropical Diseases Unit was transferred to the City Hospital on 22 July 1963 with two doctors, one ward sister, one nurse, a laboratory technician and four patients. Part of the Ex-FEPOW Memorial Library had already been installed in the Eastern General, so the remaining funds were devoted to refurbishing a sun room in Ward 20 at the City Hospital as an amenity for Ex-FEPOWs attending for tropical disease screening. The sun room was formally opened in spring of 1964 by Lt General Percival, formerly Commander in Chief of Forces in Malaya.[30]

Dr Wright was always aware of Edinburgh's long tradition in tropical medicine. In 1857 Dr A. W. P. Pinkerton, a colleague of Dr W. P. Alison, had delived lectures on 'The Effects of Climate on Health and Disease, and Hygiene',[31] but it was not until 1898 the University of Edinburgh founded a lectureship in 'Diseases of Tropical Climates'. The next year saw a Certificate in Tropical Medicine instituted and the first DTM&H course began in Edinburgh in 1905–06.[32]

Originally patients with tropical diseases were admitted to the Royal Infirmary where the Lecturer acted as Consultant. Col. Vere Hodge and later Col. Greig were responsible until Sir Stanley Davidson, Professor of Medicine, decided to bring all the patients, many of them ex-soldiers, into a newly formed Tropical Diseases Unit, at the Eastern General Hospital. Here Col. Vere Hodge continued to care for them, assisted by Dr Malcolm D MacQueen, who had worked in West Africa, and Dr E. L. Lloyd, an ex-schoolmaster wounded in the First World War and with subsequent experience in West Africa and India. Col. Vere Hodge was succeeded by Major General Sir Alexander Biggam, KBE, MD, FRCPEd & Lond who, with the continued assistance of Drs MacQueen and Lloyd, managed to combine the posts of Consultant and Lecturer in Diseases of Tropical Climates with that of Director of the Edinburgh Post-Graduate Board of Medicine and Consultant to the Colonial Office. The unit was then recognised as source of advice for those travelling overseas, a yellow fever vaccination centre and a designated centre for the diagnosis of smallpox.

Sir Alexander Biggam was succeeded in 1954 by Dr F.J. Wright. The Unit continued to look after Ex-FEPOWs and a small number of civilian patients. It also instructed candidates choosing tropical medicine as one of the 'Selected Subjects' in the Edinburgh MRCP (Member of the Royal College of Physicians) examination and it continued to run DTM&H courses.

After the unit transferred to the City Hospital in 1963, male patients were admitted to Ward 20 where there was a laboratory, examination room, and an out-patient clinic which often screened officials of the Colonial Office, and Crown Agents of the Colonies. Female in-patients were looked after in general medical wards or the Infectious Diseases Unit. Dr MacQueen retired in August 1966 after many years of service and was replaced by Dr James Carswell who had worked in South

Africa. Dr Lloyd 'retired' aged 70 but continued to teach anatomy for a further year. Also in 1966, Dr David Stevenson, a kilted devotee of the Scottish National Party, came to the unit at a time when Dr Wright was acting as Physician Superintendent of the Hospital whilst Dr Horne was Visiting Professor in Baroda.

When Dr Wright retired in 1972, the MRCPEd examination had been amalgamated with that of its two sister Colleges in Glasgow and London and became the MRCP(UK). The 'Selected Subject', formerly a feature of the Edinburgh College only, was dropped. The University felt that the Tropical Diseases Unit was no longer viable and should be disbanded. The patients then became the charge of the Infectious Diseases Unit which also continued to provide a screening programme for Ex-FEPOWs. So after a tenure of nine years at the City Hospital, the Tropical Diseases Unit closed for ever and with it the Edinburgh DTM&H course finished.

Although a small unit with very few in-patients, the Tropical Diseases Unit had provided excellent teaching, and its students achieved good results. Before he died in 1996, Dr Wright often reminisced about the 'famous' patients and students he and his unit had cared for.[33] One soldier invalided from India with epilepsy in 1905, was subjected to a craniotomy two years later by Professor Annandale in the Royal Infirmary, a procedure described by the patient as 'having done me no good but no harm'. Calcified cerebral cysticercosis was diagnosed – resulting from dissemination of a worm infestation acquired abroad. The patient was managed for many years in the unit which he in fact outlived, to die in his 99th year.

Another patient, a young Burmese doctor, had arrived in the UK with a high fever. After his amoebic liver abscess was diagnosed and drained in the unit, he went on to pass both the Primary and Final FRCSEd examinations at the first attempt. A man recently returned from Nigeria with fever and signs suggestive of meningitis was initially thought to have malaria; in fact he had Q-fever, a zoonosis he had acquired from helping with the sheep at his brother's farm in the Borders shortly after his return to the UK. A lady missionary doctor from West Africa who was to be referred to a psychiatrist for depression and headaches of dramatic onset was found by the unit to have quartan malaria. Cured of this, she resumed her postgraduate studies at the Liverpool School of Tropical Medicine without further ado.

After absorption into the Infectious Diseases Unit, ex-FEPOWs were looked after by Dr Murdoch and later myself. Their numbers slowly decreased as the years passed by but some still showed evidence of strongyloidiasis, a worm infestation, which many of them acquired on the notorious Burma-Siam Railway. Most responded to treatment with albendazole. Some of the ex-FEPOWs showed extreme irritability, emotional lability or depression as a consequence of their starvation and maltreatment by Japanese and Korean captors many years before.

As Dr Murdoch, Dr Sangster and I did not hold qualifications in tropical diseases, it was agreed that the Infectious Diseases Unit should not be renamed the Infectious Diseases and Tropical Medicine Unit even though the work carried out did include the emergency management of patients with imported diseases such as malaria and the screening of those who had been in the tropics on business or holiday. Later the unit recruited Dr Michael E. Jones, a qualified specialist in tropical medicine with extensive experience of managing third world illnesses in Tanzania. He now looks after the advice bureau for intending travellers as well as providing an expert opinion on the diagnosis and management of tropically acquired diseases. Dr Jones also looks after HIV-infected patients. His finely illustrated and enjoyable lectures on imported disease are always a *tour de force*.

The Diamond Jubilee Celebrations

In 1963, the year that the Tropical Diseases Unit came to Ward 20, the City Hospital celebrated its Diamond Jubilee. On 14 May 1963, sixty years and one day after the royal opening a commemoration service was held.[34] HRH the Duchess of Gloucester visited the hospital on 27 June 1963 which was unfortunately a day of 'very unfavourable weather'.[35] According to *The Scotsman*[36] the Duchess wore a sea green dress and jacket and a pale blue petal hat. She was welcomed by Sir Duncan Weatherstone, Lord Provost, acting as Lord Lieutenant of the County, Mr C. S. Gumley, WS, Chairman of the Regional Hospital Board, Dr D. M. Alston, Chairman of the Board of Management, and the senior medical, nursing and administrative staff of the hospital, and then she signed the visitors' book. The speeches which followed were relayed from the recreation hall to 320 of the patients. The Duchess then toured Wards 7 and 15, speaking to an 11 year old girl, Jennifer Banks, who had a collection of dolls from many countries. One disappointed patient who did not meet HRH was 82 year old Alexander Taylor, from Ross-shire, who had been in the Guard of Honour of Seaforth Highlanders at the royal opening of the hospital in 1903. Despite this and the poor weather, the visit was regarded as highly successful.

Developments in the hospital during Dr Horne's superintendentship include thoracic and ENT surgery, the Care of the Elderly Unit and the major expansion of laboratory services with the introduction of the Wellcome Research Trust Virus Laboratory. They are described next.

CHAPTER TWENTY-SEVEN

1960–74: The Surgical Units, Care of the Elderly Unit and New Laboratories; A Continuing Nursing Shortage; The Tea Room; The Bus Service

The Ear, Nose and Throat (ENT) Department

The ENT Department became firmly established in the City Hospital in the 1960s. Patients were admitted soon after it was commissioned in November 1965 and it was officially opened by the Lord and Lady Provost in 1966. The cost of the development was £260,000.[1]

Advertisements to recruit nursing staff to the ENT Department were not very successful[2] especially for staff nurses.[3] The Matron of the Royal Infirmary, however, offered to transfer six of her nurses for two or three months to help the new unit out of its difficulty.[4]

The ENT Department occupied the refurbished and now H-shaped Ward 2 downstairs. Ward 3 had its own wings linked by an upper corridor. Ward 4 was at the east end below the Wellcome Laboratory. Despite three operating theatres, the ENT waiting list grew alarmingly, peaking at 1,711 patients by January 1968.[5] By then the admission rate had risen to 300–500 patients each month. Some of the hold-up was due to the admission of patients from the Eastern General Hospital into Ward 4 in September 1966 and from Chalmers Hospital in October 1966[6] as well as the shortage of nurses. Despite the willingness of the surgeons, there never seemed to be enough operating time; the waiting list was later reduced somewhat when extra sessions were arranged in Bangour Hospital.[7]

In November 1965 there were six ENT Consultants all with affiliation to the Royal Infirmary. Dr A. Brownlie Smith also had beds at Chalmers Hospital, Drs. I. M. Farquharson, G. D. McDowall and R. A. McNeill also had beds in West Lothian and Dr K. McLay also had beds in Leith Hospital. Dr R. B. Lumsden worked almost exclusively at the City Hospital and Royal Infirmary. Two additional Consultants concentrated on paediatric ENT Surgery: Dr J. F. Birrell with beds also in the Royal Hospital for Sick Children, Chalmers Hospital and the Borders, and Dr

J. R. McCallum who also had beds in the Royal Hospital for Sick Children, the Northern Group of hospitals and the Borders.[8]

By the end of 1967 the ENT Wards were staffed as follows:[9] Ward 2 Drs I. M. Farquharson and K. McLay (with one vacancy); Ward 3 Drs A. Brownlie Smith, G. D. McDowall and R. A. McNeill; Ward 4 Drs J. F. Birrell and J. R. McCallum. Dr Farquharson was the Consultant in Administrative Charge of the ENT wards and in December 1970 he succeeded Dr J. McC. Murdoch as Chairman of the Medical Staff Committee.[10]

The Department of Anaesthetics

With its rapid throughput of patients the ENT theatres not only kept the surgeons busy but also put a strain on the anaesthetic staff under Dr Archie C. Milne. Operations carried out included surgery to the sinuses, tonsillectomies and adenoidectomies, septoplasties, ear operations such as fenestrations and stapidectomies with, at a later date, cochlear decompression and implantation. When Dr (later Professor) Arnold Maran arrived in Ward 2 parotid gland surgery and highly complicated head and neck operations were performed including pharyngectomies for malignant disease. Such procedures required great skill by surgeons and anaesthetists and a high quality of after-care. In the 1980s micro-surgical techniques were introduced for disease of the larynx and vocal cords.

From 1953 Dr Archie Milne provided much of the anaesthetic service for the hospital. Dr J. C. McIntyre was appointed as a much needed additional Consultant Anaesthetist in 1968. Other well-known anaesthetists also had sessions at the City Hospital. Besides Dr Milne there was the ever popular 'Griff,' as Dr Harold W. C. Griffiths was known, and Drs Callum McQueen, Keith Dodd, W. R. MacRae, N. A. Malcolm-Smith and G. H. Sharwood Smith. Long before the Thoracic Surgical and ENT Departments came to the hospital, the anaesthetists had been invaluable during poliomyelitis outbreaks supervising assisted ventilation for patients with respiratory paralysis. When the surgical units arrived, however, many more anaesthetic sessions were required.

Dr Milne, who served the hospital faithfully from 1953 till he retired in 1988, saw many changes. He was regarded by the surgeons as their 'physician' as well as anaesthetist for he gave much more advice and assistance than was normally provided by a 'gas man'. In the early days of cardiac surgery, a pre-requisite for some procedures was to make the patient hypothermic. This provided the surgeons with more time when carrying out complex heart operations. It was the anaesthetists' responsibility to achieve the very low body core temperatures needed in pre-operative ice-baths. Although more sophisticated cardio-vascular

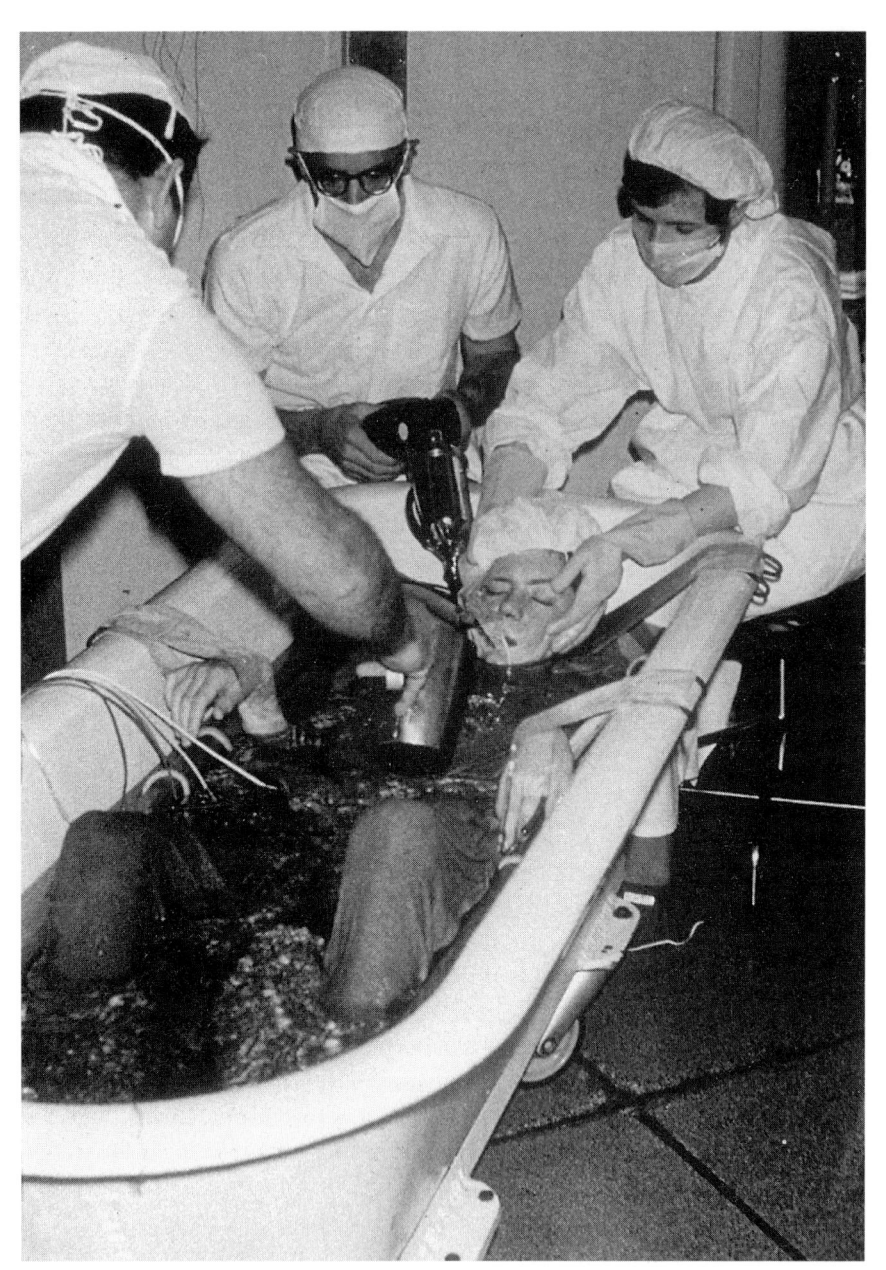

Preparing a patient for cardiac surgery. Dr A. C. Milne, Consultant Anaesthetist, at rear with Ambu bag and cannister, supervising the induction of hypothermia in an ice-bath (ca. late 1970s). (Photo: Mr Douglas Inglis, courtesy of Dr A. C. Milne and Dr G. M. Bowler)

procedures were eventually carried out such as repair of coarctation of the aorta, closing of persistent ductus arteriosus and atrial septal defects, and the correction of anomylous pulmonary venous drainage, surgery on the aortic valve did not begin until the 1960s. It was decided, however, not to pursue cardiac bypass procedures at the City Hospital.

The Thoracic Surgery Unit after 1972

When Mr Logan retired from the City Hospital in 1972, he left three consultant thoracic surgeons, Mr David Wade, Mr Bobby McCormack and Mr Philip Walbaum, and a staff of four registrars and one senior house officer. As there were currently proposals to rebuild the Royal Infirmary and Royal Hospital for Sick Children, it was decided that Mr Logan's successor should be primarily a cardiac surgeon with strong research interests. Most adult and paediatric cardiac surgery was to be done at the Royal Infirmary and Royal Hospital for Sick Children but non-cardiac thoracic work was to be done at the City Hospital. Some non-bypass cardiac surgery, however, should still be performed at both the City and the Royal Hospital for Sick Children.[11] By late 1972 Mr Philip K. Caves had been appointed Senior Lecturer in Cardiac Surgery based at the Royal Infirmary, so leaving the City Hospital a surgeon short.[12]

Work continued, however, under Messrs Wade, McCormack and Walbaum and later Messrs Evan Cameron, Christopher Sang and Ciro Campanella. Sadly Mr Bobby McCormack, who had joined Mr Logan's team in the early years of thoracic surgery at the City Hospital, died suddenly and prematurely in 1980.

The Care of the Elderly Unit

At the other end of the southern corridor of the City Hospital from the Thoracic Surgical Theatre, the Care of the Elderly Unit was formed from Wards 18–20 which had originally been upgraded in anticipation of the Burns and Plastic Surgery Unit moving into them. Even the name 'Care of the Elderly Unit' rather than 'Department of Geriatrics' reflects credit on the doctor who did so much to build it up. As a chest physician Dr James Williamson had been involved in Sir John Crofton's campaign against tuberculosis in the 1950s. In particular the mass chest X-ray campaign of 1958 had drawn upon Dr Williamson's organisational and administrative skills. As tuberculosis began to come under control, Dr Williamson appreciated that he could apply much of the experience he had derived from the campaign against tuberculosis to other branches of medicine. Feeling that care of the elderly was the next great challenge, he requested a transfer to that discipline in 1958. After tuberculous

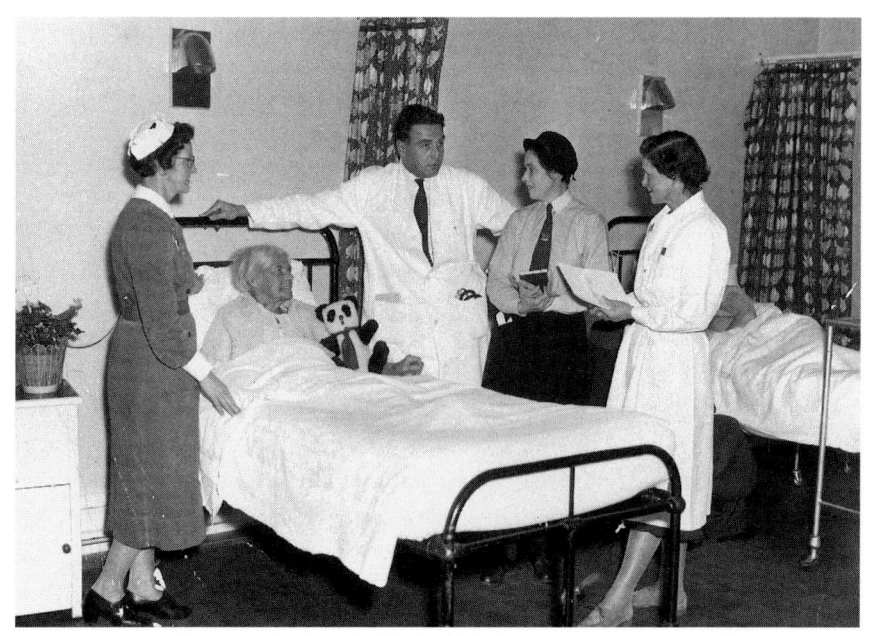

Dr James Williamson, later to hold the first Chairs in Geriatric Medicine in Liverpool, and then in Edinburgh, with his staff at Southfield Hospital (ca. 1960s) (*Nursing Mirror* Photograph, by courtesy of Professor Williamson)

patients were moved from Southfield Hospital to the City Hospital the next year, Dr Williamson was appointed a full-time Consultant in Geriatric Medicine.[13]

At that time Dr Neil MacMichael was in charge of two wards of elderly patients in the City Hospital. Drs Williamson and MacMichael respectively divided the geographical catchment area of Edinburgh into north and south of Princes Street. In addition to his commitments to north Edinburgh, Dr Williamson also covered the whole of Midlothian. In 1963 he was joined by Dr C. P. Lowther at Southfield Hospital. He next moved to the Eastern General Hospital whilst Dr MacMichael remained in charge of the long-stay unit at Southfield.

In 1972 Dr Williamson left Edinburgh to become the first Professor of Geriatric Medicine in Liverpool. During his four years absence from 1972 to 1976, two general practitioners, Drs Alistair Cruickshank and Robert Thin, looked after the City Hospital's elderly patients. On his return from Liverpool to occupy the first Chair in Geriatric Medicine in Edinburgh, Professor Williamson quickly reorganised his Department. Wards 20 and 21 became empty in 1973 when the Tropical Diseases Unit closed and, as the Burns and Plastic Surgery Unit eventually never came to the City Hospital, Wards 18 and 19 were free as well.[14]

Professor Williamson initially created a 38-bedded assessment unit in Wards 18A and 19A (upstairs) with long-stay wards below. Ward 18B later accommodated psychogeriatric patients. Wards 20 and 21, the former Tropical Diseases Unit, were converted into a rehabilitation area with a corridor link between these wards and with the physiotherapy and occupational therapy services. Professor Williamson was determined that rehabilitation services should be on site, unlike in Liverpool where rehabilitation took place several miles from the parent unit. For this reason he turned down the offer of rehabilitation accommodation two miles away in the Astley Ainslie Hospital. By 1976 he had instead established a day hospital within the City Hospital in Ward 22, the former typhus pavilion near the west gate. With this and Pavilions 18–21 he could combine on the same site his team of doctors, nurses, physiotherapists, occupational therapists, rehabilitation and social workers. The area between Wards 18 and 19 was roofed in and a covered ambulance bay created. Together with the day hospital these improvements cost £500,000.

Buildings, however, were not the only remarkable feature of Professor Williamson's new approach to the care of the elderly. He initially must have endeared himself to his general medical colleagues by relieving them of some of their so called 'non dischargeable bed blockers', a few of whom he rehabilitated so well that they got home again. He insisted on a very high standard of care with regular ward rounds rather than the pattern adopted by many contemporaneous geriatricians who merely 'popped in' to see their patients on an irregular basis. His forté was teaching and he insisted that medical students should be attached to the unit for four weeks and take part in the assessment of patients. His relations with general practitioners were excellent. Home assessments of frail, elderly patients normally took place within a few hours of the request being made. These assessments, unlike NHS domiciliary consultations, did not attract a fee, nor would members of the University team have been allowed to remunerate themselves for such practice. The day hospital had 30 places in which the frail elderly were given a full clinical examination and from which basic laboratory tests or X-rays were arranged.

Inevitably by creating an excellent new service for old people, Professor Williamson attracted staff of high calibre. Dr Roger G. Smith, an Honorary Senior Registrar at the time of Professor Williamson's return to Edinburgh in 1976, was appointed Senior Lecturer. He is an Edinburgh University graduate and former Surgeon Lieutenant, RN, FRCPEd and continued to be a University Senior Lecturer and Honorary Consultant to the Lothian Health Board. Also in 1976 Dr Colin T. Currie, another Edinburgh University graduate and also a Royal Navy Medical Officer, was appointed Senior Lecturer. He was encouraged by Professor Williamson to specialise in trauma rehabilitation, concentrating on old people who had suffered common injuries such as a fractured neck or femur. He is also well known for his regular columns in the *British Medical Journal* often with a humorous medico-political flavour, and as author of several novels about (Edinburgh) medicine, notably his first, *The Houseman's Tale*, and a longer work in 1991, *In Sickness and Health*. Dr Chris Gray, another Senior Lecturer in Professor Williamson's Department, later became Professor of Geriatric Medicine in Newcastle.

Professor Williamson retired in 1986. He had by then set up an enviable service with a fine reputation in a discipline that had previously been one of the 'Cinderellas' of Medicine. Geriatrics had not always been favoured by the then Matrons of the hospital, nor was it a specialty into which young doctors were easily recruited. Under Professor Williamson the discipline became not only respectable but attracted good staff as well.

The Microbiology Laboratories

The major developments that took place in the City Hospital's microbiological laboratories during the 1960s–80s have been admirably documented by Mr Charles J. Smith.[15] It will be recalled that the laboratory assistant, Jimmy Craig, later with William Webber, formed the original cadre of staff. They were loosely supported by a senior clinician but had good links with the Bacteriology Department at the University. There are relatively few references to named individuals in the laboratories in the Annual Reports of the City Hospital. Dr Tinne was the hospital's Bacteriologist from 1941 to 1942 when he was called up for war service. There was then a gap until Dr Archie Wallace's appointment in 1948. He was assisted by Miss Margaret Buchanan for a few years and also by Dr Nancy Conn. Dr Tinne returned briefly after the war as Dr Wallace's assistant.

On 8 March 1961 The Wellcome Research Trust Virus Laboratory was opened in the former Ward 4A,[16] after Professor Robert Cruikshank had obtained generous funding from the Wellcome Trust. For the first seven years, Dr Margaret Moffat, Virologist, worked tirelessly to build up the laboratory's services. Initially both virology and bacteriology (except tuberculosis investigations and research) were housed in Ward 4A. Mr Webber with Mr James Sutherland, then Senior Technician, was responsible for the technical administration in the Wellcome Laboratory from 1961 to 1969.

When the Bacteriology Department moved to new prefabricated premises in 1970, the virologists took over the whole of the Wellcome

Laboratory under Dr Alistair D. Macrae, who was the hospital's first Consultant Virologist. He was recruited, together with his Chief Medical Laboratory Scientific Officer (SCMLSO) since 1979), Mr David Hargreaves, from the Central Public Health Laboratory, Colindale, London. In 1974 Dr Macrae left for a post in Nottingham but Mr Hargreaves stayed on. During the next five years Dr Elizabeth Edmond was in charge and was succeeded as Director by Dr J. M. (Hamish) Inglis, who had already worked in the laboratory for about eight years. Dr Inglis' particular expertise was in respiratory viruses and he collaborated closely with clinicians in paediatric and adult medicine.

Over this time the Wellcome Laboratory, now the Regional Virus Laboratory, was proving itself in diagnostic services and research. During the 1970s Dr Winifred Thomson, later a general practitioner in Colinton, and Dr Helen Zeally, later Chief Administrative Medical Officer (CAMO) of the Lothian Health Board and Director of Public Health, both made a major contribution to the routine immunisation of Edinburgh's schoolgirls with German measles vaccine. Meanwhile Dr Heather Cubie's sophisticated research probed respiratory and human papilloma viruses.

In 1989 Dr Sheila Burns was appointed Consultant Virologist. When Edinburgh's virological services were amalgamated in 1996, she was put in charge of what then became the Regional Clinical Virus Laboratory. She was much involved with HIV antibody and hepatitis virus testing and also developed new techniques for detecting *Pneumocystis carinii*, which causes severe pneumonia in AIDS patients.

On 16 January 1986 the Regional Virus Laboratory extension, a dark red brick elevation extending eastwards from Ward 4, was opened by Sir John Crofton. There was a seminar room and staff room on the ground floor and more office accommodation above. This gave more space to help cope with the increasing amount of diagnostic work and the continuing commitment to teaching and research.

In the Bacteriology Department Dr Sheila Stewart was a great asset from 1960 onwards when she transferred from the Southfield Hospital Laboratory. She had done much of the original work on streptomycin resistance in tuberculosis. Together with Dr J. C. J. L. Bath, Dr G. Boissard, Dr Margaret Calder and Dr Margaret Moffat she investigated other pathogens of the respiratory tract, notably *Mycoplasma pneumoniae*, one of the causes of atypical pneumonia.

In 1974 Dr Alastair M. M. Wilson became Consultant Bacteriologist on the retiral of Dr Wallace. As Dr Wilson had had extensive experience overseas as Professor and Head of university departments in Nigeria and Malaya, he provided valuable insight into the diseases of travellers. Mr

Webber, who had such a long and distinguished association with the laboratory service, finally retired in 1976 and was succeeded by the efficient and amiable Mr Michael Croughan as Senior Chief Medical Laboratory Scientific Officer. Dr Calder who was Assistant Bacteriologist from 1957 to 1981 became Director of the Bacteriology Laboratory after the retiral of Dr Wilson in 1980. She was an expert in the field of respiratory pathogens, including tubercle bacilli, and particulary organisms associated with chronic obstructive airways disease. Dr Calder was also responsible for arranging the transfer to the City Hospital of the Scottish Mycobacteria Reference Laboratory after it closed in Mearnskirk in 1980.

Dr Brian Watt from the Western General Hospital was appointed in 1982 as the second Consultant at the City Hospital. He succeeded Dr Calder as Departmental Head and Director of the Scottish Mycobacterial Reference Laboratory. His particular expertise was anaerobic infections and, with the onset of the AIDS epidemic, he also provided a valuable input in diagnosing AIDS-associated, atypical mycobacterial infections. In 1993 Dr Watt became the Clinical Director of Medical Microbiology and was also Chairman of the NHS Trust Control of Infection Committee.

On 11 December 1989 Sir James Howie formally opened the Bacteriology Laboratory Extension which was built on the lawn across the driveway north of Pavilion 4. It provided much needed additional bench and office space. By 1989–90 the Bacteriology Laboratory was processing 56,432 specimens and the Scottish Mycobacterial Reference Laboratory 8,141 specimens per annum.[17] The staff complement had increased from Jimmy Craig alone, 50 years before, to two Consultants, one Registrar, 18 Medical Laboratory Scientific Officers, two part-time technicians and some auxiliary staff.[18]

The Respiratory Funtion Laboratory

Another laboratory development introduced in the 1960s was the testing of pulmonary function. Dr James Macnamara had been Senior Hospital Medical Officer (SHMO) in charge of pulmonary function studies at the City Hospital in a laboratory originally set up by Dr Andrew C. Douglas. Dr Ian W. B. Grant had looked after a similar laboratory at the Northern General Hospital. Later Drs Edward Harris and G. K. Crompton had been responsible for the service. Funds then became available from the Medical Research Council to augment the size of the laboratory and its equipment. In February 1965, backed by the Consultants in Respiratory Medicine, Professor Crofton recommended that the SHMO vacancy be filled by a Consultant Clinical Respiratory Physiologist. The appointee was to supervise the respiratory physiology laboratories at the City and

Northern General Hospitals, be the Consultant Respiratory Physiologist for the region and also have charge of eight respiratory beds at the City Hospital.[19]

Although appointed in September 1965, Dr G. J. Ross McHardy could not take up the new post for a further year during which time he was an International Post-doctoral Fellow in the US Public Health Service at Johns Hopkins University in Baltimore. Dr McHardy had trained at Oxford and the Middlesex Hospital and had held posts in the Departments of Medicine in both the Middlesex Hospital and the Royal Post-Graduate Medical School in Hammersmith. He supervised the enlargement of the Dorran-style Respiratory Function Laboratory near Ward 8 which ultimately provided blood gas analysis, pulmonary function and exercise testing.[20]

By 1973 Dr McHardy was responsible for pulmonary physiology testing at the Western and Northern General Hospitals as well as at the City Hospital. Five years later he took over the laboratory at the Royal Infirmary that had been set up by Professor D. C. Flenley. By 1981 he had created an area-wide Pulmonary Function Service with staff trained to uniform standards who could work throughout the whole network. Dr McHardy also played an important role in the confusing and rapidly changing medical administration of the time. He was successively Chairman of the Division of Medicine of the South Lothian District, Chairman of the South Lothian Division of Medicine and was then appointed the first Chairman of the Area Division of Medicine from 1989 to 1992. He retired in 1993.

The Medical Residency and Other Departments

During Dr Horne's Superintendentship, there were moves to regularise medical student teaching. Dr Murdoch encouraged overseas and local students to carry out clerkships during the summer vacation and requested free board and lodging for them.[21] The Board of Management felt accommodation for 25 living-in medical students was required and resolved to ask the Regional Hospital Board to consider a new building.[22] When this was agreed, Eric Hall & Partners were asked to design the new medical residency.[23] It was to be brick built with three 3-storey blocks each of nine bed-sitting rooms and one single-storey, rectangular block containing lounge, breakfast room, television room and kitchen.[24] A new roadway and car park for 20 vehicles was also planned.

Although it eventually cost £75,000, the original estimate of £58,000 for the new medical residency was accepted by the Regional Hospital Board. Later it was agreed that the cost be shared, the NHS contributing 26/36ths and the University the remaining 10/36ths.[25] The on-call surgical

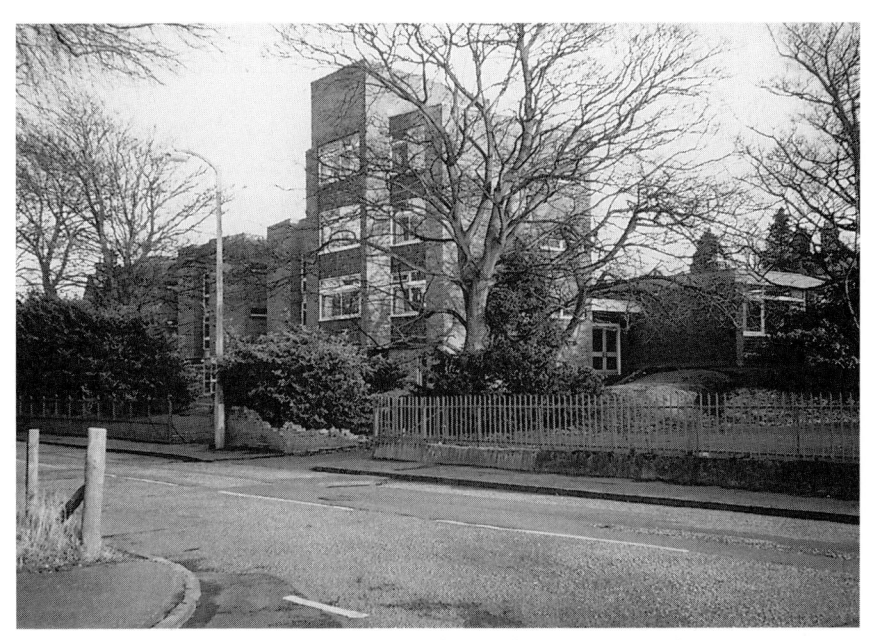

City Hospital medical residence from the north west. Doctors' quarters are on the left, students' tower block in the centre and dining and sitting rooms on the right. (Photo J. A. Gray)

teams were to be accommodated in the new residency as well as the resident doctors. The students would occupy the block with smaller bedrooms. Dean of Guild approval was granted in 1963 and John Dennis & Co. of Dalkeith were awarded the contract.[26] The building was completed and commissioned in November 1965.[27]

There followed a spirited battle between the resident doctors, the catering department and the Regional Hospital Board regarding dining facilities for living-in medical staff. Because of the distance from the kitchens and the increased costs of transporting food, the Regional Hospital Board decreed that only breakfast be served in the residency; all other meals were to be taken in the hospital canteen. Dr Horne strongly supported the resident doctors.[28] The British Medical Association's Central Consultants and Specialists' Committee resolution was quoted:

> The doctors should have their own dining room. The doctors' dining room has traditionally provided a forum for the exchange of opinions on clinical matters and for the discussion of difficult cases.[29]

Even though the Regional Hospital Board was asked to supply extra funds for staffing and transporting food to the residency for the evening meal, they only gave permission for dinner to be served in the residency until April 1966.[30] By November 1966 costing for a ramp to take trolleys to the residency and the extra costs of staffing were put to the Regional Hospital Board with appropriate justification[31] and, later still, the cost of a hoist for the trolleys in place of a ramp.[32] The arguments, however, dragged on. As late as March 1968 the residents would not accept an offer to have a screened-off area of the staff canteen set aside for them rather than their own residency dining room.[33] Eventually, however, the dining facilities in the residency were withdrawn despite the protestations of Dr Horne and the house doctors.

Another sad event at this time was the retiral of Miss Marion Miller after 45 years of service. This delightful lady of strict moral principles had mothered generations of residents at the City Hospital.[34] She was the residency maid or waitress and always wore a starched white apron. Her hair was tied in a tight bun with a long white ribbon. It was said that she originally came from the Isles as a teenager seeking service. Being teetotal, she strongly disapproved of some of the young doctors' habits. When a firkin of ale for a mess party was introduced into the old residency dining room, then in the general offices, Miss Miller would shake her head and 'Tut, tut' but smiled genially when requested to supply plenty of drinking straws for the barrel of 'lemonade'. The morning after the party she served breakfast to those residents who had to be on duty. Attending to one such doctor, who usually had a generous helping of bacon and two fried eggs, she looked closely at his drawn face and bloodshot eyes on the morning after the night before and declared 'No, no. I'm thinking just one small egg would do this morning, and that very lightly poached'. Miss Miller was just able to see her doctors into the new medical residency before she retired in December 1965. Meals would never be the same again without her devoted attendance.

The major new developments in capital building in the 1960s with their dates of completion and approximate final cost were the non-resident staff changing accommodation (1964) £56,000, new medical residency (1965) £75,000, stores and pharmacy block (1966) £60,000 and the ENT Department (1966) £260,000. Besides there had been the major upgrading of wards. In 1960 the Regional Hospital Board gave permission to upgrade Pavilion 8 at a cost of £27,500.[35] Other wards were to follow.

The former servants' home was converted into the X-ray Department, and Medical Out-patients' Department with offices above for the Respiratory Medicine Unit and Department of Geriatrics. This New Medical Block was officially opened in September 1961 by Mr Gumley on the same day as the nurses' Prize Giving.³⁶ The construction of the new kitchens and open plan staff dining room took place later, being opened in February 1971. The fine hardwood floor to this dining room so increased noise levels that normal dining-room conversation became impossible and it was soon carpeted to dampen the sound. After much campaigning by the thoracic surgeons, their theatre was upgraded on the site of former Cottage 11 to the east of Pavilion 5.³⁷

Three prefabricated, Dorran-design teaching rooms were erected in 1965, along the covered corridors, one each for Infectious Diseases and Tropical Medicine and the third for Respiratory Medicine and the Chest Unit. These were paid for by the Regional Hospital Board³⁸ and were used regularly each month by undergraduates attached to the different units. Postgraduates also continued to attend as part of the Internal Medicine Course and later its summer and autumn clinical courses run by the Postgraduate Board for Medicine. Clinical examinations for Part II of the MRCP (UK) diploma were also held regularly in the infectious diseases and respiratory medicine wards.

Dr Murdoch and his medical colleagues always pressed hard for the teaching status of the hospital to be recognised and maintained.³⁹ Both the building of the medical residency incorporating student accommodation and, in 1963, the provision of a medical library on the first floor of the New Medical Block helped maintain the teaching tradition. The library contained standard textbooks and journals reflecting the special disciplines in the hospital (except for ENT Surgery which had its own library in the ENT Unit). The cost of the fitting out of the library for the hospital was accepted by the Regional Hospital Board and the running costs shared between the Board and Edinburgh University, the latter also providing the part-time services of a trained librarian.⁴⁰ Opposite the medical library was the Medical Records Office. In 1965 Mr Jimmy Knowles was appointed Group Records Officer⁴¹ with responsibility for the case notes, X-rays, and admission and discharge documentation for the hospital group.

For administrative management, social and medical meetings (without patients) a conference room was built in 1963.⁴² It was equipped with attractive wooden panelling and furnishings and was situated at the east end of the infectious diseases corridor on the site of the former hospital visitors' interviewing room. For many years the Board of Management and its satellite committees used the conference room for their monthly meetings.

On 20 September 1967 the Board of Management recorded the untimely death of its Chairman, Dr Douglas M. Alston. He had joined the Board at its inception in 1948, was elected Vice-Chairman in 1955 and had been Chairman for more than eight years when he died. He was a popular and hard working official as this testimony from the Board suggests.

> Although modest and quietly spoken, he was nevertheless always in complete command of affairs. His knowledge of medical matters was of inestimable value to the Board and he was able to absorb the specialised knowledge and experience of other Board members and of officials and meld it all with a wisdom and purpose that was unique. He was Chairman of the Board during almost the whole period of great development which had taken place in all the hospitals in the Group – the City Hospital transformed in function, enhanced and extended in buildings, the Royal Victoria Hospital, Southfield and Loanhead Hospitals changed in function and greatly developed to serve the people of Edinburgh in the expansion of geriatric services. He guided everyone through it all with wisdom, foresight and dedication. For him, the healing, the comfort and the safety of the patient in hospital and clinic were foremost in his thoughts. On official occasions, when the formal business was over, it was not long before he had left the platform to mingle with members of staff of all grades. He enjoyed the complete confidence and affectionate respect of the administrators with whom he worked.[43]

Dr Alston was succeeded as Chairman by the Vice-Chairman, Mr C.J. Phillips; Dr J.McC. Murdoch then became Vice-Chairman.[44]

Opposite the conference room a small suite was created for the use of visitors who wished to spend the night when a relative was dangerously ill or dying.[45] Other services to visitors, patients and staff came with the provision of a hospital shop, Sub-Post Office and a branch of the Bank of Scotland. Initially the bank was housed in a prefabricated hut and opened for two hours each weekday and later also for two full days at the end of the month.[46] The bank then moved to the gate lodge and eventually to the central block which it shared with the hospital shop.[47] This did not happen, however, until the much delayed new pharmacy and stores block was built on the site of the former reception block and Cottage 13, the original X-ray Department.[48] Other improvements included the tarmacking of the spaces between pavilions to provide car parking. The 'boxing in' of the sides of the covered corridors between Pavilions started in 1963 at the Respiratory Medicine Department and Chest Unit[49] and only included the infectious diseases corridors after Dr Murdoch retired in 1983. He had objected to this 'boxing in' procedure, on the grounds of the spread of infection but patients transported in winter weather from wards to the X-ray Department would not have agreed with him.

One sacrifice made to improve the roads was the removal of the elm tree planted in 1903 by Queen Alexandra just east of general offices. The 'King's tree' to the west of the offices was preserved inside an iron railing for many more years until it too had to be removed.[50]

In June 1962, the Department for Health for Scotland and the Scottish Home and Health Department were dissolved and the new Scottish Home and Health Department and Scottish Development Department were formed. That same month, the Secretary of State approved the change of name from the 'City Hospital for Infectious Diseases' to the 'City Hospital'.[51] This more satisfactory title encompassed those new disciplines, either already established or proposed, which came to join the hospital (e.g. chest and respiratory medicine, thoracic and ENT surgery, geriatric medicine, etc.).

The Nursing Shortage

In the early 1960s Edinburgh hospitals suffered the national shortage of beds for emergency patients. The City Hospital had 612 staffed beds in March 1960.[52] In addition to the patients normally accepted into the specialist units, general medical admissions became routine. In March 1964 Dr Horne reported to the Board of Management that he had recently been asked by the Bed Bureau to find accommodation for 25 general medical patients and Dr Murdoch had already admitted five the previous evening to the Infectious Diseases Unit.[53]

Finding accommodation for acutely ill general medical patients put a strain on the medical staff. An even greater limiting factor to the hospital's functioning, however, was the shortage of nurses. This became particularly apparent when the admission figures rose dramatically as the ENT Department became established. During the summer of 1965 the monthly number of hospital admissions was in the upper 300s. The figures for 'infectious diseases' were augmented each month by 40–50 patients accepted into the Pyelonephritis Unit bringing the total there to 150–190. The Tropical Diseases Unit admitted about 10–20 each month, the Chest and Respiratory Diseases wards took in 110–150 with a further 10–20 with tuberculosis. The thoracic surgeons admitted 40–60 patients monthly and a handful of admissions labelled 'chronic sick' came into the long-stay wards. In November 1965, with 123 ENT admissions, the hospital's monthly intake rose hugely to 548,[54] from the upper 300 mark earlier that summer. Once the ENT Unit was fully operational, its monthly intake rose quickly. For instance in March 1971 there were 509 ENT admissions, pushing up the hospital's admissions that month to a total of 926.[55] The monthly admission figure for the hospital rarely fell below 700 in the later 1960s and early 1970s.

Despite the devotion of the ward sisters, nursing recruitment could be difficult particularly to the ENT and Care of the Elderly Units.

As early as December 1960[56] there were few applicants for senior nursing posts. despite all the entrants to the Preliminary and Final State Examinations being successful. Features discouraging recruitment were the heavy nursing, the increased turnover of patients, the introduction of the 44-hour week and the continuing dilution of trained staff by untrained nurses. Many recommendations were made, but the national advertising of vacancies was condemned. It was felt that this would pin-point the less attractive hospitals if they were frequently seen to be looking for staff.

Everything possible was done to enhance the lot of nurses. In 1961, the Matron, Miss Adams, asked for £15 for nurses' prizes and £3 for the C. B. Ker Memorial Medal which was still being presented annually. The Board of Management generously voted a total of £25 to cover both.[57]

In 1961, the Nursing Committee reported a disappointingly low number of Enrolled Nurses completing their training.[58] 1962, however, saw better facilities for pupil nurses in the upgraded infectious diseases wards where student and pupil nurses were to train together. Their work was to include respiratory diseases and tuberculosis. Out-patient duties would replace the unpopular ambulance duties. Mr A. R. Chase, who had just passed his Clinical Instructor's Examination, was to give in-service training to nursing auxiliaries.[59] Later that year Dr Horne proposed a staff nurses' course at the City Hospital in 'Infectious Diseases, Thoracic Medicine and Surgery'. This offered free lodging for candidates who agreed to work in the hospital for three months after the course or else enroll as staff nurses for six months.[60]

The paratyphoid outbreak in 1963 put a further strain on staff. Late that year, Miss Cordiner, Matron at the Royal Infirmary, recommended that some of her nurses should be seconded to the City Hospital for 'special experience' as the Group Nursing Training Scheme had been unsuccessful.[61] In late 1963 the Registered Nurse Training Committee agreed to second nurses from the Royal Infirmary, Dunfermline and West Fife and Peel Hospitals because of the 'excellent experience available in control of infection' at the City Hospital.[62] For six-week periods, up to 25 student nurses would be seconded. A further 10 nurses from the training school in south Edinburgh were to come to the City Hospital instead of going to Bangour General Hospital as formerly.[63] Dr Murdoch also pushed for the secondment of student nurses to train in the Pyelonephritis Unit.[64] One interesting initiative to improve conditions for nurses sadly did not materialise. The idea was to build a new nurses' home complex on the City Hospital site along the lines of corporation housing and equipped for both resident nursing and medical staff. It would also provide some accommodation for married staff.[65]

In October 1964 Miss Adams announced that she would cease to recruit nurses to the Fever Register. There were currently only nine nurses undergoing training in infectious diseases but they would be encouraged to complete the course. The possibility of a postgraduate course in infectious diseases to replace fever nurse training was to be explored.[66] The last official fever examination was set for October 1968. Any nurse failing at that time would not be allowed to resit.[67] As it happened the remaining three nurses M. McAulay, B. Watson and P. McKinney completed the course well before schedule. At a sad farewell ceremony on 1 June 1966 Lady Haddow presented them with their certificates, badges and prizes at the Board of Management meeting. She congratulated them on the smartness of the new pilot scheme uniforms they were wearing for the occasion. Dr Alston, the Chairman, also wished the nurses well. He reminded the meeting that fever nurse training had begun in 1919 and that an unknown but very large number of nurses had completed their training since then, including 460 since 1948.[68] With the disappearance of fever nurse training, however, another nail was driven into the recruitment coffin.

Other initiatives either proved only partly successful in aiding recruitment or else were not implemented. These included a comprehensive nursing training to include ENT surgery, a combined secondment for control of infection and paediatric nurse training, and a postgraduate course in infection control.[69] Miss Adams however, did designate 20 State Enrolled Nurse posts at the City Hospital to help staff Wards 5, 5A, 6, 8A, 18A and 19.[70]

The new nurses' uniforms to which Lady Haddow had referred (and which she had been instrumental in choosing) were tried out at Southfield and the City Hospitals.[71] There was to be a one-piece garment, changed daily, over which a barrier gown would be worn for ward duties. Linen aprons were abolished. Caps were to be similar for all staff, and seniority was to be denoted by coloured bars. Sisters and staff nurses were to wear black stockings and shoes and all other grades white shoes with light coloured stockings.[72]

Miss M. I. Adams, who had been appointed Matron in 1944, retired in September 1965 after very nearly 21 years in office. She had been particularly active in nursing training and committee work at Board, Regional and National levels.[73] She was succeeded by her Deputy Matron, Miss J. K. Taylor who became Matron Designate from 1 August 1965 and Matron a month later. This gap was to allow Miss Taylor to have a refresher course and visit other hospitals with problems similar to those at the City.[74] This included a fortnight at the Victoria Hospital, Belfast.[75] Miss A. E. Christie was appointed non-resident Deputy Matron to Miss Taylor.[76]

In 1965 a new title, the South Edinburgh School of Nursing, was conferred on the nurse training school, and agreed by all Boards of Management and the General Nursing Council.[77] Miss Taylor attributed the nursing shortage partly to the closure of the Fever Register, the fact that seconded nurses were only coming in their first and not subsequent years of training and, finally, the unpopular extra shifts worked by Preliminary Training School nurses when their colleagues were on 'block teaching'.[78] Miss Christie then reported a further drain by trained staff when three sisters and seven staff nurses left without replacements in June 1966.[79] On a happier note, however, at the Prize Giving ceremony of the South Edinburgh School of Nursing on 25 May 1966, Miss Keddie gave an excellent address and amongst those receiving certificates and prizes from Lady Birsay were four pupil nurses trained at the City Hospital.[80]

In January 1966 the Nursing Committee[81] recommended that the transfer of ENT beds from the Eastern General Hospital be delayed until March to allow more time to recruit nurses. Even in April 1966, Ward 4 could not be opened because of the nursing shortage.[82]

The next problem confronting the beleaguered nursing services was the Salmon Report in the 1966–67 period. This recategorising of grades of nursing staff was initially discussed at the Medical and Allied Services Committee on 6 July 1966, although the actual recommendations of the Salmon Report were not implemented until 1968. It was felt that the Matrons of smaller hospitals would lose control to more senior management and their 'figurehead image' would be destroyed. Middle management grades could be difficult to fill. The grouping together of schools of nursing was, however, greeted with favour.[83] Inevitably many nurses, felt that to 'leap up the Salmon ladder' above No. 6 grade (ward sister/charge nurse) and lose clinical input was not what they had become nurses for in the first place. An interesting (but perhaps nowadays commonplace) comment came from the Regional Hospital Board in 1971 regarding the implementation of the Salmon Report. It was reiterated by the Finance Convener who expressed the Board's:

> very considerable concern that a scheme that was encouraged by a Government Department and which inevitably cost additional money should not receive an allocation. There was evidence that Nursing Staff were extremely discouraged in this matter.[84]

In 1969 there was anxiety again about the number of nurses leaving.

The thoracic surgical theatre list had to be cut by 50 per cent. There were only 12 full-time staff nurses for 17 wards. Although the problem was a national one, it meant that, if there was an infectious epidemic, the City Hospital could no longer cope.[85] Ward 15A was closed temporarily. Rarely thereafter could it be staffed sufficiently to keep it open for any length of time. A reduction of more than 20 per cent in staff nurses seemed likely to continue over the winter of 1969–70.[86] This prompted a meeting between Miss A. E. Christie, Dr Horne and Mr Welstead with Dr Hugh Raeburn, Senior Administrative Medical Officer, and his Deputy Dr Ian Campbell, Mr Douglass, Secretary of the Regional Hospital Board, and Miss Brayton, Regional Nursing Officer. Unfortunately the result of their deliberations was not recorded.[87]

After only four years as Matron, Miss J. K. Taylor retired at the end of 1969. She had been trained at the City Hospital and her life was the hospital to which she had devoted many years of service. No one could have taken a kinder or more understanding view of staff problems than she did. She was the last Matron to live in the nurses' home. Miss I. S. Willox replaced her as Matron and, as well as not living in the nurses' home as her predecessors had, she discarded the uniform of Matron for a business suit.[88] In December 1970 she reported on the continuing nursing shortage at the City Hospital stating that the present establishment, including student and pupil nurses, was 325 but should be 363.[89] Shortly afterwards Miss Willox left the City Hospital having been promoted to Principal Nursing Officer of the Group.[90]

In April 1971 Miss A. E. Christie, the Deputy Matron, became the City Hospital Matron (Senior Nursing Officer, Salmon Grade 8). A year later she was able to report a slight improvement in the nursing establishment on the ENT Unit but was unable to guarantee how long it would last.[91] In 1973, however, despite wide advertising, including Northern Ireland, the nursing shortage was such that agency nurses were routinely employed to make up the deficit.[92] In September 1973 there were six staff nurses and two enrolled nurses employed at the City Hospital on an agency basis.[93] In planning the future of the hospital in 1974 it was repeated that a serious epidemic could not be managed in the face of the nursing staff shortage.

That the welfare of patients and their visitors deeply concerned the staff and administrators can be illustrated by two developments during Dr Horne's Superintendentship: the Tea Room and the bus service.

The City Hospital Tea Room

An outstanding example of voluntary service by the congregations of Greenbank Church and neighbouring churches was the provision of a

1960–74: New Clinical Units and Laboratories

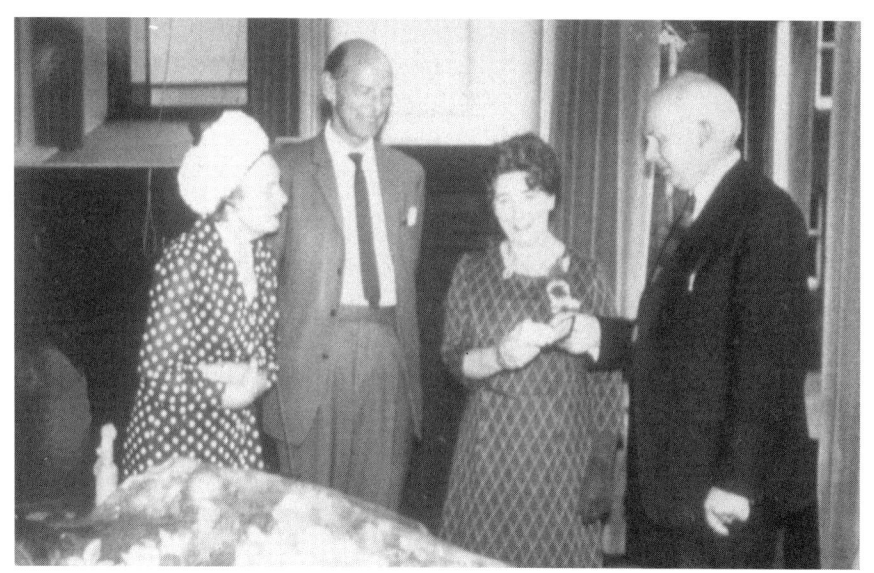

Miss J. K. Taylor's farewell presentation, 1969. Left to right: Lady Haddow, Mr A. G. Welstead, Miss Taylor and Dr N. W. Horne. (By courtesy of Miss J. K. Taylor)

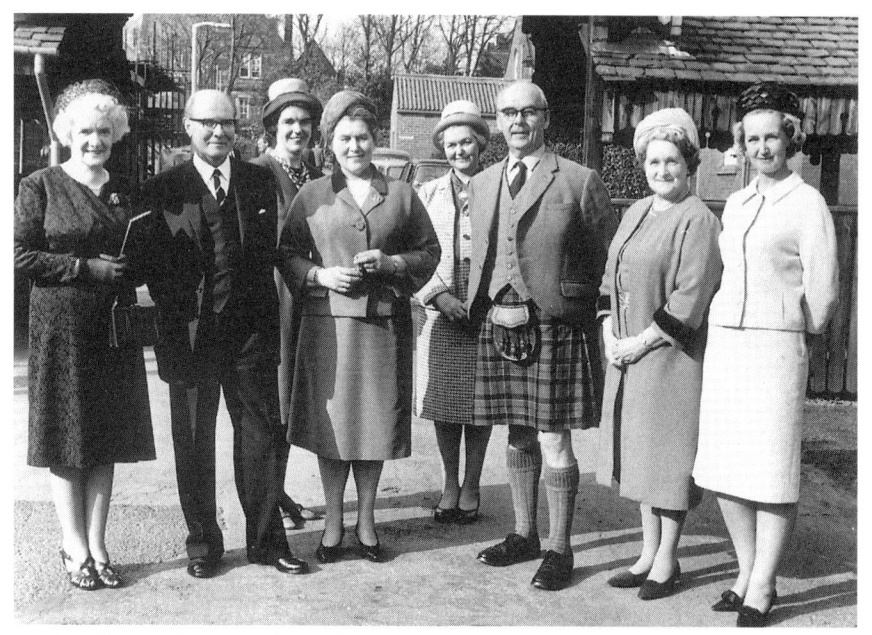

Opening of the City Hospital Tea Room, 2 April 1965. Left to right: Miss M. I. Adams, Matron; Dr Douglas Alston, Chairman, Board of Management; Mrs Joyce Tulloch; Mrs Elsie Dickerson; Mrs Lora Craw; Sheriff Harold Leslie (later Lord Birsay) who performed the opening ceremony; Mrs Christian Mitchellhill and Mrs Ruth Dundas. (Photo John K. Wilkie, by kind permission of Mrs Wilkie)

Tea Room for ambulant patients, visitors and staff. In 1965 Dr Horne, an elder of Greenbank Church, had put forward the idea of a Tea Room to the then Minister, the late Rev. Mr Donald Mackay. The concept received enthusiastic support and on 1 April 1965 a prefabricated building between Ward 18 and the New Medical Block was formally opened by Sheriff Harold Leslie. Teams drawn from 250 devoted volunteers not only provided a welcome service but donated their profits to the hospital. Generous annual contributions from the Tea Room have financed the upgrading of wards and waiting rooms and provided new furnishings and comforts for patients. The Tea Room would still be running successfully and probably would have continued indefinitely were it not for the imminent closure of the hospital. With much reluctance, after its 32 years service, it was decided that the Tea Room must close. A farewell party was held before its doors shut for the last time in October 1997.

The Bus Service

A second initiative, which became a long drawn out struggle, was the hospital's fight to improve the bus service. In the early years of the hospital, when visiting was actively discouraged, it perhaps did not matter that the trams and buses came no nearer to the east side of the hospital than Comiston Road. However it was, even then, a problem for non-resident staff. In May 1960, Councillor M. R. Mackenzie, a member of the Board of Management, agreed to recommend to the Town Council that the 39/41 bus service should be extended at least as far as the top of the hill in Greenbank Drive at the east end of the hospital.[94] By July 1960, Councillor Mackenzie had prevailed upon the city authorities to get the bus to run as far as a point between the engineer's house and the coal entrance, provided that a reversing bay was made there within the hospital grounds.[95] This bay was completed in September 1961 and was granted on a 20 year lease to the Corporation.[96] The service started running to that point the following month.

Nonetheless, the Corporation was criticised for not extending the service to the main gate, which would especially help elderly visitors coming to the hospital in bad weather. Worse was to come. In December 1962 the Corporation withdrew the service altogether and substituted a special bus to run from Comiston Road on visiting days.[97] By February 1963, even this special visitors' bus was withdrawn despite strong objections by the Board of Management and Regional Hospital Board.[98] In November 1963 it was intimated that the No. 39 bus service would be withdrawn altogether but the No. 41 would run quarter-hourly instead.[99]

The Town Clerk and the Corporation Transport Committee stated in 1965 that no additional City Hospital bus could be agreed upon [100] but later that year Councillor Mrs N. Mansbridge and Councillor Fitzpatrick proposed to the Transport Manager that the only satisfactory solution would be to run a route through from Firrhill to Morningside. [101] This was put to the Highway Committee [102] but without result. In 1967, with no further solutions in sight, the *Edinburgh Evening News and Dispatch* reported on the bus transport problems for the large number of visitors and out-patients attending the hospital. [103] This may finally have stimulated the Transport Manager to review the possibility of the bus running to the main gate [104] and a sum of £2,300 was quoted for this. [105]

The saga continued. The frequency of service dropped in 1968. Councillor Mrs Mansbridge was asked to reinvestigate the possibility of extending the service to the west end of Greenbank Drive, [106] and the City Transport promised to reappraise a turn-around at the west end of the Drive. [107] Two months later, in June 1968, agreement was reached for an enlarged turn-around, the cost to be shared between the local authority, the NHS and the General Post Office (GPO) as this would also provide better access to its nearby radiomast. [108]

No progress was made until almost 18 months later. Dr Horne was asked to invite the Transport Manager to the next Board Meeting and an 'Action Wanted' piece was to be submitted to the *Edinburgh Evening News*. [109] Next month the Corporation put out tenders for the enlargement of the turning area. [110] Work started on this in June 1970 [111] and was completed by July 1970 [112] when the Transport Manager also agreed to help towards the cost of a bus shelter. The Board of Management must have sighed with relief knowing the 10 year long battle had been won. In September 1970 it was informed that the extended No. 41 bus service to the hospital's main gate was at last a reality.

Social and Sporting Events

Besides improving amenities for patients, visitors and staff with the extended bus service, the hospital bank, shop and Tea Room, there was the lighter side to hospital life as well. In the summer of 1964 Dr (later Professor) Barry Kay produced a fine open-air performance of *A Midsummer-Night's Dream* with members of staff as Oberon, Titania, Bottom, Puck and the fairies flitting in and out of the Corsican pine trees to the south of the Respiratory Medicine wards. It was a great success.

Cricket also became a passion for some members of staff and their friends. The adaptation of two rooms in a workshop close to the cricket pitch was approved by the General Purposes Committee in May

1965 [113] and £60 was voted for changing room accommodation.[114] Dr Graham K. Crompton, who became a locum Consultant Chest Physician at the City Hospital whilst Dr Horne was in Baroda in 1966, was one of the leading cricket enthusiasts, as well as Dr Horne (when not overseas). Dr Crompton later became a Consultant in the Northern General Hospital with Dr I. W. B. Grant. Other notable cricketers were Mr Alec Welstead, Group Secretary and Treasurer, and Mr Robert Fairley, Deputy Secretary of the Board but also Honorary Secretary of the City Hospital Cricket Club. In August 1968 Bob Fairley asked the Board's permission to lift and relay part of the recreation ground as a cricket pitch. Professional advice was taken and some money came from the Welfare Fund, but the Club members themselves provided the labour. The Board acquiesced and 'noted with pleasure the success of the C. H. C. C during the past four seasons'.[115]

Preparing for a Reorganised Health Service

In addition to his skills on the cricket pitch, Mr Welstead was the epitome of a Group Secretary and Treasurer. Events were moving quickly towards the 1974 reorganisation of the health service in Scotland when he decided to move to the Borders rather than be incorporated into the South Lothian District of the new Lothian Health Board. His departure after 22 years of unstinting service was a great loss to the City Hospital. He could look back on many achievements. Despite all the changes which had taken place his maxim, 'Any system can be made to work if the staff concerned want it to – No system will work well if the staff have no faith in it'[116] still holds good today. He took up his new appointment as Secretary to the Borders Health Board on 1 April 1974.

As far as the City Hospital itself was concerned, there was much disquiet in the Medical and Allied Services Committee of the Board of Management in November 1973.[117] Despite requests over the previous five years, the Board of Management and the Regional Hospital Board had not discussed the future of the City Hospital in times that were changing rapidly and demands on the service were different from what they had been even ten years before.[118] The Chairman of the Board of Management wrote to the Chief Medical Officer at the Scottish Home and Health Department regarding the lack of any fruitful discussion with Regional Hospital Board.[119] The Regional Board regretfully acknowledged that forward planning was unlikely to take place until the new Lothian Health Board, which was to replace the relevant part of the South-Eastern Regional Hospital Board (Scotland), had taken charge of the health services in Lothian with effect from 1 April 1974.

The Board of Management, however, made the following six points regarding the City Hospital.

1. The full potential of the Hospital was not being used.
2. Staffing difficulties were already serious and would became disastrous if any further specialties were introduced.
3. The lack of use of this nurse training ground would lead to a further effect on recruitment in the future.
4. The Regional Board was to be informed that the Hospital was no longer in a position to meet the demands of an epidemic should it arise.
5. The lack of purpose and knowledge of the future was seriously affecting morale.
6. Present considerations such as the possible transfer of the Bacteriology Laboratory (to the Western General Hospital) would only worsen the situation.[120]

In December 1973 the Regional Board in turn expressed its concern that the City Hospital could not cope with an epidemic. Wards simply could not open at short notice because of the staff shortage.[121]

Three days before the South-Eastern Regional Hospital Board (Scotland) was to cease functioning and the City Hospital came under the auspices of the South Lothian District of the new Lothian Health Board, the last meeting of the Board of Management was informed that its Chairman Mr C. J. Phillips, Dr N. W. Horne and Mr A. G. Welstead had at last met with Mr Eliot-Binns and others of the Scottish Home and Health Department in St Andrews House. A little more hope was given to the City Hospital staff. They were told future development at the Hospital would take place. They were informed that there was no immediate solution to the medical and nursing staff shortage but that no new medical or surgical beds were likely to be introduced. The 40 acres of ground still available for building would provide a persuasive argument in deciding if the City Hospital would become the new district hospital for the south side of the city.[122] Perhaps there was after all a glimmer of hope for a rebirth of the hospital to reward all the efforts that had been made to build it up over the previous 14 years.

Staff changes were also imminent. Dr Archie Wallace retired from the hospital after 26 years of service, and Mr Alec Welstead after 22 years of service. Dr Horne would no longer be Physician Superintendent but agreed to take on the Chairmanship of the Medical Staff Committee in succession to Dr I. M. Farquharson. Times were indeed changing but many more changes were to come in the next two decades.

CHAPTER TWENTY-EIGHT

1974–94: A Reorganised Health Service; Infectious Diseases and AIDS; the Fire in the Nurses' Home; Milestone House

Reorganisation of the Health Service
Although I worked as a clinician before, during and after the 1974 reorganisation of the NHS in Scotland, I am is still sometimes bemused by its complexity and aftermath.[1] Administration and management changes followed fast upon each other. Who would be responsible, to whom, or to which committee? Old positions vanished; some reappeared in a different guise; new ones were created. Both familiar and unknown faces filled the new posts. Some well-known clinicians struggled bravely on within the rapidly changing administrative and managerial hierarchy and adjusted to their new roles with a good grace. Had it not been for their determination to ensure that a workable system emerged each time a change was imposed, chaos would have reigned and much of the previously cherished goodwill in the NHS could have been lost forever.

This account attempts to summarise the organisational changes from 1974 to 1994, as far as they concerned the City Hospital.[2] Until 1 April 1974, the City Hospital was administered by the Royal Victoria and Associated Hospitals Board of Management which in turn was responsible to the South-Eastern Regional Hospital Board, Scotland. This Regional Hospital Board covered hospital services in Fife, Lothians and the Borders. Resulting from 'Reorganisation of the NHS in Scotland' in 1974, these Regional Hospital Boards were replaced by Area Health Boards such as the Lothian Health Board. Although the new Area Boards were geographically smaller, they were responsible not only for each hospital in their area but also for providing health services previously administered by local authorities and executive councils. So far as the hospitals were concerned, the three-tier system of Regional Hospital Boards, Boards of Management and hospitals was replaced by another three-tier system of Area Health Boards, Health Districts and then the individual hospitals. Consensus style management was introduced at all levels.

The Lothian Health Board had three Health Districts: North, South and West. The City Hospital came under the South Lothian Health District which geographically covered clinical services in Midlothian and the City of Edinburgh south of Princes Street. It included hospitals and clinics as disparate in size and function as the Royal Infirmary, the Simpson Memorial Maternity Pavilion, Queen Mary Maternity Hospital, Chalmers Hospital, the Princess Alexandra Eye Pavilion, the Royal Hospital for Sick Children, the Princess Margaret Rose Orthopaedic Hospital, the Astley Ainsle Hospital, Bruntsfield, Deaconess, Longmore, Southfield, Liberton, Loanhead, Rosslynlee and Gogarburn Hospitals and the Royal Victoria Dispensary – as well as the City Hospital.

By January 1974 a proleptic South Lothian Health District Executive Group had formed with Dr A. H. Duncan as District Medical Officer, Mr W. J. Farquhar as District Administrator and Mr D. G. Nicolson as District Finance Officer. Over the next few years Dr Harry Duncan was succeeded by Drs Roger Barclay and Rosamund Gruer as District Medical Officers. Miss M. S. Laing was appointed District Nursing Officer.[3] Simultaneously Professor J. D. Roberston (Anaesthetics) and Dr A. A. Brown (General Practice) became respectively Chairman and Vice-Chairman of the new South Lothian District Medical (Advisory) Committee.[4] An advisory Division of Medicine for the South Lothian District respectively appointed as the Chairman and Vice-Chairman of its Executive Committee, Dr N. W. Horne (former Physician Superintendent of the City Hospital) and Dr J. D. Matthews (Consultant Physician in the Royal Infirmary).[5]

By the mid-to-late 1970s, the new consensus management style and multi-tiered administration was felt to be impeding decision making, the development of new medical strategies and the fostering of good relations with local authorities and union representatives. A Royal Commission was set up therefore in 1976:

> to consider in the interests both of the patients and those who work in the NHS the best use and management of the financial and management resources of the NHS.

It reported in 1979.[6] After much consultation, the Secretary of State decided that the Area Health Boards themselves had functioned satisfactorily, but that those Boards which contained several Districts should abolish them in favour of forming a unitary district within the area. This it was hoped would remove one tier of management. In Lothian this was implemented by setting up hospital management groups (each comprising several hospitals) which reported to an Area Executive Group. Between 1984 and 1987, therefore, the City Hospital with the Bruntsfield, Deaconess, Liberton and Longmore Hospitals came under one of these

Lothian Health Board Units of Management. Mr Jack Burton, its Unit Administrator, proved to be likeable and efficient. He had come to the City Hospital via the Astley Ainslie Hospital and Royal Infirmary. His two assistants were Mr Stuart Docherty, and Mr Malcolm Wright, who later became Chief Executive of the Royal Hospital for Sick Children NHS Trust. During his time as Unit Administrator, Mr Burton supervised the closing of the Deaconess and Bruntsfield Hospitals. When Unit General Management replaced the District system in 1987–88, Mr Burton returned to the Astley Ainslie Hospital as an Assistant Manager.[7]

No sooner was the new system established in 1985 than a businessman, Mr Roy Griffiths, published the recommendations which the Government had asked his team to provide regarding the best way to manage manpower and other resources in the NHS. This Griffiths Report introduced the concept of general management in *all* tiers of administration with tight budgeting control in each unit. Clinicians were also to become budget holders. They were to allocate the manpower, staffing and resources consistent with their workload and within specified financial constraints.

Following the introduction of general management, Mr Winston Tayler was appointed as the first General Manager of the Lothian Health Board in 1986. He was succeeded, following an inter-regnum when Professor Frank Clark was General Manager, by Mr John Lusby and then in 1995 by Mr Trevor Jones.

By 1987, seven units had been created within the new Lothian Health Board structure. The Royal Infirmary, the Simpson Memorial Maternity Pavilion, Elsie Inglis Memorial Maternity Hospital and the Dental Hospital were reunited as a single unit after four years of separation. Other units were the East and West Units, the Mental Health Unit, the Royal Victoria, Western and Northern General Hospitals Unit, the United Hospitals Unit and finally the Primary Care and Community Unit. Each unit was the responsibility of a Unit General Manager, a post that was open to managers and professionals.

The City Hospital became part of the United Hospitals Unit together with Princess Margaret Rose Orthopaedic Hospital, the Royal Hospital for Sick Children, the Astley Ainslie, Bruntsfield, Longmore, Liberton, Southfield and Loanhead Hospitals, the Royal Victoria Dispensary, the Mass Radiography Unit and the Area Sterilising Service. The General Manager of this conglomerate United Hospitals Unit was a Consultant in Community Medicine, Dr Sheena Parker.[8] She was particularly welcome as a medically qualified manager, married to a Consultant Haematologist in the Royal Infirmary, and as someone who could appreciate the problems of clinicians trying to adjust to the changes that were taking place.

The Operational Services Manager at the City Hospital was Mr Jim Smith who has continued to serve the hospital in a friendly and efficient manner. He had worked previously at Princess Margaret Rose Orthopaedic Hospital from 1971 to 1980, then in administration at the Royal Hospital for Sick Children and the Simpson Memorial Maternity Pavilion before being deployed to the City Hospital in 1987.[9]

In 1990 Mr Ken Dobson succeeded Dr Parker as Unit General Manager of the United Hospitals Unit. The City Hospital's local Manager from 1990 to 1993 was Mr Robert (Bob) Purves. Having previously been the City Hospital's Principal Nurse he was appointed in 1993 to be in charge of Operations, Nursing and Quality in the new Royal Infirmary NHS Hospital Trust.

The formation of NHS Trusts was the result of a White Paper, 'Working for Patients (Scotland)'. It introduced the new concept of the purchaser-provider system and an internal market. This was yet another major change in the organisation of the NHS to which everyone had to adapt quickly. Basically the Health Boards purchased the services they required for the community they served from the Trusts which usually comprised one large hospital or a group of hospitals. From the seven Units established in Lothian in 1987, there emerged six NHS Trusts. The first was West Lothian whose services were accepted by Lothian Health Board in 1992. The other five followed in 1993–94: the Royal Infirmary, of which Trust the City Hospital was part, the Western General Hospital, the Royal Hospital for Sick Children, the East Lothian and Midlothian Trusts and finally Edinburgh Health Care Trust.

The Royal Infirmary NHS Trust's Chairman was Professor Cairns Aitken, with experience in psychiatry and rehabilitation before he became Vice-Principal (Planning and Budgeting) of the University of Edinburgh. The Chief Executive was Mr John J. Owens and the first Medical Director at the Royal Infirmary was Dr Iain A. Davidson, a Consultant Anaesthetist with a flair for administration, followed later by Dr Charles Swainson, a renal physician.

At the City Hospital Arnold G. D. Maran, Professor of Otolaryngology, a noted head and neck surgeon and later President of the Royal College of Surgeons of Edinburgh, became the Head of Service. He worked closely with Mr Mike Pearson, Business Manager, with Mr Jim Smith and with Mrs Maureen Lees, who became Principal Nurse after Mr Purves had left for the Royal Infirmary. Collectively they have had the unenviable task of presiding over a hospital in its declining years and providing its staff with much needed boosts to their morale.

Because of their complexity, the administrative and managerial changes in the organisation of NHS from 1974 to 1994 have deliberately been described in sequence. It is now appropriate to consider the condition of the City Hospital at the time of 'Reorganisation of the NHS in Scotland', 1974.

The Hospital Review [10] had reported on 31 March 1973 that the City Hospital was regarded as a 'General Hospital with some teaching units but not necessarily wholly teaching'. Of its 573 beds, 181 were for infectious diseases (with a further 80 in reserve or unclassified), 95 for chest medicine, 93 for ENT surgery, 46 for respiratory tuberculosis, 42 for thoracic surgery and 36 for geriatric medicine. There were 25 staffed wards and two isolation cottages, four operating theatres and three endoscopy rooms. The X-ray Department had two functioning rooms, a 'skull room', two mobile and three portable X-ray machines.

In 'whole time equivalents' (WTE) at the City Hospital, there were 312 nurses, 196 domestic and ancillary staff, 54 laundry workers, 44.3 medical and dental staff, 32 craftsmen, 26 professional and technical staff, 23 administrative and clerical staff and seven 'others' making a WTE staff complement of 694.3.[11] The net annual running costs of the hospital were £1,155,161. All the major departments, except geriatric medicine, had busy out-patient clinics with annual attendances ranging from 440 for respiratory tuberculosis to 26,390 in physiotherapy.

The Hospital Review listed the major additions and upgrading in the period of new building and refurbishing during Dr Horne's Physician Superintendentship from 1960 to 1974.[12] Adverse comments were made on the poor quality of accommodation for resident nursing staff. In the nurses' home, in fact, only 40 of the 132 bedrooms had been upgraded and attractively decorated but a further 20 were about to be modernised. It was unusual for more than 100 nurses to live in at any time and 12 of the bedrooms had already been allocated to resident domestic staff. The two flats consisting of 5 and 4 rooms each (for Matron and Assistant Matron or Home Sister respectively) were empty in March 1973. The bed-sitting room accommodation for eight living-in sisters was considered substandard.

The Hospital Review commented favourably on the new changing room accommodation for non-resident staff and on the modern residency for medical staff and students. The wooden huts, which had once been temporary wards and later occupied by the social workers, physiotherapists and occupational therapists would be replaced. The physiotherapists and occupational therapists would move to the new central block [13] and the social workers eventually to the lodge at the main gate.

In addition to re-siting the Departments of Physiotherapy, Occupational Therapy and Social Work, the Regional Board, before being disbanded, promised that a Sterilising Centre, Sterile Infusion Production Centre and Area Pharmacy should be developed at the City Hospital.[14] During the actual building of the new Department of Dermatology at the Royal Infirmary Lauriston Building, skin patients would be temporarily housed at the City Hospital.[15] The City Hospital also supplied services to many other hospitals outside its own requirements. These included the use made by other hospitals of the Regional Virus Laboratory, the Bacteriology and Respiratory Physiology Laboratories, the Group Pharmacy and Stores.[16] Moreover, the newly upgraded laundry catered for 15 other hospitals besides the City Hospital,[17] and the Personnel Department for 10 hospitals was run by Miss Mary Weir from the former Medical Superintendent's home at the City Hospital from October 1975 until she retired in 1986.

Most importantly before the Regional Board disbanded, it agreed that the City Hospital should continue to be the isolation hospital for the whole area formerly covered by the South Eastern Region south of the Firth of Forth.[18] Cameron Hospital at Windygates in Fife and King's Cross Hospital in Dundee would provide the required isolation accommodation immediately north of the Forth. It, therefore, seemed in 1974 at the time of the reorganisation of the NHS in Scotland that the future of the City Hospital was secure.

The Regional Infectious Diseases Unit (RIDU)

In 1975 the population in Lothian was estimated to be about 754,000. Of the classical infectious diseases, notifications of measles had doubled in the previous year up to 1,452.[19] Figures for whooping cough were also high at 375, rising to 611 in 1978 and 888 in 1982.[20] This probably reflected a lack of confidence in pertussis immunisation because of the combination of reports of vaccine induced encephalopathy and the erroneous impression that whooping cough was no longer a serious disease. In 1982 only about 50 per cent of pre-school children in Lothian were receiving measles and whooping cough immunisation.[21]

In 1975 no cases of diphtheria or poliomyelitis were reported in Lothian[22] and only one of each in the whole of Scotland that year suggesting that, despite the far from perfect uptake of immunisation, these diseases were being conquered. Rubella remained a common cause of notification with an outbreak in Lothian in 1979 of 4,302 cases.[23] When boys as well as girls were routinely immunised against German measles with the introduction of MMR (measles, mumps and rubella), notifications of rubella dramatically dropped.

In 1975 viral hepatitis was the third commonest disease notified in Lothian with 298 cases.[24] This may have reflected the introduction of hepatitis type B although the various types of hepatitis were not then differentiated for statistical returns. Increasingly food poisoning came to oust dysentery as a more common cause of gastrointestinal infection. The proportion of *Shigella sonnei* dysentery cases dropped and the number of reports of food poisoning rose to 1,127 in 1981.[25] Of these 630 were of the recently recognised camplylobacter organisms and 439 of various salmonellae. Thereafter the food poisoning notification figures appeared to drop but this was due to the change in recording whereby only outbreaks of food poisoning were reported, not isolated, sporadic cases on their own. Scarlet fever, which had required 320 beds to be set aside in the City Hospital in 1903, was still being notified but with a peak of only 201 cases in the whole of Lothian in 1980.[26] It was also a much milder illness without the serious complications of previous years.

At the City Hospital the total bed complement dropped from 569 in 1975 to 523 in 1986.[27] The number of beds for infectious diseases progressively fell from 199 to 103 with an average of only 70 staffed beds. The mean length of stay in the Infectious Diseases Unit fell from 10.6 days to 7.9 days during this period. The annual number of discharges, deaths or transfers, however, remained fairly constant between 1,738 (1983) and 2,042 (1985) confirming there was still a need for isolation facilities. The low average daily bed occupancy of 42 in the Infectious Diseases Unit was explained by the need to keep some beds empty to allow for the rapid intake of patients in the event of an outbreak. In response to the Health Board's request for more beds to be made available for general medical patients in the winter of 1974–75, 17 beds were allocated from the Infectious Diseases Unit.[28]

By 1977 the beds in Ward 17, previously occupied by men with infectious diseases, had been converted into beds for women with acute general medical illnesses and were looked after by Dr Sangster. Dr Murdoch objected strongly to the suggestion that beds upstairs in Ward 17A should also be used for general medical cases.[29] In fact they never were, more because of nursing shortages than because of the demand or the type of patient that was to occupy them.

In 1974 the senior medical staff of the Infectious Diseases Unit – later called the Regional Infectious Diseases Unit (RIDU) – were Dr James Murdoch, Dr George Sangster and myself. Dr C. Christopher Smith, the Senior Registrar of the Unit, and noted cricketer, had been appointed in 1973 to a consultant post with general medical beds in the Aberdeen Royal Infirmary and infectious diseases beds in the Aberdeen City Hospital. He was followed as Senior Registrar in March 1974 by Dr Sam Pickens, who afterwards became a Consultant Physician in Burnley. Dr Raymond P. Brettle was the next Senior Registrar from 1979 to 1983 when, after his visit to North Carolina, he was appointed Consultant in Infectious Diseases in the City Hospital to replace Dr Murdoch. Dr W. T. Andrew Todd, a well-liked Registrar in the Unit from 1979 to 1981, returned from medical experience in Harare, Zimbabwe, to become the next Senior Registrar in 1983. He spent nine months of his rotation with Dr J. D. Matthews at the Royal Infirmary. In October 1985 he left to take up a Consultant position at Monklands and Bellshill Hospitals. Dr Todd's successor was Dr Graham Douglas, Senior Registrar 1985–86, who had already trained in respiratory medicine. He was afterwards appointed to a Consultant post with Dr C. C. Smith in Aberdeen Royal Infirmary and the Infection Unit at Urquhart Road, Aberdeen. Dr A. (Tony) J. France who followed Dr Douglas had also been trained in respiratory medicine. He came to the Unit for experience in infectious diseases and HIV infection from January 1986 to September 1989 when he was appointed to King's Cross Hospital in Dundee with responsibility for HIV and AIDS patients in Tayside. Dr Peter J. Flegg, who had worked with Dr Brettle as a research fellow in HIV infection, followed Dr France as Senior Registrar. Dr Flegg held the DTM&H and had previously obtained tropical medicine experience in his native Zimbabwe. He became a Consultant in Blackpool in 1997.

During this time a rotation scheme between the RIDU and the Genito-Urinary Medicine Unit at the Royal Infirmary had led to Dr Carolyn Thompson and Dr Jonathan Ross coming to the City Hospital for further training in the management of HIV infections whilst Senior Registrars from the City Hospital in turn acquired experience in the field of sexually transmitted infections at the Royal Infirmary.

By 1980, Dr George Sangster had retired after 32 years of service to the City Hospital. He was missed as a clinical teacher and as one of the Unit's much loved characters. He was succeeded by Dr Philip D. Welsby, FRCPEd, who had trained at the Royal Free Hospital School of Medicine in London, graduating in 1970. Dr Welsby subsequently trained in Surrey, Aberdeen and then returned to the Royal Free Hospital in London for more experience with infectious diseases. He is an inveterate commentator on the local and international medical scene and the keyboard of his word processor hardly ever rests. He is author or co-author of several books on infectious diseases. He illustrates his medical lectures with masterpieces of clinical photography. He swims almost daily. With his clarinet he leads a small group of wind instrument players who entertain both colleagues and patients at the hospital, and old folk in their nursing homes.

The next change in senior staff in the RIDU came about when Dr Murdoch retired aged 60 in 1983 after 23 years as the senior consultant. He died in 1996 but will be long remembered for his enthusiastic 'larger than life' approach, his contributions to the study of urinary infection and antibiotics and his close links with the pharmaceutical industry and medical colleagues all over the world.

HIV Infection

The unit's Senior Registrar, who had been working for two years in North Carolina, was appointed to replace Dr Murdoch. Dr Raymond P. Brettle had been identified as a bright, hard working, research-oriented doctor who would not let the grass grow under his feet. He graduated from the University of Edinburgh in 1974, passed the MRCP (UK) examination in 1976 and became FRCPEd in 1986. He was invited to give three named lectures and later, as a consultant, held the Abbott Research Travelling Fellowship, the Winston Churchill Trust Fellowship and the WHO/Council of Europe Fellowship which he used to study models of AIDS care in Europe and the USA. He has worked both in Manchester and the Royal Postgraduate Medical School in Hammersmith.

While nominally a Senior Registrar in the Regional Infectious Diseases Unit, Dr Brettle was in fact a Fellow in Infectious Diseases in North Carolina. There he gained experience in HIV disease which was to become his special interest. HIV infection was spreading rapidly in the USA about three years ahead of the UK. Dr Brettle was later to write

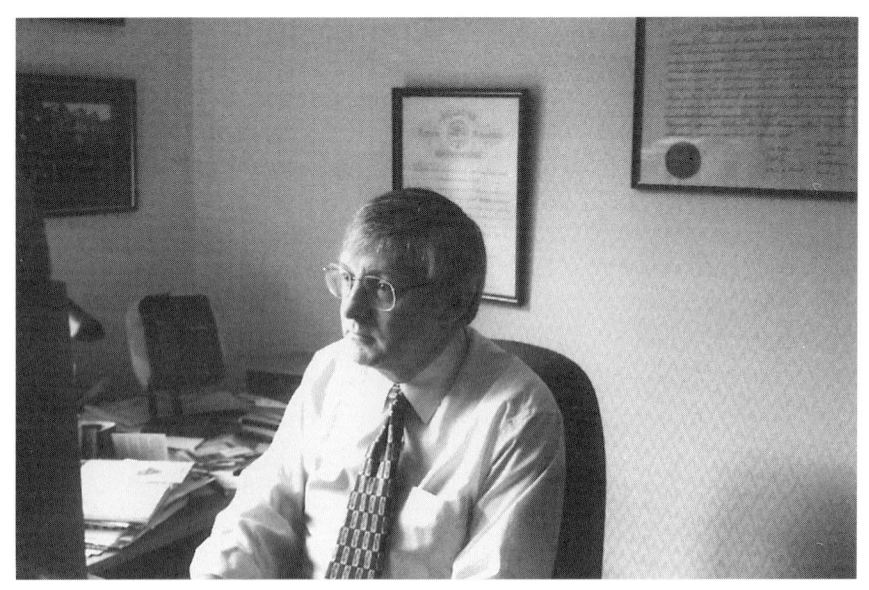

Dr Ray P. Brettle, 1998, Clinical Director of the RIDU and expert in HIV infection. (Photo by courtesy of Mrs Helene Brettle)

his two-volume gold medal MD thesis on this subject and the associated drug misuse in Edinburgh. He became an international authority on HIV infection and an adviser to countries like Malaysia which had similar problems of intravenous heroin misuse and HIV disease. His research and the new services he set up for screening, treating and preventing HIV infection were recognised by the University of Edinburgh in 1995 when he was made part-time Reader.

The increased workload caused by HIV infection was such that a fourth consultant became necessary for the RIDU. In May 1989 Dr Clifford (Lam Shang) Leen was appointed. A native of Mauritius, he studied in Edinburgh, qualified MB, ChB in 1978 and passed the MRCP (UK) examination in 1982. He trained in the Royal Infirmary of Edinburgh and then as Senior Registrar in the Infectious Diseases Unit at Monsall Hospital, Manchester. The subject of his MD thesis (1987) related to research work he had previously carried out with intravenous immunoglobulins and immunotherapy in the Scottish Blood Transfusion Service with Dr Brian McClelland. This experience was to be valuable in his Consultant post at the City Hospital where he took particular interest in HIV infection.

When I retired in 1995 after 26 years in the RIDU, I was replaced by Dr David Wilks, who held the MB, BChir (Cambridge 1983) and who gained the MA, MD in 1991. He passed the MRCP (UK) examination in 1986 and the DTM&H in 1987. He had been Senior Registrar in Infectious Diseases at Addenbrooke's Hospital, Cambridge and, before that, a Research Registrar in Immunology at the Clinical Research Centre, Harrow, Middlesex. He is co-author of *The Infectious Diseases Manual* (Blackwell Scientific 1995).

In 1986 viral hepatitis was still responsible for a continual stream of admissions to the RIDU, fewer with hepatitis type A but more with drug-misuse-associated hepatitis type B. Hepatitis virus type C may have been responsible for some hepatitis admissions although its identification and that of the other non A, non B forms of hepatitis virus was not then routinely possible. Staphylococcal endocarditis and hepatitis type B, infections commonly associated with injecting drug misuse, were prevalent in the 1970s and early 1980s. They were indicators of the forthcoming heroin-associated HIV epidemic which was to have a major impact on the work of the RIDU from then on.

To put the Edinburgh HIV epidemic in the world perspective, the early story of HIV infection bears retelling. In 1981 a report in *The Lancet* described a very rare tumour, Kaposi's sarcoma, in eight young homosexual men in the USA.[30] When the Centers for Disease Control in Atlanta, Georgia, in 1981 and 1982 reported the combination of oral thrush, Kaposi's sarcoma and the previously rare *Pneumocystis carinii* pneumonia in other gay groups, it seemed likely that some transmissible agent was responsible.[31] In 1983 the Paris laboratory of Dr Luc Montagnier reported the isolation of the responsible virus and in the USA Dr Robert Gallo succeeded in propagating the virus in a cell line in 1984.

This virus was originally named Human T-cell lymphotrophic Virus III (HTLV-III) as it attached itself to T4 lymphocytes (CD4 cells) an important part of the body's cellular defence mechanism. An alternative name was the Lymphadenopathy Associated Virus (LAV) because of the enlarged lymph glands found in the disease. Later both these terms were replaced by Human Immunodeficiency Virus type 1 (HIV–1). It was shown to have originated in East Africa and to cause the Acquired Immunodeficiency Syndrome (AIDS). The similar virus, HIV–2, from West Africa has not spread to the same extent. In sub-Saharan Africa the route of infection of HIV–1 is predominantly heterosexual but, when introduced to the Western world, the virus was disseminated initially by male homosexual practices and injecting drug misuse and to a lesser extent by heterosexual intercourse.

After the virus has established itself in the body, normally over a period of years the victim remains well but may be infective. The symptomatic stage of the disease begins with fever, lethargy and enlarged lymph glands. This in time may progress to full blown AIDS when the individual is abnormally susceptible to viral, fungal, protozoic and some bacterial infections and may also develop malignant diseases such as lymphomas and Kaposi's sarcoma. Although modern treatment of HIV infection prolongs life, most patients with AIDS ultimately die. At any time the number of deaths in a cohort of patients with AIDS is about 50 per cent. By mid-1996 21,000,000 adults and 830,000 children had been infected with HIV globally and the estimate of AIDS cases was 7,700,000 (77 per cent in Africa) with a cumulative mortality of 4,500,000 adults and 1,300,000 children. The problem continues to grow.

In his gold medal MD thesis 'Human Immodeficiency Virus, The Edinburgh Epidemic',[32] Dr Ray Brettle describes HIV infection in the Lothians and how it differed from epidemics in other parts of the UK and in other Western countries. By 1989, 82 per cent of AIDS notifications in the UK involved homo- or bi-sexual practices alone and only 2 per cent implicated injecting drug misuse alone as the risk activity. At that time only 3.8 per cent of all AIDS reports were from Scotland and 11 of them were in drug misusers. In the UK as a whole, only 16 per cent of notifications of HIV infections were among drug misusers. By contrast in Scotland those infected with HIV through drug misuse comprised 54 per cent of whom 60 per cent were from Edinburgh.

An early indication of the problems Edinburgh was to face came from the tragic news that 15 out of 34 (44 per cent) haemophiliacs in Edinburgh had become HIV-antibody positive between 1983 and 1984 having received treatment for their bleeding tendency with the clotting agent Factor VIII derived only from local blood donors.[33] This suggested significant levels of infection among those donating blood in Edinburgh up to October 1985 after which the Scottish National Blood Transfusion Service routinely screened all its donors.

At the same time Dr Roy Robertson of the West Granton Medical Group was investigating the numerous drug misusers in his 18,000 patient general practice in a deprived part of Edinburgh. Together with Dr Bucknall and colleagues in clinical and virology disciplines, the report he wrote was startling.[34] Among 164 intravenous heroin misusers in his practice, Dr Robertson found 83 (51 per cent) positive for HIV antibodies. About 70 had acquired the infection during the 15 months after midsummer 1983 and the remainder by the end of 1985. The 83 HIV-positive drug misusers were young, with a mean age of 24.1 years, and 23 of them were women.

It was later found there had been some intravenous heroin misuse as early as 1965.[35] Intense needle sharing amongst heroin users took place in the early 1980s after an Edinburgh surgical supply shop closed and police activity discouraged drug users from carrying potentially incriminating syringes and needles on their person. This led to groups of 10–20 people congregating at the drug supplier's address and sharing equipment which at best was rinsed with tap water between users. During this time, cheap brown heroin from Pakistan became readily available, thus adding to the problem.

An increasing number of people started to inject between 1975 and 1983 in which year the figures peaked, subsequently declining rapidly. Unfortunately this period of intense needle sharing in 1983–84 coincided with the introduction of HIV infection into Edinburgh. The virus probably came in through a few mobile misusers who had shared needles in European capitals like Amsterdam and in other parts of the UK.

When Dr Brettle returned from North Carolina to take up his Consultant post at the City Hospital in 1983, he was acutely aware of the problems in the USA where the HIV epidemic was a few years ahead of that in the UK. With considerable foresight he approached the Scottish Home and Health Department for funding to set up the UK's first self-referral HIV screening clinic for those who preferred to attend an infectious diseases unit rather than their own GP or a sexually transmitted diseases unit.

This pilot study clinic set out to determine the extent of the infection among those attending and to provide data to show whether there was a demand for such a service. It was also hoped that the City Hospital Screening Clinic (CHSC) would reduce the risks to the Blood Transfusion Service which might otherwise be used dangerously as a diagnostic screening facility by those who donors felt they were at risk. Indeed the opening of the CHSC on 16 October 1985 was purposely timed to coincide with the introduction of routine testing of all blood donors. The services of the CHSC were announced in the press, the Blood Transfusion Service, Scottish AIDS Monitor, Gay Switchboard and in drug abuse agencies. All local GPs were circulated. Data collection and the protection of the Blood Transfusion Service from high-risk donors, however, were not the only objects of the CHSC. It also offered assistance to those found antibody positive, and targeted health education at high-risk individuals whether positive or not.

The clinic was made user friendly with its own confidential telephone line and answering machine informing callers of clinic hours. Initially the CHSC operated every afternoon from Mondays to Thursdays, each session staffed by a doctor and a nurse counsellor with appropriate AIDS counselling training. Most patients were given an appointment within 24–48 hours and adequate time was given for pre- and post-test counselling with the offer of a full medical examination and follow-up to those found positive. Both verbal and written advice were features of the clinic irrespective of risk factors or whether the client agreed to testing and, if so, irrespective of the result. Clients were encouraged to let the CHSC inform their GPs of test results but, if they did not agree, the patient alone was given the result. Those considered at high risk despite a negative test were offered a further appointment some months ahead.

In his 'Preliminary Report of Progress (October 1985-March 1986)' Dr Brettle showed that despite 'no shows' numbering 107, a total of 204 had attended in the first six months. Although patients came from as far afield as London, Glasgow and the north of Scotland, and nine gave no address, 161 (80.5 per cent) were from the city of Edinburgh. Of all those attending, 67 per cent were either intravenous drug misusers or their sexual contacts. The prevalence of antibody to the AIDS virus was high (65 per cent) among drug misusers but low (5 per cent), at that time, among their sexual contacts. Only 7.5 per cent of homosexuals or bisexuals were positive. The mean age of the drug misusers was 25 years, 22.9 years for those antibody positive and 29.25 years for those antibody negative. Those starting to inject younger (mean 17.5 years) were more likely to be positive. Ninety-eight per cent of drug misusers admitted needle sharing, a habit which correlated closely with positivity for antibodies to the AIDS and hepatitis B viruses.

The expected high primary default rate made staffing difficult. Most of those who did attend once, however, were motivated to reattend and did so. Imprisonment on drug related charges or the distance of the CHSC from their homes were reasons for some not attending. Both of these considerations were to some extent met when Dr Brettle opened a screening clinic at Leith Hospital and later another in Saughton prison.

Dr Brettle, therefore, amply justified the continuation of the clinic on its first six months' showing. He projected from this the costs of the in-patient and out-patient services that would ultimately be required to care for the large number of antibody positive drug misusers in the community. The CHSC became the focus for health care workers, social workers, occupational health nurses, foster parents and a source of local and national information.

The staff increased as more funding became available: Dr Alison Richardson, Top Grade Clinical Psychologist, Dr W. Anne Tait, Consultant Psychiatrist, Dr Bal Dhillon, Consultant Ophthalmologist, to advise on the toxoplasma and cytomegalovirus eye infections in AIDS patients, Mr Gordon Bolas and colleagues to care for the shocking dental decay and poor mouth hygiene of drug misusers, Dr (later Professor) Robert Will and then Dr Robin Grant on the neurological problems. Dr Claire Benton, Consultant Dermatologist now provides expertise on the skin manifestations of HIV disease.

Dr Sami Moussa gives valuable advice on the radiological aspects of AIDS diagnosis. Professor J. Best and Dr Brettle obtained generous funding from the Medical Research Council and University of Edinburgh to provide an HIV-patient dedicated MRI scanner which occupied a custom-made brick building between Wards 16 and 17. The scanner's high quality imaging assisted in the differential diagnosis of HIV-associated brain atrophy, multi-focal leucoencephalopathy, cerebral infections such as toxoplasmosis and *Herpes simplex*, and tumours such as lymphomas.

As these services were developing, out-reach nurses were appointed to provide care in patients' homes and their collaboration with social workers and drug misuse agencies became very important.

In 1986 Dr Jacqueline Mok, a Consultant Community Paediatrician, was appointed to look after antibody positive pregnant women and their babies together with Dr Frank Johnstone, Consultant Obstetrician at Simpson Memorial Maternity Pavilion. Together they assessed the risk of infection in newly born babies born to HIV-antibody positive mothers. In the early days, when it was thought many babies were truly infected rather than being transiently positive with maternal antibody, termination was often advised. Later as a result of the work of Dr Mok and Dr Johnstone, the factors predisposing to true neonatal infection were better appreciated and terminations were rarely advised. Besides, the recommendations that the mother take the anti-HIV drug, zidovudine (AZT), in her last trimester of pregnancy, that she be delivered by caesarean section and discouraged from breast feeding were shown to decrease significantly the risk of transmitting HIV from mother to baby.

Pneumocystis pneumonia frequently caused death in patients with AIDS in the early days. Then it was shown that high doses of cotrimoxazole given at the onset of the illness often provided effective treatment, and lower doses of cotrimoxazole or inhaled pentamidine could be used for prophylaxis. Nonetheless isolation of *Pneumocystis carinii* was difficult without invasive procedures such as the open lung and transtracheal biopsies employed in the USA or diagnostic lavage of the airways through a bronchoscope. Hence a close liaison was maintained with the chest physicians, and Dr (later Professor) W. MacNee was particularly helpful at that time in carrying out emergency bronchoscopies on these ill patients.

Because of the particular interest of Dr Sheila Burns, who became Director of the Regional Virus Laboratory in 1989, the diagnosis of pneumocystis pneumonia became easier. Highly sensitive monoclonal antibody techniques replaced silver staining for the identification of the organism. Satisfactory specimens were obtained after the more acceptable, and safer, saline inhalations and coughing performed by specially trained physiotherapists were introduced and so replaced the previous unpleasant procedures. The new diagnostic techniques would still yield positive results even up to a day or two after cotrimoxazole treatment had been started. There was therefore less urgency in proving the diagnosis and bronchoscopy was no longer needed. Any hypoxic AIDS patient suspected of pneumocystic disease could be treated at once without awaiting microbiological confirmation. The prognosis improved dramatically as a result.

Dr J. (Hamish) M. Inglis, Director of the Regional Virus Laboratory, had been very active in the development of HIV testing techniques when the epidemic started. He, Dr Burns and their colleagues, Dr Heather Cubie and more recently Dr N. Hallam, with the Senior Chief MLSO Mr David Hargreaves have contributed greatly to the rapid diagnosis of HIV infection, pneumocystis pneumonia, and associated viral illnesses such as cytomegalovirus, *Herpes zoster* and *simplex* and the newer hepatitis viruses.

Similarly the bacteriologists, Dr Brian Watt and Dr Xavier Emmanuel, provided new methods for diagnosing opportunistic bacterial infections in AIDS patients. Dr Watt, as the Director of the Scottish Mycobacteria Reference Laboratory, developed rapid diagnostic techniques and sensitivity tests for the atypical mycobacteria (TB-like bacteria) which often invaded patients with advanced AIDS.

Dr Helen E. Zealley, Chief Administrative Medical Officer to the Lothian Health Board became Director of Public Health in December 1989. Her report 'Health in Lothian 1974–89'[36] summarised the events which had occurred since the last of the Public Health Department's Annual Reports in 1974. She filled in the gaps created by the absence of any really satisfactory account of those years during which the HIV epidemic became established. The Standing Conference on Drug Abuse (SCODA)[37] had reported that the number of new narcotic addicts notified to the Home Office by the Lothian and Borders Police increased rapidly in the 1980s, that the three-fold increase of drug related offences between 1979 and 1984 had remained at a high level, that there were proportionately more hard drug seizures in Edinburgh than in Glasgow, the young age at which Edinburgh's misusers started injecting and the concomitant increase in hepatitis B infections in the 1980s. More women reported for treatment of drug misuse in 1984 (45 per cent) than in 1981 (33 per cent). The Community Drugs Problem Service (CDPS) under the care of Dr Judy Greenwood, Consultant Community Psychiatrist, had seen 314 drug abusers by the end of 1989 and estimated that there were between 1,500 and 2,000 injection misusers in Lothian. Dr Greenwood was awarded the OBE for her work in this field and for liaising with the general practices that were affected by patients with drug related problems.

Dr Zealley's report[38] showed that, by late 1989, 70 people in Lothian had full blown AIDS and 1,036 were HIV infected. Each week in 1989 showed one new case of AIDS and two newly diagnosed with HIV infection. Of those infected in Lothian, 52 per cent had shared needles and only 13 per cent were homosexual. By complete contrast in the rest of the UK only 15 per cent were infected by drug misuse and 49 per cent were infected by homosexual practices. This accorded well with Dr Brettle's findings.[39] In Lothian the HIV-infection rate was 141 per 100,000 compared with only 21 per 100,000 in the rest of the UK.[40]

Funding for HIV infection in Scotland was initially divided equally among all the Health Boards so that Orkney and Shetland with no notified cases received the same as Lothian which had the most. Later this funding maldistribution was corrected to reflect more equitably the number of HIV-infected people in each Health Board. The Lothian Health Board's General Manager's Report 1987–88[41] commented that, during the first year that funding had been given by SHHD specifically for dealing with AIDS, the Board would be able to meet the first year of costs of a 15-bedded AIDS unit to be established at the City Hospital.

Dr George Bath, who was tragically to die young of cancer, was appointed AIDS Coordinator. He estimated in the 1987–88 Report[42] that 1,000 people in Lothian had been infected with HIV by drug misuse and that the total infected in Lothian from all causes was between 1,500 and 2,000. By 1991 he predicted there would be two or three new cases of HIV infection reported every week. He applauded the funding for the new AIDS Unit at the City Hospital. A needle exchange was already in operation and the Community Drugs Project was proposed. The Lothian Health Board's Annual Report for 1991–92[43] confirmed that the new 15-bedded AIDS Unit at the City Hospital and outreach clinics at Saughton Prison and Leith Hospital had been established. There was also funding for the MRI scanner through the Medical Research Council and the Department of Radiology of the University of Edinburgh.

The new AIDS Unit in Ward 14 at the City Hospital was specifically not labelled as a ward concerned with HIV infection so that no stigma should be attached. Besides, its well-appointed intensive care room could be used for both AIDS and non-AIDS patients. There were 11 single rooms (with television, integral shower and toilet) and a 4-bedded area for less ill patients. The extra space needed was made by a 'bubble' projecting westwards from the side of the ward which then enclosed a small courtyard patio with potted plants. The privacy of the single rooms was much appreciated by patients but involved extra nursing and increased the difficulty of observing patients who persisted with drug misuse in hospital.

A dedicated nursing team, admirably led by Sister Shirley Parker and later by Sister Sheena Boyle, coped courageously with the emotional stresses of the ward as well as physical and verbal abuse from drug misusers. The Rev. Dr R. (Bob) C. M. Mathers, the Hospital Chaplain, gave much needed spiritual comfort to relatives, patients and staff. He even officiated at the marriage of some patients. After attending the funeral service Dr Mathers had conducted for a fellow patient, one AIDS sufferer poignantly told him how beautiful it had been and would he please see her into her own grave when the time came.

At the far end of the Infectious Diseases corridor in Ward 17 Dr Brettle and his colleagues masterminded a brand new out-patient clinic with a reception area, new waiting space, treatment and consulting rooms. In 1992 an adjacent extension to the records office was built at the blocked-off end of the corridor. Above in Ward 17A were counselling rooms for Dr Kate Bissett and her staff, a room for Mrs Anne Chisholm and Mr Vince Egan carrying out auditory evoked responses and psychological testing to predict HIV encephalopathy, and rooms for research staff, secretaries and meetings. Miss Pauline Douglas (later Mrs Burns) coordinated the secretarial staff upstairs while Ms Barbara Hamilton was active on the research front.

The reception staff in Ward 17 were the ever courteous and reliable Mrs Maureen Boddie and Mrs Anne Scott. Sister Mina Begg quickly stamped her memorable, couthy, and firm mark on the out-patient clinic. Her blunt spoken but friendly manner and sense of humour, despite all the difficulties of running a clinic coping with ID and HIV infected patients, set an example to all who worked there; she quickly earned the respect of patients and staff. She had succeeded the jovial, larger than life, Sister Cossar whom the RIDU inherited as out-patient sister, on the amalgamation of Tropical Diseases Unit with the RIDU.

Dr Brettle held meetings on Monday mornings to coordinate in-patient and out-patient care, research work and new initiatives into HIV infection. Among those who worked closely with him were Dr Michael Jones, Dr Jim Bingham, Mrs Sue Davidson, Mrs Claire MacCallum and Drs Linda MacCallum, Gwyneth Jones, Robert Laing, Peter Flegg, Valerie Hayhurst, Sue McHardy and P. Hughes.

On Friday afternoons the medical, hospital and district nursing, occupational and physiotherapeutic staff, social workers, counsellors, Mrs Sue Maxwell, representatives of the Community Drugs Problem Service (CDPS), Milestone House and the Chaplain all met in the Conference Room to discuss the current in-patients and coordinate their further medical care and welfare. These totally confidential meetings helped to up-date staff on patients' progress and provided a forum for inter-disciplinary exchanges.

Milestone House

Milestone House opened in February 1991 as the first, purpose-built, AIDS hospice in the United Kingdom. Founded by Lothian Health Board, Lothian Region Council and the Waverley Care Trust, it became a model for the accommodation, facilities and staffing arrangements required. An attractive, single-storey, brick and wood building with much light and airiness, Milestone House stands within the fringe of pine trees which are all that remain of the Coronation Wood that had been planted in 1953 at the hospital's west gate. Dr Linda MacCallum and Ms Ruth Murie (Mrs Ruth McCabe) and later Dr Jennesse Cameron must take credit for the usually smooth running of the hospice. Consultants from the RIDU could be called in to see their own patients who were in respite or terminal care at the request of the Milestone House team which was otherwise self-sufficient. A Milestone House representative always attended the Friday afternoon meetings in the City Hospital Conference Room. In 1991 the House was visited by Diana,

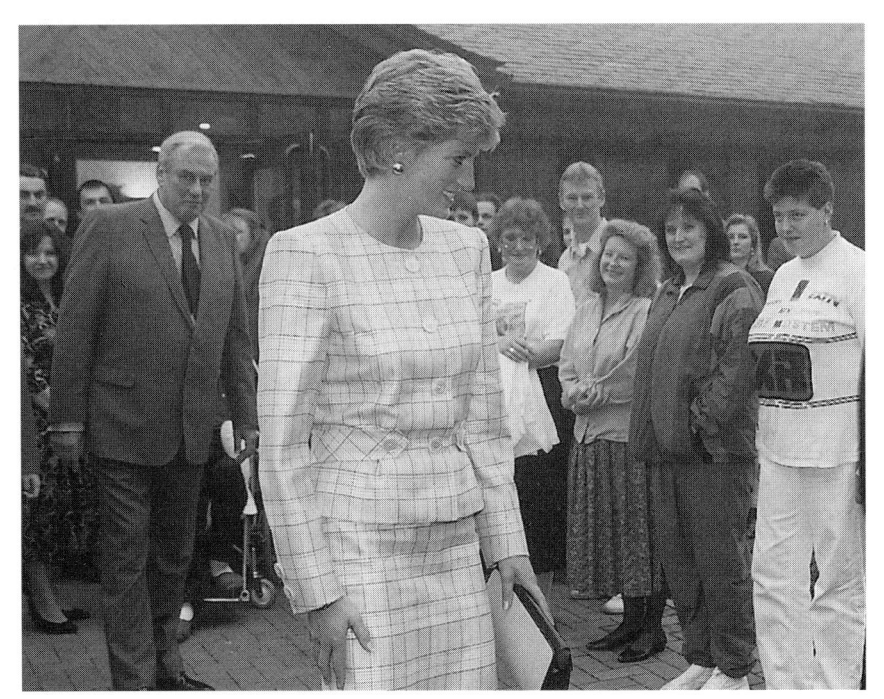

Diana, Princess of Wales, visits Milestone House, 21 October 1991, with Mr Roger Kent, Waverley Care Trust behind her. (By courtesy of Scotsman Publications Ltd)

Princess of Wales and by Sean Connery both of whom helped to boost the morale of patients and staff.

The Fire in the Nurses' Home

During the building of the new HIV and AIDS facilities in the hospital the RIDU was temporarily lodged in Ward 7A. Viewed from there one sunny November afternoon in 1988, what was initially thought to be a large bonfire of fallen leaves behind the nurses' home was soon appreciated to be a fire actually in and not simply behind the home. It rapidly spread through the upper floor and roof space of the south east wing of the building, emerging with spectacular plumes of flame and smoke from the ventilation towers. The Fire Brigade attended promptly with numerous appliances and eventually brought the blaze under control. Fortunately no one was killed or hurt. The fire and water damage meant that the two upper floors had to be abandoned as unsafe. No satisfactory explanation for the cause of the fire was found.[44] The lack of use of the whole building as a dormitory led to its demolition a few years later leaving a gap behind the New Medical Block which was then afforded a fine view of the Pentland Hills.

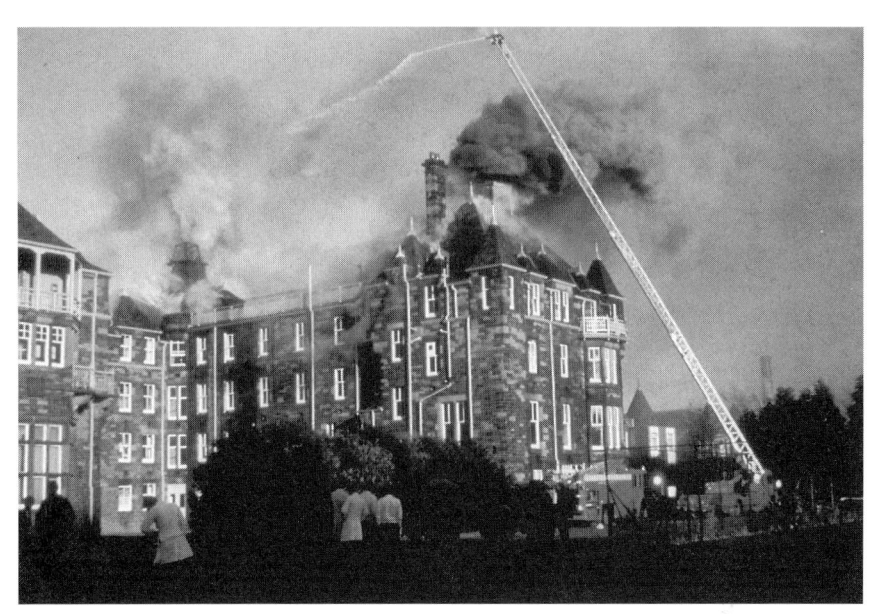

Fire in the nurses' home fire, November 1988 (Photo by courtesy of Dr M. E. Jones)

Dr Michael Jones, who had first noted the nurses' home fire from Ward 7A, was an important member of the RIDU team. He had joined the Unit as a locum Consultant in 1983 after Dr Murdoch retired and remained until Dr Brettle was appointed. He had formerly been a medical missionary in Tanzania but had to return to the UK because of illness in his family. With his wife Elizabeth, a trained counsellor, he set up a respite centre in Berwickshire for missionaries on leave from overseas. Dr Jones still works with Dr Brettle's HIV-infected patients. He was also instrumental in setting up the tropical disease advice centre in Ward 17 which provided intending travellers with immunisations, malaria prophylaxis and recommendations on how to keep well abroad.

The Findings of Dr Brettle's HIV Research Team

Dr Brettle and colleagues continued working with and researching their HIV-infected patients. By March 1990 contact had been made with 470 HIV-infected people of whom 77 per cent were infected through drug misuse, 13 per cent were male homosexuals and only 8 per cent appeared to have acquired the infection heterosexually.[45] Once contact had been made and care initiated for the HIV-infected drug misusers, the emphasis was placed on harm reduction with methadone substitution, needle exchanges, counselling of patients and relatives, and health education.

Dr Brettle was clear that methods of harm reduction without counselling were unlikely to succeed.

By the end of 1992, 624 HIV sero-positive people had attended the out-patient clinic at the RIDU of whom 70 per cent were intravenous drug misusers. Sixty per cent of all these out-patient attenders had been admitted at some point and 154 had developed AIDS.[46] The services of the HIV team at Saughton prison were much in demand as Dr Brettle reckoned that at any one time 10 per cent of his clinic population were in prison. Dr Jacqueline Mok's family clinic which started on 1 January 1986, had by the end of September that year counselled and examined 23 mothers and babies at risk.[47]

Research has involved the follow-up of this unique cohort of patients most of whom had acquired the virus at about the same time. Rates of progression from the estimated time of infection to the development of AIDS were measured. The older patients — and also the very young in Dr Mok's study — progressed most quickly. Advancing disease was predicted by clinical and laboratory testing and latterly by calculating the virus load by polymerase chain reaction. Transmission of HIV by the heterosexual and perinatal routes was also closely monitored.

Studies on the phamacokinetics of zidovudine in drug misusers taking methadone showed their increased susceptibility to the nucleoside analogues. The effect of zidovudine on the platelets and blood cells was monitored. Dr Brettle participated actively in the international studies on anti-HIV therapy such as Concorde. Various drug combinations with nucleoside analogues, transcriptase and protease inhibitors now offer genuine hope for HIV-infected people. Management of opportunistic infections such as pneumocystis pneumonia, cytomegalovrus retinitis, atypical mycobacterial and fungal diseases are other areas of research, together with the investigation of the effect of dual infections with hepatitis viruses and HIV which are common in drug misusers. Much is still awaiting investigation.

That these HIV-infected drug misusers were particularly difficult to manage was endorsed by Dr Brettle and by his fellow consultants, the nursing staff and all the paramedical support personnel who came in contact with them. Many of the patients carried out criminal activities in pursuit of their drug habit. They manipulated statutory agencies, distrusted official organisations and utilised poorly, if at all, any existing health services. Many came from deprived home environments and generally exhibited a chaotic behaviour pattern.[48] Unlike the gay groups, there was little self-support among the drug misusers.

Dr Brettle and his colleagues must take credit for winning the confidence of so many of these difficult patients and families, and for providing them with continuing care. Counselling seemed to be the key factor, together with harm reduction advice. Only in this way was an epidemic of truly disastrous proportions prevented from developing. A plateau was achieved in the number of new cases of HIV infection instead of the previously predicted steeply rising curve on the graph. This resulted from a dramatic reduction in needle sharing and an overall lessening of injecting drug misuse. These changes were a remarkable achievement. Although much remains to be done, it seems Dr Brettle was indeed the right man at the right time.

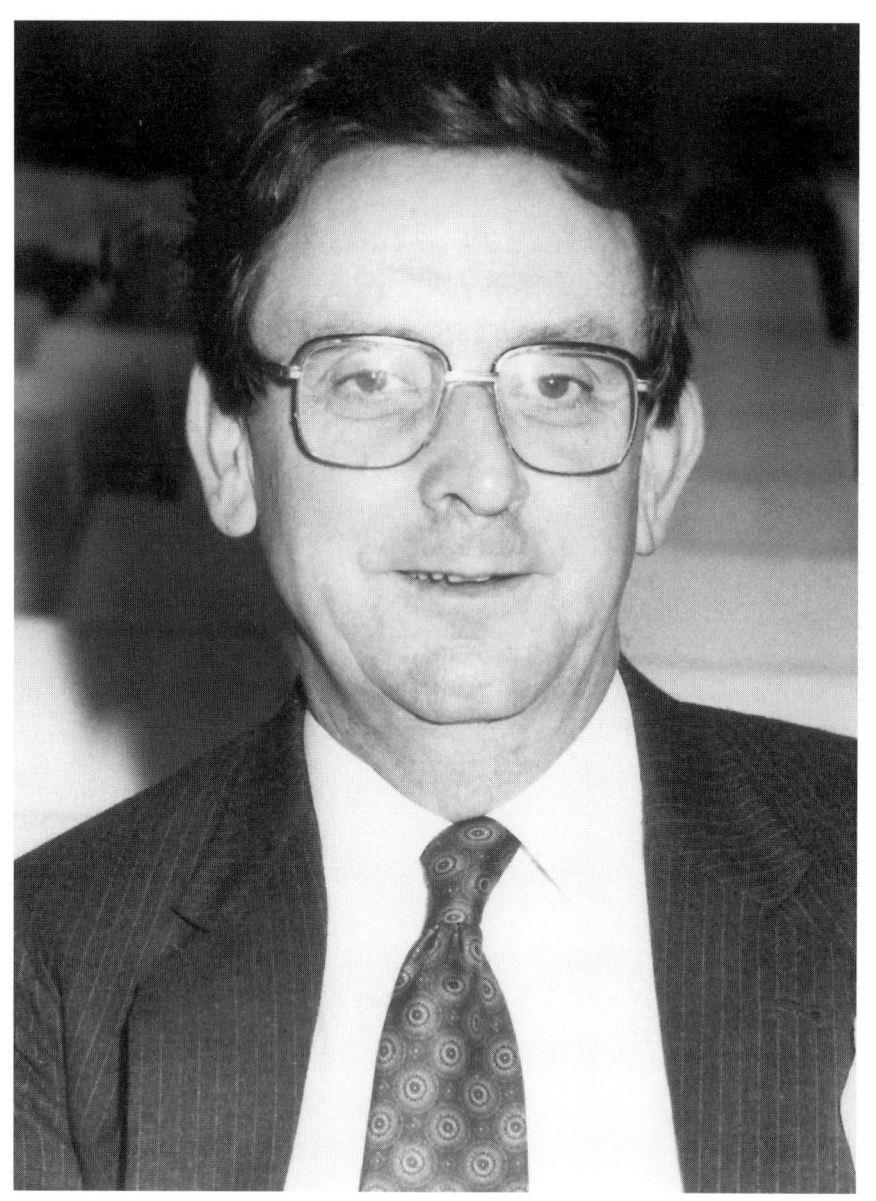

Professor David C. Flenley, Head of the Respiratory Medicine Unit, 1978–89. (Photo: Fotocronache 'Olympia', Milan)

CHAPTER TWENTY-NINE

1974–94: Respiratory and Chest Medicine; the Rayne Laboratory; Thoracic, ENT and Maxillofacial Surgery; Care of the Elderly Unit; the X-ray Department

Respiratory and chest medicine; the Rayne Laboratory
If Dr Ray Brettle of the Regional Infectious Diseases Unit was the man to control the spread of HIV infection in Edinburgh, similarly but earlier, Professor David Flenley of the University Department of Respiratory Medicine, proved to be the man to investigate the pathophysiology of lung disorders and devise the modern treatment of chronic obstructive airways disease (formerly chronic bronchitis) and emphysema. The department of which he became Senior Lecturer and Honorary Consultant Physician in 1969, Reader in 1974 and then Professor from 1978 to 1989 was originally the University Department of Tuberculosis. It thereafter changed its name from the Department of Tuberculosis and other Respiratory Diseases to the Department of Respiratory Diseases, then to the Department of Respiratory Medicine and finally to the Unit of Respiratory Medicine.

David Caton Flenley was born in 1933 son of a Lancashire general practitioner and never lost his blunt, to the point, Lancastrian approach to life.[1] From Baines Grammar School he obtained a Ministry of Education State Scholarship on entrance to the University of Edinburgh in 1950. From then on he distinguished himself academically with a First Class Honours Degree in Physiology (1954), an Honours MB, ChB (1957) winning the Ettles Scholarship and Leslie Gold Medal as the most distinguished medical graduate of his year. He became MRCPEd (1962) and MRCP London (1965) and was elected a Fellow of both Colleges in 1970 and 1972 respectively. In 1967 his PhD thesis entitled 'The Chemical Control of Respiration in Chronic Ventilatory Failure' presaged his subsequent research.

After holding posts as house surgeon and physician in professorial departments in the Royal Infirmary of Edinburgh, he spent 1958–60 in the RAMC using this time abroad to study the physiology of acclimatisation to heat. Following his army service he rose progressively from Assistant Lecturer (and Honorary Registrar) to Lecturer and Reader to become the Professor of Respiratory Medicine in 1978, following Professor Sir John Crofton. Professor Flenley had also held an MRC Travelling Fellowship which took him to San Francisco in 1967 and to McGill University and the Royal Victoria Hospital in Montreal in 1968.

Professor Flenley was the first Vice-President (1981–82) of the European Society of Pneumology and, during his Presidency (1982–83), he organised the Society's Second Convention in Edinburgh. He was for a time Editor of *Recent Advances in Respiratory Medicine* and Chairman of the Editorial Board of *Clinical Science and Molecular Biology*. He published 78 original papers in peer-reviewed journals and wrote 106 communications in the form of reviews, leading articles and chapters in books and 157 abstracts. The second edition of his *Concise Medical Textbooks: Respiratory Medicine*,[2] published posthumously in 1990, was regarded as the best undergraduate book on the subject.[3]

Professor Flenley also took an active part on university and NHS committees where he was noted for his fair, honest and often bluntly spoken views. He was a memorable teacher and delivered clinical dictates eloquently and enthusiastically at the bedside.

Envious colleagues of Professor Flenley spoke of him as the man with the Midas touch for obtaining research funding. Overall he acquired for the university, sometimes in collaboration with colleagues, over £2.3 million of research money. With this he set up important investigations in respiratory physiology and increased greatly our knowledge about obstructive airways disease and its treatment.

Professor Flenley was justly proud of the Rayne Laboratory funded generously by the Rayne Foundation.[4] He won this for Edinburgh in competition with all the other Scottish medical schools. The single-storey, red brick clad, building situated between Ward 8 and the New Medical Block was constructed rapidly and was functioning by August 1982. It was formally opened by Sir David Steel on 12 May 1983. The opening ceremony was a rather less grand affair than had been expected, the BBC, ITV and the other media who had been invited preferring to cover the forthcoming general election, which had just been announced by Prime Minister Margaret Thatcher.

The Rayne Laboratory was run by Dr Patricia Warren, BSc, PhD, who moved there from the Respiratory Function Laboratory where she had been working with an MRC grant. Dr Patricia Tweeddale then moved from the Western General Hospital to the City Hospital's Respiratory Function Laboratory to work with Dr G.J.R. McHardy. She replaced Miss Sylvia Merchant who in turn moved from Dr McHardy's laboratory, also in early 1983, to the Rayne Laboratory where she became responsible for its day to day administration.

The Rayne Laboratory was devoted to several studies. There was a sleep laboratory with three bedrooms and a control room which became the province of Dr (later Professor) Neil Douglas, an exercise laboratory with treadmill, a catheter room with an X-ray facility and a mechanical laboratory with plethysmograph. The original underfloor trunking for the satellite visual display units (VDUs) in each room became redundant later with the arrival of minicomputers. One room was devoted to cell biology where Dr Andrew Greening developed his interests. Later three rooms in the Rayne Laboratory were taken over for cell biology by Professor Haslett who succeeded Professor Flenley and was to investigate the pathophysiology of the adult respiratory distress syndrome (ARDS).

After the respiratory medicine clinicians had left the City Hospital wards for the Royal Infirmary in December 1993, the Rayne Laboratory moved in April 1994 to the Medical School in Teviot Place where the cell biology arm of the laboratory became linked with Edinburgh University's Department of Pathology. This was assisted by further funding from the Rayne Foundation, this time in the name of Professor Haslett.

Another major research grant won by Professor Flenley came from the Norman Salvesen Emphysema Research Trust in 1984, with subsequent generous funding over the next five years. This was devoted to investigating the pathophysiology and cellular factors causing emphysema. These funds contributed to the salary of the clinical Senior Lecturer, Dr Andrew Greening, who coordinated the Emphysema Research Group programme, and also paid for a computer-aided tomography (CT) scanner and CT lung density histogram for use in emphysema research.

Such funding, together with his scientific and clinical skills, enabled Professor Flenley to build a formidable research team with Drs Neil Douglas, W. (Bill) MacNee (both later Professors), Drs Andrew Greening, George Rhind, and Patricia Warren and also with Miss Sylvia Merchant and an electronics engineer for the Rayne Laboratory. His department also attracted many research fellows from overseas who were often guests at the Flenleys' home. The Professor's wife, Hilary, a graduate librarian, was a charming and generous hostess. The overseas links were mainly with China and India and several of the fellows Professor Flenley encouraged subsequently became professors in their own countries.

Despite his clinical work, teaching, academic and research pursuits, David Flenley was a keen hillwalker, gardener and fisherman. On social occasions in his home his staff were sometimes invited to feast on a salmon which their chief had caught. He was fond of music, read widely, and was an excellent raconteur. Above all he hated humbug and excessive bureaucracy. These he would counter in his forthright Lancastrian style, sometimes laced with a flare of anger which was always short-lived and never bore permanent malice.

It was therefore a shock and tragedy that a man with so much still to offer should suddenly die in his prime at Easter 1989. The tributes paid to him at his funeral, the obituaries in national newspapers and in many medical and scientific journals bear testimony to his great contributions to medical knowledge and to the University of Edinburgh. His widow, Hilary, who had always been so supportive, later unveiled an inscribed brass plaque as a memorial to him at the City Hospital Lecture Theatre which thereafter bore his name.

Professor Flenley was succeeded in the Chair of Respiratory Medicine by Professor Chris Haslett who came to the City Hospital in July 1990. Professor Haslett trained at the University of Edinburgh acquiring a BSc and then in 1977 MB, ChB with Honours winning the Ettles Scholarship and Leslie Gold Medal for being, as was his predecessor, the most distinguished medical graduate of his year. After working in residency posts with Professor James Robson and Sir David Carter in the Royal Infirmary, and a post at the Eastern General Hospital, he moved as Senior House Officer to the Respiratory Medicine Unit at the City Hospital under Professor Flenley. Like Professors Flenley, Douglas and MacNee before him, Professor Haslett was awarded the Dorothy Temple Cross Travelling Fellowship by the MRC which took him to Denver to study inflammatory cell biology. He was appointed a Senior Lecturer at the Royal Postgraduate School and Hammersmith Hospital before he applied successfully for the chair in Edinburgh after the death of Professor Flenley. In the Rayne Laboratory at the City Hospital, his research continued on macrophage responses in ARDS.

Between the death of Professor Flenley and the appointment of Professor Haslett (1989–90) Dr Neil J Douglas acted as Head of Department. Dr Douglas qualified MB, ChB from the Univeristy of Edinburgh in 1973, passed the MRCP Examination in 1975 and was later elected FRCPEd. In 1985, like his colleagues in Respiratory Medicine, he was awarded an MRC Travelling Fellowship and he also studied at Denver in the University of Colorado in 1980–81. He was later the Chairman of the Editorial Board of *Clinical Science* and Honorary Secretary of the British Thoracic Society.

The subject of Dr Douglas' MD thesis in 1983 had been the control of ventilation in chronic bronchitics during sleep. In 1995 he was given a personal chair as Professor of Respiratory and Sleep Medicine. He is now the Director of the Scottish National Sleep Laboratory, which has 1,100 new patient referrals each year, approximately one third from

Lothian and two thirds from the rest of Scotland. The provision of continuous positive airways pressure (CPAP) to control sleep apnoea remains under-funded yet is essential to prevent tragic accidents, characteristically in overweight men who snore all night and then nod off during the day, perhaps when driving on a motorway. CPAP is delivered by a simple device at night, the cost of which in pecuniary and human terms is tiny compared with the disaster of a motorway pile-up. Professor Douglas is also much involved with Continuing Medical Education and is Dean in the Royal College of Physcians of Edinburgh.[5]

Another doctor in the Respiratory Medicine Unit recently appointed to a personal Chair is Professor W. (Bill) MacNee. He qualified MB, ChB from the University of Glasgow in 1975 and later was awarded the MD and elected FRCPG and Ed. He came as a registrar to the City Hospital in 1979. He next worked in the Chest Unit with Dr N. W. Horne and Dr (later Professor) A. Seaton, then in the Respiratory Medicine Unit as a MRC Research Fellow and next with Dr Andrew C. Douglas and Professor James Robson in the Royal Infirmary. At this time he was studying with Dr Pat Warren the hypoxic drive to breathe in mine rescue workers exercising on a treadmill. In 1982–83 he studied for his MD thesis under Dr (later Professor) A. L. Muir investigating the hearts of patients whose chronic chest disease had caused right heart failure (cor pulmonale).

Like his contemporaries, Professor MacNee won an MRC Dorothy Temple Cross Travelling Fellowship which took him to Vancouver. The University of Edinburgh has awarded him a personal chair as Professor of Respiratory and Environmental Medicine and he now works closely with scientists at Napier University where the effects of dust in the atmosphere are studied in their Edinburgh Lung and Environment Group Institute.[6]

Dr A. Gordon Leitch was another prominent member of the respiratory medicine team. He gained an Hons BSc in 1961 and Hons MB, ChB in 1970 both from the University of Edinburgh. He subsequently obtained his MD, PhD and FRCPEd after working in the Royal Infirmary and City Hospital with both Professors Crofton and Flenley. He spent a year studying in Cincinnati and his MRC Travelling Fellowship took him to Boston. When Dr N. W. Horne retired in 1982, the four physicians in Pavilion 5 at the City Hospital were Drs G. J. R. McHardy, Anthony Seaton, Colin Soutar and Gordon Leitch. Dr Leitch then took over much of the work in monitoring tuberculosis in which he, like Dr Horne before him, was meticulous and conscientious. Some of his time was spent researching medical history especially about tuberculous. When he died tragically in a drowning accident in Cyprus in August 1996, he had been writing the story of the Scottish Thoracic Association. He is much missed.

After Dr Leitch died, Dr Michael F. Sudlow shouldered the responsibility for tuberculosis. He had graduated MB, BS in 1964 through St Thomas's Hospital, London, and is regarded somewhat as a medical intellectual by his colleagues. Besides studying respiratory physiology and chest medicine in the Brompton Hospital, he was for a time a lecturer in aeronautical engineering at Imperial College. He holds the FRCP of London and Edinburgh. After coming to Edinburgh in 1972, he worked both in the City Hospital and then the Royal Infirmary. He was appointed Consultant Physician and Honorary University Senior Lecturer in 1980 and is now Associate Dean in Postgraduate Medicine. His expertise ranges from tuberculosis to the chemotherapy for bronchial cancer.[7]

In October 1993, Professor Haslett transferred the Respiratory Medicine Unit to the Royal Infirmary as he wished it to be part of a big general hospital and the future of the City Hospital was becoming increasingly uncertain (see Chapter 34). When he left the City Hospital he took with him a worthy team of researchers and clinicians to join Dr Sudlow and others already working in the Royal Infirmary. This did, however, mean that the viability of the City Hospital was further compromised by losing of the Unit of Respiratory Medicine and the Rayne Laboratory.

Thoracic Surgery

As the closure of the City Hospital became imminent (see Chapter 34), the Thoracic Surgery Unit became one of the last departments to be transferred to the Royal Infirmary in Lauriston Place rather than go directly to the new Royal Infirmary at Little France. It left the City Hospital in December 1997 vacating Pavilion 6 and the thoracic theatre at the east end of the south corridor.

By the late 1950s Mr Logan and Mr Wade had been concentrating their cardiac surgery at the Royal Infirmary. Mr McCormack and Mr Walbaum must take credit for developing the service in thoracic surgery at the City Hospital where they also carried out some closed cardiac surgery. There was not, therefore, a complete separation in cardio-thoracic surgery between the two hospitals. It did mean, however, that looking after patients at two separate sites became increasingly difficult for the surgical team.

In 1972 when Mr Logan retired from the NHS, Mr Philip Caves was appointed Senior Lecturer in cardiac surgery, based almost entirely at the Royal Infirmary. When he moved to Glasgow in 1976 he was replaced for approximately the next four years by Mr David Wheatley who also left for Glasgow when he was appointed Professor. In turn,

Mr Wheatley was replaced by Mr Kenneth Reid who concentrated largely on cardiac surgery at the Royal Infirmary. He left for Saudi Arabia in the late 1980s and was succeeded by Mr Ciro Campanella who then became the new Senior Lecturer in cardiac surgery.

Mr McCormack and Mr Walbaum did most of the cardio-thoracic work at the City Hospital until Mr McCormack's untimely, sudden death in 1980. Mr Wade had retired in 1978 and he was succeeded by Mr Evan W. Cameron.[8] Mr Cameron carried out most of the chest surgery at the City Hospital but also operated at the Royal Infirmary on cardiac patients. He is an Edinburgh graduate of 1966 who later gained experience in Wentworth and King George V Hospitals in Durban. Mr McCormack was succeeded in 1982 by Mr Chris Sang who qualified in Edinburgh in the same year as Mr Cameron. Both surgeons hold the FRCSEd. Mr Cameron additionally is a BSc graduate of Edinburgh University and Mr Sang has been elected FRCPEd. Mr Sang's lists are mainly in cardiac surgery in the Royal Infirmary but he also performed thoracic surgical operations at the City Hospital.

When Mr Philip Walbaum retired he was succeeded by Mr William (Bill) S. Walker, MA (Cambridge 1978), MB, BChir (1977), FRCS Eng and Ed. He was appointed in 1988 and, like Mr Cameron, had operating sessions in cardio-thoracic surgery at the City Hospital and Royal Infirmary. During the early 1990s, Mr David Hamilton held the Professorial Chair and for four years concentrated his expertise in paediatric cardiac surgery at the Royal Hospital for Sick Children. When he retired, the Chair was ablated and Mr Pankaj Mankad was appointed as an NHS Consultant in adult and paediatric cardiac surgery. Mr Ciro Campanella converted from Senior Lecturer with the university into NHS Consultant.

These frequent changes within the staff and between the Royal Infirmary and the City Hospital did not mean that the Thoracic Surgery Unit was underachieving. Rather the reverse was true. Having been established for so many years, the unit could justifiably boast of a continuity of practice. From its inception to the present day, it has been spear-heading innovations in surgical technique. In the early years Mr Logan had pioneered mitral valvotomy inventing a novel instrument for enlarging the valve diameter in hearts diseased from previous rheumatic fever. With cardioplegic arrest many exciting new procedures could be carried out on the heart, although most of that work was done at the Royal Infirmary rather than in the City Hospital. Mr McCormack carried out over 300 operations to repair atrial septal defects, usually under hypothermia which, by chilling the patient, gave the surgeon the precious extra time necessary to carry out the procedure. This required the utmost cooperation between the surgeons and anaesthetists such as Dr Archie Milne.

More recently Mr Cameron has specialised in the surgical relief of upper gastrointestinal cancer in addition to cardio-thoracic operations. About 10 per cent of all the oesophagectomies carried out for cancer in the United Kingdom are now performed in the unit.[9]

Mr Walker's arrival in the unit in 1988 heralded a new era in thoracic surgery. Previously pulmonary surgery was often a traumatic experience for patient and surgeon alike. It usually required an extensive incision and rib resection to gain access to the lungs, resulting in much discomfort, a prolonged post-operative convalescence, and slow return to work. With minimal access surgery, of which Mr Walker has become a world leader, even a total pneumonectomy can be carried out through a relatively small thoracoscopy wound leading to only minor trauma to the patient, greatly increased safety, shortened convalescence and a more rapid return to work. The unit is involved in training courses run by the College of Surgeons in Ireland, the European Association of Cardio-Thoracic Surgeons in the Hague and in the Minimal Access Therapy Training Unit Scotland (MATTUS) based at Ninewells Hospital, Dundee. The unit also scored a 'first' in 1994 having operated successfully on the youngest patient in the United Kingdom to undergo puemonectomy by minimal access surgery.[10]

The unit remained busy throughout the 1990s with 1,200–1,400 discharges and between 1,400 and 1,700 out-patients per annum. In 1992 the Tea Room volunteers provided funds to refurbish the patient areas of Ward 6A and artwork on the ceiling of the theatre's corridor to help relax patients lying on trolleys awaiting operation.

In April 1995 Sir David Carter chaired a Lothian Health Board working party which reviewed the delivery of clinical surgical services. Apart from short-term measures to improve the environment for patients, it was recommended that the Thoracic Surgery Unit be relocated as soon as possible in the existing Royal Infirmary.[11] This move, completed in December 1997, relieved the justifiable anxieties of the surgeons who felt it was totally unsatisfactory to have their clinical work and operation sessions split between the two sites. Nonetheless there was a sense of loss to those remaining at the City Hospital at the departure of another prestigious department.

ENT Surgery

In the meantime one of the largest units at the City Hospital, the Ear, Nose and Throat Department, had been active. As described in Chapter 27, Edinburgh's disparate ENT surgical units coalesced in 1965 at the

City Hospital. The Eastern General Hospital ENT Department was closed and, to accommodate a boiler house at the Royal Infirmary, the ENT surgeons moved *en bloc* from their pavilion there to the City Hospital. Although originally an unpopular move with some of the surgeons, the concentration of ENT surgical expertise at the single City Hospital site ultimately proved an advantage. In time it led to the creation of 'one of the biggest, best and most active' ENT Units in the UK.[12]

The layout of the new City Hospital ENT Department remained much the same over the years, concentrated on Pavilions 2, 3 and the downstairs ward of Pavilion 4. In May 1991 when the maxillofacial surgeons transferred from the Royal Infirmary, theatres were shared. Their interrelated interests meant that the two disciplines settled in happily together.[13] In 1992 the waiting areas for patients and visitors in Ward 2 were carpeted, and artwork, specifically designed to amuse children, was applied to the corridor ceiling of Ward 4 theatre and on the doors of the anaesthetic room. Attractive murals appropriate to the corridors in the Care of the Elderly Unit and the children's Ward 15 in the RIDU were also created.[14]

Various initiatives helped to reduce the waiting time to a maximum of one year.[15] The following year after Ward 3 was upgraded the length of stay in the ENT wards fell.[16] In September 1994 the opening of a purpose designed, eight-bedded, ENT day surgical unit greatly increased the throughput of patients, with 600 ENT day case operations in the first six months. Better facilities were arranged for children undergoing ENT surgery and a more spacious area for ENT and maxillofacial out-patients. A two-bed high dependency unit for adults undergoing major head and neck or ENT surgery was also opened.[17]

The number of ENT in-patient discharges between 1992 and 1996 ranged between 4,000 and 6,000 thousand annually, the day case figures nearly doubled to 1,118 in 1995–96 and about 20,000 out-patients were seen each year. Maximum use was made of the operating theatres. The surgeons were assisted in attaining these figures and in performing complicated and extensive surgery by the capable anaesthetic team. This was led in the early days by Dr Archie C. Milne and later by Drs J. Clark McIntyre and William R. MacRae, the latter becoming Vice-President of the Royal College of Anaesthetists.

Of the original team of doctors who came to the ENT Unit at the City Hospital in 1965, none were there in the closing years of the hospital. Dr Bill Newlands, in the unit briefly from 1975 to 1977, left for Saudi Arabia. Dr J. A. M. Murray left in 1995 after nine years to undertake private practice in Bermuda. The present clinical director is Dr Alastair I. G. Kerr, a Glasgow graduate who later trained in Edinburgh and is the author of several textbooks on adult and paediatric otolaryngology. Dr Bryan A. B. Dale, a recently retired Edinburgh graduate, was both a neuro-otologist and ENT surgeon who demanded very high clinical standards. He specialised in the management of tinnitus. His dry wit has enhanced many lectures and committee meetings. Dr David L. Cowan, an Edinburgh graduate, has most experience in paediatric ENT surgery having worked as a Consultant at Bangour General Hospital, the Royal Hospital for Sick Children, and the Western General Hospital in addition to the City Hospital. Dr William E. Grant came to the City Hospital via Dublin and London to concentrate especially on rhinology. Dr Robert Sanderson trained with Professor Maran in head and neck surgery and continues to work in this field.

One uniting feature of almost all the ENT surgeons is their prowess on the golf course. They have frequently defeated the golfers of the Royal College of Physicians of Edinburgh in the annual Royal Colleges' Golf Outing.

No exception to this rule is Professor Arnold Maran, a member of several golf clubs, not least the Royal and Ancient in St Andrews. He is also a classical and jazz musician who plays the flute, piano and percussion instruments. His interest in music and the human voice led him to build a unique voice laboratory at the Royal Infirmary. In conjunction with Colin Watson, who has dual input through opera singing and knowledge of fast computers, voice analysis has become routine. Their joint expertise is widely sought by professional singers, especially during the Edinburgh International Festival of Music and Drama.

Professor Maran qualified MB, ChB from the Univeristy of Edinburgh in 1959, FRCSEd in 1963 and MD in 1965. He is a Fellow of Surgical Colleges in Australia, England and South Africa, of dental surgery of Edinburgh and is also a FRCPEd. He has worked in Iowa University and has been Professor of Otolaryngology of West Virginia, a member of the Senate of Surgery of the UK, a Fellow and President of the Laryngological Section of the Royal Society of Medicine and President of the British Association of Academic Otolaryngology. He is currently a Professor of Otolaryngology of the University of Edinburgh and an Honorary Consultant in the Royal Infirmary and City Hospitals. He has progressed from Fellow of the Royal College of Surgeons of Edinburgh in 1963 to be the College's Treasurer, elected Council Member, Secretary, Vice-President and in October 1997 was elected President.[18]

Besides his special interests in the larynx and voice, Professor Maran is an expert in head and neck surgery and author of a textbook of that title published in 1994. Over the years the City Hospital's various

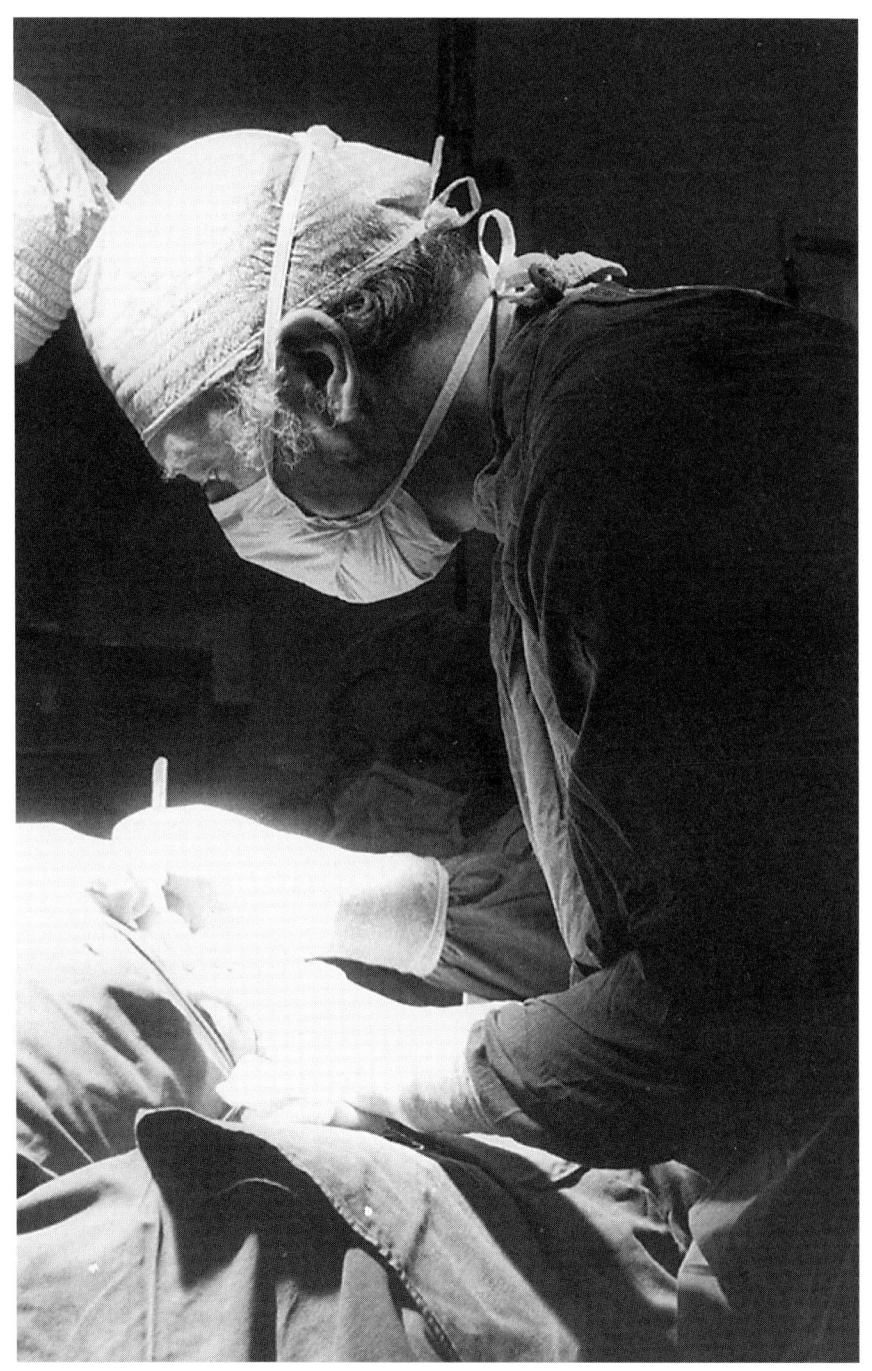

Professor Arnold Maran operating (Photo Jimmy Patience. By courtesy of Professor A. G. D. Maran)

departments have seen several illustrious professors including Arnold Maran who, in addition to his other obligations and high offices, became Head of Service of the hospital in 1993. Sadly, with only the Scottish Mycobacteria Reference Laboratory, and the Regional Clinical Virus Laboratory, and some temporary day case surgery left, the ENT Department will soldier on alone in the relatively deserted City Hospital from 1998 until accommodation becomes available in Phase I of the new Royal Infirmary about 2001 or 2002.

Maxillofacial Surgery

Closely allied to ENT surgery was the Department of Maxillofacial Surgery. After 25 years in the Royal Infirmary it moved to the City Hospital in May 1991. Since then the outpatient accommodation, which was initially inappropriate for the service, was upgraded and the theatre and ward facilities were improved.

At the time of transfer, the department consisted of 1.5 full-time NHS Consultants with a support staff of nine people in total. Mr Glenn Lello, NHS Consultant and university Senior Lecturer, reported a doubling of the staff over the next four years in keeping with more than doubling of the work throughput. The City Hospital department then encompassed virtually the entire spectrum of maxillofacial and oral surgery.[19] With this has come the improvements in operating theatre and office equipment, the attractive artwork adorning the anaesthetic room and theatre (shared with ENT) and the provision of an X-ray room re-equipped to the requirements of the maxillofacial surgeons.[20] In 1993 the facilities in Ward 3 [21] were upgraded and in 1994 new imaging equipment was introduced for examining the temporo-mandibular joint.[22] Undergraduates from Guy's Dental School and Hospital in London attended during the winter months, a testimony to the unit's high reputation.

Mr Lello graduated MB, ChB (Sheffield) in 1978 after his BDS degree five years earlier. He also holds the FRCS, FDSRCSEd in 1975 and a PhD (Witwatersrand, 1989). He has been a Senior Lecturer at the University of Manchester and also Professor and Head of the Department of Maxillofacial Surgery of the University of South Africa.

Mr Lello's fellow consultant in Edinburgh is Mr Roy Mitchell, BDS (Sheffield in 1969) and MB, ChB (Edinburgh in 1975). He also holds the ChM (Edinburgh), FRCSEd and FDSRCSEd. His particular expertise is in the use of biological implants to repair deficits in the reconstruction of the face and jaw.

The throughput of work in maxillofacial surgery steadily increased after it arrived at the City Hospital. In particular the combined figures for in-patient and day case patient discharges rose from 1,418 (1992–93) to 1,467 (1995–96) with a much increased use of the day case compared with inpatient facilities during that time. The outpatient attendances rose from 2,769 to 5,670.[23] The Maxillofacial Department transferred to St John's Hospital at Howden, West Lothian, in the summer of 1998.

The Care of the Elderly Unit

In the Care of the Elderly Unit (see Chapter 27) founded by Professor James Williamson, changes were also taking place. The new holder of the Chair of Geriatric Medicine from 1 September 1986 was Professor William (Bill) J. MacLennan, MD, FRCP London, Edinburgh and Glasgow. He was born in Glasgow, educated at Hutcheson's Boys' Grammar School and at the University of Glasgow. He was a Hansen Research Scholar, then from 1965–69 Assistant Lecturer and then Lecturer at Glasgow University Department of Materia Medica. After Senior Registrar posts at Stobhill Hospital and the Western Infirmary in Glasgow, he was appointed Senior Lecturer in geriatric medicine at the University of Southampton in 1971. He returned to Scotland in 1980 to become Senior Lecturer in geriatric medicine at Dundee University and was promoted to Reader in 1984. Two years later he was appointed Professor of Geriatric Medicine at the University of Edinburgh succeeding Professor Williamson. He has written several books on the clinical care and drug treatment of the elderly, and on bone, metabolic and endocrine disease in old people. After 10 years in the Chair, he retired in 1996.

At the end of 1996, after more than 20 years in the City Hospital, Dr Colin Currie (see Chapter 27) left to join Edinburgh Health Care. He had considerably advanced the important sub-specialty of trauma rehabilitation in the elderly. Dr Brian J. Chapman, BSc, MB, ChB, FRCPEd, who had been appointed as Consultant Geriatrician to the Royal Infirmary and City Hospital in 1989, became employed solely at the Royal Infirmary from June 1996. He had been particularly active in rehabilitating the elderly after stroke disease. Dr Nicola R. Colledge BSc, MB, ChB, FRCPEd another Edinburgh graduate who had previously worked at Milesmark Hospital, Dunfermline, and then as Senior Registrar and Senior Lecturer (1991) at the Edinburgh City Hospital, resigned her post at the end of 1996 to become a Consultant Geriatrician at Liberton Hospital.

Most of these changes in 1996 were brought about because of the imminent closure of the Care of the Elderly Unit. By 31 March 1996, five of the eight continuing care wards at the City Hospital were closed in keeping with the terms of the Community Care Act of 1991. The remainder were to close by the end of the year. This, together with the previous departure of the Respiratory Medicine Unit in 1993 and the projected departure of the Thoracic Surgery Unit by the end of 1997, meant the City Hospital site was no longer viable. Permission to close the whole hospital was then sought from the Scottish Office.[24]

Nonetheless the Care of the Elderly Unit remained a highly active and progressive department. For instance in 1992–93 the Assessment Unit's in-patient discharges rose to 584, the number of day cases was 5,211, and 239 out-patients were seen. The number of in-patient discharges from the geriatric long-stay (continuing care) wards fell progressively from 299 in 1992–93 to 216 in 1994–95 and thereafter these beds were emptied and the wards closed. Similarly the number of in-patient discharges from the psychogeriatric ward fell progressively from 76 in 1992–93 to 43 in 1994–95 after which this ward too was closed.

In 1995–96, however, the new unit at the City Hospital, which had opened in 1993–94 for the rehabilitation of stroke patients over the age of 75, recorded a dramatic 91 in-patient discharges. Most of these patients who might otherwise not have got home had been transferred to the City Hospital following their initial admissions to the Royal Infirmary. The Report for 1993–94[25] recorded that, in collaboration with the local Directorate for the Psychiatry of Old Age at the Royal Infirmary, a monthly memory clinic had been instituted.[26] Twelve respite beds based on the continuing care wards at the City Hospital and Astley Ainslie Hospital were introduced to provide support for carers by admitting old people for periods of from a few days each year to periods of up to a fortnight every six weeks.[27] A research project on Pressure Sore Prevention and Care resulted in the provision of a link nursing network designed to improve the nursing practice and the training of nurses in this area.

The throughput of the Geriatric Assessment Unit increased between 1993 and 1994 and the average length of stay fell below three weeks. The Annual Report 1994–95 showed that, despite the closing of beds, the new Stroke Rehabilitation Unit succeeded in getting over half of the 77 patients treated in that year back home.[28] The Annual Report 1995–96 emphasised the importance that was placed on ensuring the maintenance of good relations with patients, relatives and service providers in the community when transferring elderly people home. Also in a difficult year for staff, the Report claimed 'Every effort has been made to provide alternative posts for the staff'.[29]

The once prestigious Care of the Elderly Unit at the City Hospital was closed and had its windows boarded over and made secure against vandals. Ever since Professor Williamson pioneered the then new discipline of geriatric medicine, much has been achieved which is now taken for granted but which was new territory in the 1970s. It was Professor Williamson who promoted the concepts of liaison with general practitioners and community services, rapid domicilliary and day care assessments, the concentration of all geriatric medical, para-medical and social work services on the same site, the promotion of the developing discipline through excellence in teaching and clinical example which led to the attraction of good staff. Latterly, the triumphs of the unit were the trauma and stroke rehabilitation programmes and seeing the recommendations of research projects such as Pressure Sore Prevention and Care being put into practice. One member of staff likened Professor Williamson's influence to that of Field Marshall William Slim in that he 'commanded affection and communicated energy'. There can be few higher tributes.

X-ray Department

It was not until the end of 1948 that patients in the City Hospital could be X-rayed on the site. Only then was part of the hospital's electricity supply changed from DC to AC, allowing Dr Cummack to supervise the fitting out of the City Hospital's first X-ray Department (see Chapter 24). Dr D. Hunter Cummack, the Consultant Radiologist in Administrative Charge at the Western General Hospital, qualified from the University of Edinburgh in 1936 and held the FFRCSI, DMR and FRCSEd. He had been a specialist radiologist with the rank of Major in the RAMC and he was expert in gastrointestinal radiology about which he published a *Descriptive Atlas* in 1969.

Mr E. Jimmy Rawlings, Group Superintendent Radiographer, who has kindly supplied much of the following information, came to the City Hospital in September 1956 and remembers the first X-ray Department set up by Dr Cummack. From 1948 to 1965, it occupied Cottage 13, situated between Pavilion 14 on the west and the central block on the east. Cottage 13 was a three roomed bungalow unconnected with the wards by any of the roofed corridors. The X-rays and reporting were carried out in one of the two large rooms, the other being the waiting area. The small room in between became the dark room, staff room and office. After its demolition in the 1960s, Cottage 13 was replaced by the Group Pharmacy and stores.

Mr Rawlings recalls the original staff of three radiographers and a dark-room technician. As Group Superintendent Radiographer he had to supply cover for the Royal Victoria Dispensary and Hospital, Southfield Hospital and the City Hospital. Two porters who doubled as ambulance drivers delivered the patients for X-rays in an ancient ambulance 'which gave about 5 mpg, 10 mph and produced clouds of smoke from its exhaust'. One of the drivers, called Tommy, was also the hospital 'runner' who took bets at unusual times and places.[30] Most requests at that time were for chest X-rays for the thoracic surgical and respiratory diseases wards and fewer for the infectious diseases wards.

The X-ray Department moved in the mid-1960s from Cottage 13 to the ground floor of the former servants' home, now the New Medical Block. Here there were two X-ray rooms but there was only enough money to furnish one. A year after moving to the New Medical Block, however, the second room was equipped with an old X-ray unit from the Royal Infirmary. When Southfield Hospital closed, its tomogram unit was transferred to the City Hospital. It was of the latest multi-section type which could offer seven films of different sections with one exposure. Manual processing was laborious and difficult but was later done automatically in seven minutes with a Kodak X-omat machine. A third room was added next providing better staff accommodation and offices. New, powerful mobile units were provided, one for each of the four hospital corridors, and one radiographer was detailed each day to carry out portable X-rays on the wards.

The staff of the X-ray Department integrated well into the social life of the hospital, partaking of strawberry teas on Wednesday afternoons in the summer and several of them participated in Dr Barry Kay's outdoor production of *A Midsummer-Night's Dream* in 1964. Some evenings were enlivened by barbecues and bonfires. Mr Rawlings bitterly recalls being excluded from the 1956 Christmas dance, then held in the dining room in the central block. These annual dances were only open to hospital staff who had been in post for at least six months. He missed it by one month but in those days rules were enforced strictly. Mr Rawlings and a colleague were later volunteer drivers of the ancient brown bus which took elderly patients from the Geriatric Medicine Department out for runs in the country. Colleagues whom Mr Rawlings particularly remembers were Mrs Christine Baillie, a radiographer at the hospital for many years, and Mr Tony Fital the ECG technician. Mr Rawlings also worked closely with Mr Girvan, the Head Porter, who was responsible for transporting patients to and from the X-Ray Department.

Extra work was generated from 1960 onwards by the Pyelonephritis Unit in Pavilion 14 once Dr Murdoch had begun investigating the aetiology of urinary infections in women. Intravenous pyelography (IVP) was then the standard investigation to image the urinary tract. It usually required the services of the senior house officer of the Pyelonephritis Unit to attend the X-ray Department several times a day in order to inject the intravenous iodine contrast material. Fortunately there were few reactions. Later a plain film of the abdomen and the safer ultrasound scan largely replaced the IVP.

Patients with blood in the urine or recurrent infections unresponsive to antibiotics required cystoscopic examination and retrograde pyelography which was carried out on Tuesday afternoons in Ward 14A's theatre by Mr Selby Tulloch, Mr Jack Newsam, Mr G. Foster, Mr Jack O'Brien, Mr G. Carswell, Mr J. Hindmarsh and their successors. Retrograde pyelography was done during cystoscopy by squirting radio-opaque contrast up the ureters to the kidneys. The X-ray unit was bolted onto the cystoscopy theatre wall and operated from a control panel in the adjacent dark room. Mr Rawlings remembers that the other radiographers were unhappy about operating this antedeluvian and potentially dangerous machine, so it was left to him personally to make the exposures. Despite these difficulties, the films of kidneys, ureters and bladder were surprisingly good.

During the 1980s the radiographers were much in demand in the Rayne Laboratory where they found the scanning of liver, bone, brain and lungs with a Siemens' gamma camera and links computer particularly interesting.

One of the earliest Consultant Radiologists appointed to the City Hospital also worked at the Eastern General Hospital. From the early 1950s till 1975 when he was moved to the Royal Infirmary, Dr W Norman Thomson was in charge. He graduated in medicine from Aberdeen University in 1944 and held both the DMRD Eng and FFR. He had served as a radiologist in the RAMC, and had been Assistant to the Department of Radiology in Aberdeen Royal Infirmary. Before his appointment to the City Hospital he was Chief Assistant to the Radiodiagnostic Department at Guy's Hospital in London. He is remembered for several new developments during his time at the City Hospital, his slow, calculated sense of humour and his love of old automobiles.

Dr Thomson was succeeded in April 1975 by Dr A. J. A. Wightman as Consultant Radiologist. Dr Wightman graduated MB, BS (London 1967) through St Mary's Hospital and also holds the DMRD Eng, FFR and FRCR. After being House Surgeon and Senior House Officer in medicine at St Mary's Hospital, he became Senior House Officer in radiotherapy at the Hammersmith Hospital where he later was the registrar in diagnostic radiology. He also held a similar appointment at King's College Hospital. His Senior Registrar post was in the Royal Infirmary of Edinburgh. He is a co-author of *Clinical Radiology* (Butterworth Heinemann) first in 1983 and, by 1994, it its fourth edition. He has also written papers on ENT and chest radiology. Dr Wightman has particular expertise in the interpretation of chest films.

In September 1988 Dr Wightman was joined by Dr Sami A. Moussa as Consultant Radiologist both at the City and Western General Hospitals. He qualified MB, BCh (Alexandria 1971) and holds the FRCSEd, FRACS, FRCR and DMRDEd. Before coming to Edinburgh Dr Moussa was Senior Registrar at Northwick Park Hospital, Harrow, Middlesex. He is an expert in ultrasound and MRI scanning and interpretation. He also works closely with the urological surgeons at the Scottish Lithotripter Centre in freeing patients of kidney stones by non-surgical means. His informal seminars on interpreting X-rays and scans are always enlivening and educational.

Despite the closure of much of the hospital, some X-ray facilities will continue to serve the ENT Department until it moves to the new Royal Infirmary. Part of the development of the western side of the City Hospital site will be delayed because of the MRI scanner between Pavilions 16 and 17. Only when it goes to a new home will work begin on the scanner site, Pavilion 17, Cottages 23 and 24 and the Geriatric Day Hospital.

CHAPTER THIRTY

Changes in Nursing Management and Practice; Nurses' Medals and Badges

Miss E. L. Sandford, Lady Superintendent of Nurses at the second City Hospital, who had presented Queen Alexandra with a bouquet during the opening of the third City Hospital in 1903, retired the same year (see Chapter 16). It is likely she supervised the changeover from the Infirmary Street site to Colinton Mains.

Miss Sandford's three immediate successors held office between them for a remarkable total of 62 years. First came Miss I. Thomas who had trained in fever nursing at Infirmary Street. Possibly as early as 1903, but certainly by 1907,[1] she had taken the title of Matron rather than Lady Superintendent. Miss Thomas, therefore, was the first Matron of the third City Hospital, a post she held from 1903 till 1925. Her successor was Miss Mary Pool, Matron from September 1925 till May 1943. She died in March 1944. The next appointee was Miss M. I. Adams who was Matron from November 1944 till September 1965.

Two of Miss Adams' Assistant Matrons subsequently also became Matrons of the City Hospital: Miss J. K. Taylor, Matron from 1965 to 1969[2] and Miss A. E. Christie, Matron from 1971 to 1983.[3] Miss Christie was also deputy to Miss Taylor during her time as Matron. Miss Taylor (often called 'Neen') was a very popular Matron whose whole life was devoted to the service of the hospital. She carried out her fever nurse training at the City Hospital, and her general training at the Royal Infirmary before returning as a ward sister and then Assistant Matron at the City Hospital. After she retired in 1969 to Newton Stewart, she still kept a lively interest in her old hospital.

Miss Taylor was followed by Miss Willox, Matron 1970–71, who had been a Sister Tutor in Glasgow. She became Group Senior Nursing Officer covering both the Princess Margaret Rose Orthopaedic Hospital and the City Hospital. She introduced a trial in nursing training whereby nurses spent much longer in the classroom and so anticipated the present Project 2000.

From about 1974, senior members of the nursing hierarchy occupied offices at the City Hospital for various periods. These included Miss Agnes 'Nan' Grieve who came from Bangour General Hospital and

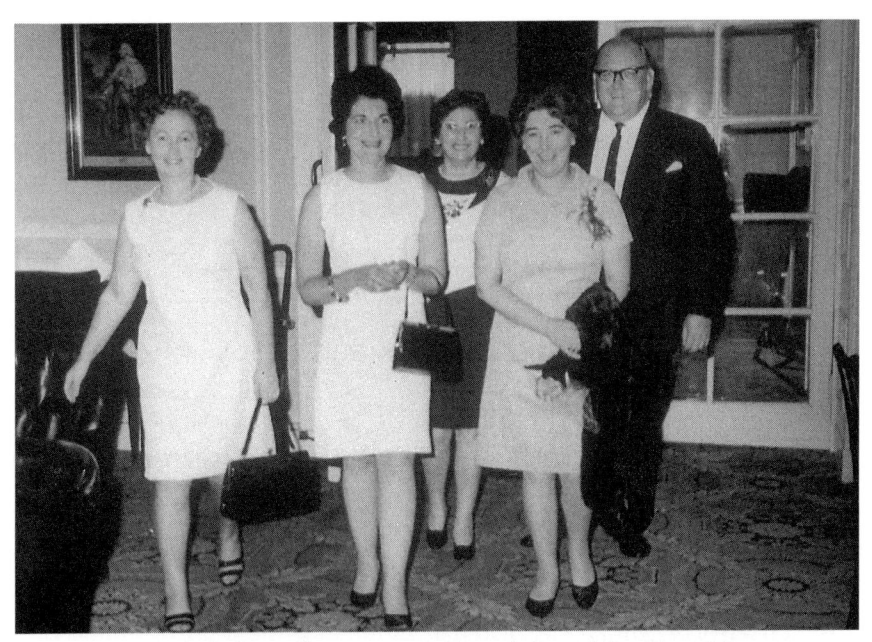

Miss J. K. Taylor's farewell party, 1969. Front left to right: Sister Mary Sibbauld, Miss A. E. Christie and Miss J. K. Taylor. Back left to right: Miss Turner and Mr George Wilson. (By courtesy of Miss J. K. Taylor)

became Group Nursing Officer for the City, Princess Margaret Rose Orthopaedic, Liberton and Southfield Hospitals before she left to become Director of Nursing Services in Stirling. Mr (C.) Larry Mackie was Group Nursing Officer and then Divisional Officer until June 1983. For a short period too Miss Marion Buchanan also worked from the City Hospital. She had trained at the Western General Hospital where she also became ward sister and Assistant Matron, and she was later appointed Matron of the Royal Hospital for Sick Children. Whilst at the City Hospital she was the Director of Nursing Services for the United Hospitals Group. Throughout this time, radical changes in nursing training and management structure were taking place, titles of posts altering and the hospitals grouping, separating and regrouping frequently.

Miss Christie, Assistant and later Deputy Matron to Miss Taylor and then herself Matron (Senior Nursing Officer) from 1971 to 1983 was a stabilising force for the City Hospital even through she also held a series of other senior appointments. Miss Christie trained at the Western General Hospital, then moved to the Northern General Hospital which specialised in neurology, chest medicine and rheumatic diseases. She then studied midwifery at Aberdeen Royal Infirmary and Simpson Memorial Maternity

Pavilion in Edinburgh where she became a staff midwife. She worked next in the Hammersmith Hospital in London and later overseas in Rhodesia and Iran. After an administrative course at the Royal College of Nursing Miss Christie came to the City Hospital in 1965 where she rose rapidly to become Matron in 1971. Miss Cowan became Miss Christie's Assistant Matron.

From February to May 1983, Miss Christie was Acting Divisional Nursing Officer for the unit and, from June 1983 to May 1984, the substantive Divisional Nursing Officer. When the Districts were abolished and everyone's title changed in 1984, Miss Christie became Director of Nursing Services until she retired in August 1987. From 1971, however, she was always responsible for the City Hospital directly or indirectly and so provided a valued continuity of nursing management despite the frequent changes taking place during this time. After Mr (C.) Larry Mackie, the Divisional Nursing Officer based in the old Superintendent's house at the City Hospital, moved on in 1981, another senior nurse who gave useful continuous day-to-day management for the City Hospital was Mrs Maureen Lees.

After Miss Christie retired in 1987, Mr Robert (Bob) Purves[4] was appointed in 1988 with the new title of Principal Nurse for the City Hospital. Mr Purves had trained at Stracathro Hospital in Brechin and moved to Edinburgh Royal Infirmary and then Dundee before coming to the City Hospital. He showed a particular flair for administration and management during his time as Principal Nurse and from 1992 to 1994 was appointed the hospital's Business Manager. For those two years, Mrs Lees was Acting Principal Nurse.[5]

Mr Purves had to provide appropriate nursing cover when Wards 14 and 17 opened for HIV-infected patients, and he was responsible for recruiting and training suitable personnel. Some of the nurses in Milestone House had an introductory training in the City Hospital wards. Mr Purves also presided over the transfers in the continuing care Wards 7A, 8A and 15A, which were upgraded and recommissioned in August 1991. Only three years later he arranged the transfer to nursing homes of those elderly patients who could not be looked after in their own homes after discharge from hospital. Nurses were recruited in 1991 for the recently arrived Maxillofacial Surgery Unit and to work in the ENT surgical out-patient department which moved to Ward 8 in December 1993.

With the assistance of Mrs Dyer, play coordinators for paediatric patients in Ward 15 and the ENT Department were arranged by Mr Purves through Action for Children in Hospital and Play in Scottish Hospitals. The entrance and internal corridor of Ward 15 were painted with attractive, child-friendly, decorations of circuses and beach scenes.

It was during Mr Purves' time too that the fire occurred in the south east wing of the nurses' home in November 1998. Fortunately no one was injured but a lot of personal and hospital property was destroyed or damaged. Some years later that whole building was demolished, being in part unsafe and too old fashioned to fulfil its original purpose. Besides most nurses, even in training, preferred to live out.

As the Royal Infirmary gained NHS Trust status, Mr Purves was appointed as its Director of Operations, Nursing and Quality. When he left the City Hospital, Mrs Lees, who had been Acting Principal Nurse from 1992 to 1994, became Principal Nurse for the City Hospital from 1994 until she retired in 1998. Mrs Lees had occupied several senior posts at the Hospital before this, including sister in the paediatric, infectious diseases Ward 15A. Before she retired in March 1998, she had the thankless task, together with Professor Maran, the Head of Service, Mr Pearson, the Business Manager and Mr Jim Smith, Service Manager, of trying to maintain staff morale during the difficult closing years of the hospital.

During the early decades at the Hospital, nurses were subject to very strict discipline. Some of the teenage nurses recruited and most of the domestic staff would have had only a basic education and had to be inculcated with the rules to prevent cross-infection. The authoritarian regime relaxed somewhat in the 1960s at the same time as limited hospital visiting was permitted, though even then not encouraged. Yet the Matron and her Deputy were held in awe. All would rise in the hospital dining room when they entered for lunch and none left the room before they did.

The nursing in great fever hospitals became more uniform in 1911 with the introduction of the Fever Nurse Certificate by the Local Government Board for Scotland. External examiners from different parts of Scotland tested the nurses. For example, the certificate granted to a Nurse Isabella Gibson of Ruchill Fever Hospital in Glasgow was signed on 25 May 1914 by very senior doctors from Glasgow and Dundee, including an MOH. They were assisted in the practical part of the examination by Miss I. Thomas, Matron, City Edinburgh Hospital and Miss F Merchant, Matron of the Eastern District Hospital, Glasgow.[6] The coveted badges issued to successful candidates later showed a traditional white on blue enamelled saltire surrounded by silver lettering REGISTERED FEVER NURSE, SCOTLAND.

The original City Hospital medal was a svery small silver ellipse pointed at top and bottom and decorated with an alternating bead and bar edge. The City of Edinburgh coat of arms and motto, NISI DOMINUS FRUSTRA, appeared at the top with EDINBURGH CITY HOSPITAL below

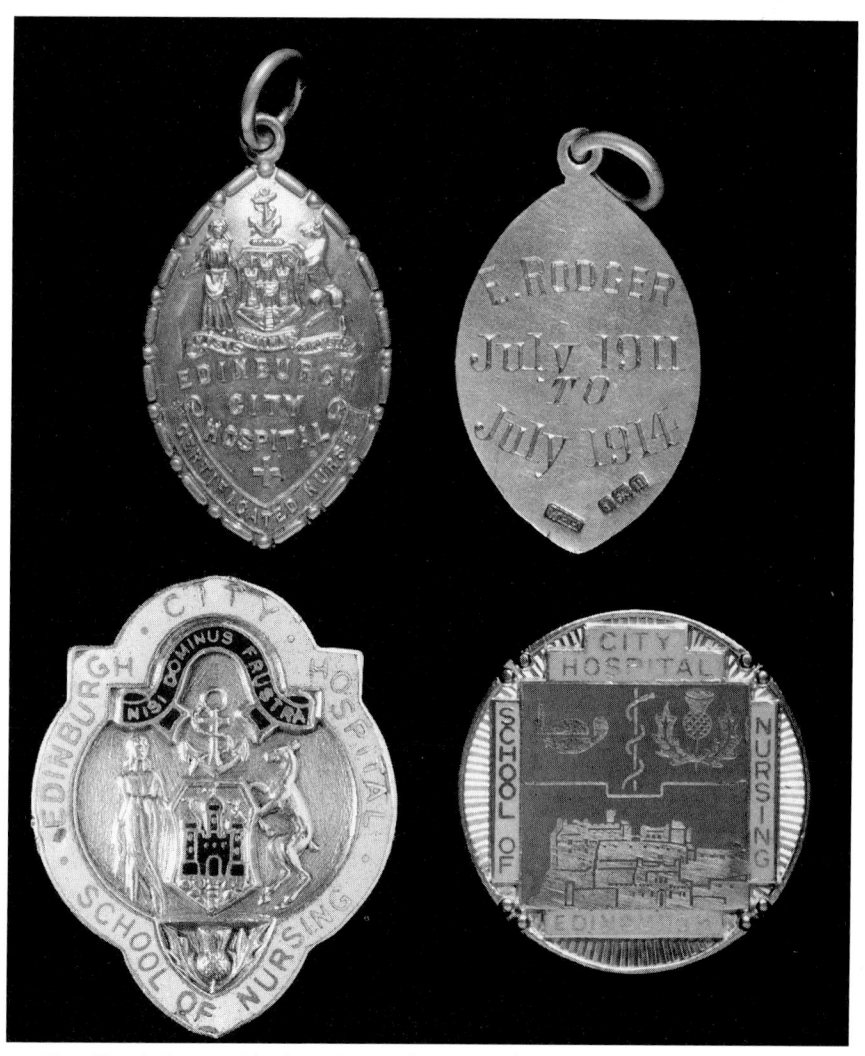

City Hospital nurses' badges. Top: The original medal given by Bailie Russell in December 1890 but still in use in 1914. Obverse on left, Reverse on right (by courtesy of Miss A. E. Christie). Bottom left: Badge in use in 1938–41 (By courtesy of Mrs Pat Hunter). Bottom right: Badge of 1961 (By courtesy of Mr Ron Munro). (All photos by Medical Photography, Royal Infirmary of Edinburgh)

which there was a simple cross and at the foot and the words CERTI-FICATED NURSE.⁷ On later medals the reverse was engraved with the nurse's name and the dates she started and finished her training.

A larger, more sophisticated badge was introduced probably in the 1930s. It bore the city coat of arms in the centre with a thistle below and, in silver and red enamel above, the city motto. The whole was surrounded by silver lettering: EDINBURGH CITY HOSPITAL SCHOOL OF NURSING on a pale blue enamelled ground.⁸ The reverse was similar to the earlier medal.

By the early 1960s when the Hospital was no longer under the local authority, the city arms were removed from the badge. The new circular, silver, sun-ray badge had an internal squareish format showing in silver on blue enamel a lamp of learning on the left, a caduceus in the centre and a Scottish thistle on the right with Edinburgh Castle below, the whole surmounted by: CITY HOSPITAL SCHOOL OF NURSING, EDINBURGH in silver on yellow enamelling.⁹ Mrs Lamont is credited with its design.

One nurse, Mrs Mina Begg, the RIDU's out-patient sister¹⁰ started training at the City Hospital in 1958 and was awarded her Registered Nurse Certificate and Badge in October 1961. She recalls the starched white caps and blue crossover military style uniforms with buttons down one side. No aprons were issued but 14 barrier gowns instead. At each bedside or cubicle the barrier gown hanging there was donned over the nurse's own gown and replaced on leaving. The doctors wore a fresh white coat at each bed. Hand washing was strictly enforced for all staff.

In 1960 Ward 2 still had scarlet fever patients and a young woman with respiratory paralysis was also nursed there in an 'iron lung'. Ward 2A was for dysentery patients. Ward 3 was the only cubicle ward but it closed in 1960 and its patients were transferred to Wards 16 and 16A, the cubicles in those wards being completed about 1962. Mrs Begg recalls during her training the several rounds a day in Ward 3A cleaning the eyes and noses of measles patients. There was also a weekly inspection of all heads for lice. Ward 4 was closed and 4A became the Wellcome Research Trust Virus Laboratory. Ward 14 accommodated patients with gastroenteritis.

In those days of poor home hygiene and sanitation, patients with infectious diarrhoea were required to submit three negative stool cultures, each 72 hours apart, before discharge home. For school attenders or patients referred on to another hospital, a minimum of six stools, failing which rectal swabs, were needed. Inevitably this delayed the patient's discharge and considerably lengthened the duration of hospital stay. A middle-aged man with respiratory paralysis from poliomyelitis was eventually transferred from Ward 14A to be nursed in a cuirasse by the ever conscientious Mr James Marshall, charge nurse in Ward 17. Wards 15 and 17 became adult male infectious diseases wards with adult female patients in Wards 15A and 17A. Puerperal sepsis was still treated at the City Hospital which accommodated mothers and babies either in Ward 15A or 16A.

Mrs Begg carried out 'ambulance duty' until it was discontinued about 1961. This meant responding to a call, day or night, to accompany the ambulance to the patient's home to assess the infection, complete a form detailing a child's feeds, immunisation status and any benefits being received. All the patient's clothing was taken into hospital with the patient for return later after appropriate disinfection. The nurses on ambulance duty wore conspicuous, red capes which often set wagging the tongues of inquisitive neighbours.

Visiting was actively discouraged until the early 1960s at which time the newspaper bulletins detailing patients' progress were discontinued (see Chapters 17, 18). Until then anxious relatives could attend between 2 and 3 p.m. at what became the conference room. They entered 'horseboxes' from the roadside, handed in sweets and chocolates (which were later shared in the ward) and could talk briefly with the appropriate ward sister or charge nurse.

As telephones were still not universal, a postcard was sent to parents in advance of a child's discharge home and a further three went off at two-day intervals if there was no response. Failing this the police were asked to contact the relatives. It was not uncommon for parents or grandparents wanting a holiday on their own to give children syrup of figs hoping to get their offspring admitted to hospital on the pretext of gastroenteritis. Even in the 1970s one disadvantaged parent, whose child was offered his discharge on Christmas Eve, asked for him to stay in the ward where she claimed he would have a much better time than at home.

Mrs Begg recalls the busy time she had in training. Sometimes only two nurses would be deployed in a whooping cough ward of 20–30 babies some of whom required immediate and repeated attention for apnoeic episodes. Before oral penicillin was available, scarlet fever patients received intramuscular penicillin injections every six hours. Part of the fever nurse's training also involved the management of tuberculosis. Frequently up to 45 intramuscular injections of streptomycin (in 1 g and 750 mg cartridges) had to be given daily before the ward breakfasts were served.

About 1962 Mrs Begg, with Night Superintendent Sister Binnie, both recently revaccinated, volunteered to look after a smallpox suspect isolated in Cottage 26. The patient was a turbaned Sikh, off a plane from India. He eventually turned out not to have smallpox but needed observation and strict isolation, until the tests proved negative. Sister Binnie and Mrs Begg wearing overall 'siren suits' zipped at the back stayed with the patient for several days until he was cleared. Food was left in the cottage vestibule and all outgoing crockery was washed, then disinfected with potassium permanganate before being uplifted by outside staff. A bill was run up for sweets and cigarettes at the hospital shop. Mrs Begg recalls the kindness of Miss Adams at this time and also members of staff like William Webber of the bacteriological laboratory who left piles of magazines for them to read.

More recently the devotion of the nursing staff in caring for patients with highly infectious or dangerous diseases has been remarkable. Latterly some of the emotionally distraught or frightened patients with hepatitis and/or HIV infection could be verbally or physically abusive to the nurses and resistant to simple requests designed to reduce the risk of spreading their infections to staff or other patients. The quiet courage, determination and patience of nurses in these difficult situations deserves to be recorded.

CHAPTER THIRTY-ONE

The Pharmacy; the Professions Allied to Medicine; the Dietetic and Social Work Departments

The Pharmacy

The original plans of the hospital show two large rooms labelled the dispensary and drug store on the east of the red-brick central block.[1] Immediately to the north of the dispensary, occupying the north east corner of the central block was the maids' work room and close by this the mattress and clothes room. The dispensary had separate entrances and counters for the scarlet fever nurses and the other nurses picking up medicines for their respective wards, mirroring the segregation in the nurses' dining room already referred to.[2] In 1907 Dr C. B. Ker mentioned a Lady Dispenser, Miss Duncan, one of whose duties was to teach and examine nurses on 'Medicine'[3] and in 1919 he reported that Miss Bell, Dispenser, was continuing to do 'excellent work in her beautifully kept department'.[4]

Much of the following information has been kindly supplied by Mr Andrew B. H. Hunter, BA, MPS who was successively Group Chief Pharmacist and then Principal Pharmacist from 1973 until he retired in 1994. In the period up to 1965 Miss Brindle, MPS, was responsible for preparing and dispensing medicines within the original drug store and dispensary. She imposed strict requisitioning procedures because even then the containment of the hospital's drug and general pharmaceutical expenditure was the Pharmacist's responsibility. She supplied the City Hospital and some other local hospitals with drugs, dressings and pharmaceutical products.

When Miss Brindle retired in 1965, Miss Rosemary Railton became Group Chief Pharmacist to the Edinburgh Royal Victoria and Associated Hospitals. About this time the recommendations of the Grosset Report to the Scottish Health Services Council stressed the need to group hospital pharmacies efficiently together instead of continuing with small, often isolated, hospital departments. Miss Railton adopted the new expanded role and became responsible for the Royal Victoria Hospital and Dispensary, Princess Margaret Rose Orthopaedic, Southfield and Loanhead Hospitals besides the City Hospital itself. In May 1966 she and her department moved into the purpose-built new pharmacy and stores between the central block and Ward 14, on the site of the former Cottage 13 and original X-ray Department.

The Group Pharmacy and store were responsible for the purchase and supply of a wide range of pharmaceutical products for wards and departments in the hospital group as well as drugs, dressings, disinfectants, intravenous fluids, surgical instruments and other sundries. Locally produced and prepared medicines were also dispensed and Miss Railton was justly proud of her new autoclave and aseptic preparation facilities.

The Group Chief Pharmacist also controlled the expenditure on drugs by contract buying, physically monitoring ward stocks and encouraging a policy of prescribing approved drugs rather than brand named (and often more expensive) medicines. The Pharmacy Committee, chaired by Dr James Murdoch, reported to the Medical Staff Committee and tried to educate staff in correct prescribing. This committee was the first in the Lothians and was the forerunner of the drug and therapeutic committees which are now commonplace in all large hospitals. April 1968 saw the first of the *City Hospital Pharmacy Bulletins* which were funded by the Group's Board of Management and distributed biannually to coincide with each intake of new residents. It kept everyone abreast of the committee's deliberations and encouraged cost-effective and responsible prescribing.

Miss Railton was promoted in 1972 to become the District Pharmaceutical Officer in Cumbria. Her place was taken by Mr Andrew B. H. Hunter as the new Group Chief Pharmacist in 1973. He takes up the story:

> Almost immediately the Department was affected by a series of events which influenced its day to day function and physical layout as well as its relationship with the hospitals and wards for which it provided a service. These were the enforcement of the Medicines Act affecting medicine classification and the separation of dispensing from manufacturing procedures; the Misuse of Drugs Act and its application in relation to storage and security of drugs, and the Health and Safety at Work Act. A period of reorganisation and restructuring ensued resulting in even larger groupings of hospital pharmacies stemming from the recommendations of Sir Noel Hall. The post of Group Chief Pharmacist was abolished only to be replaced by the title of Principal Pharmacist.

Mr Hunter soon became responsible for the pharmaceutical service for 1,600 beds comprising the South Lothian District which included the

City, Princess Margaret Rose Orthopeadic, Loanhead, Southfield, Liberton, Longmore and Astley Ainslie Hospitals, the Royal Victoria Dispensary, the Royal Hospital for Sick Children and Queensberry House. Mr Hunter continues:

> Such enlargement naturally led to delegation and specialisation within the Pharmacy. An efficient purchasing and supplies team was developed under the direction of Mary Kay and John McCulloch whose knowledge of sphygmomanometers, auroscopes and tracheostomy tubes was legendary.
>
> With the introduction of the Medicines Act and its requirements for licensing and manufacturing procedures together with the condemning of the autoclave under the Health and Safety at Work Act, more emphasis was placed on medicine purchase from commercial sources, leading to more restricted buying, stock control and prescribing policies. This could only be achieved optimally by the use of computer technology which eventually developed to cover individual wards and departments.
>
> The domino effect continued. Medical and nursing staff sought more pharmacist input at ward level and so Clinical Pharmacology came into being. The City Hospital Pharmacy was soon a leader in the installation of new computer technology, initially dedicated to purchasing and supply but latterly in the production of broadsheets, histograms, pie charts etc. detailing and forecasting expenditure by ward, specialty and hospital. Such factual and graphic material later proved invaluable when the Principal Pharmacist and his team gave a 'Grand Round' presentation.
>
> By the late 1980s the Pharmacy Department was at the peak of its contribution to the functioning of the City and the remaining associated hospitals. A new aseptic suite had been commissioned about 1984 further strengthening the clinical aspect of pharmacy. This initially provided aseptically prepared feeds and infusions and the occasional clinical trial material for the RIDU, later expanding into the other specialties with total parenteral nutrition and intravenous infusions.
>
> However, further organisational change was soon to reverse this expansion. When I retired from the City Hospital in 1994 after 21 years of service, the Unit had contracted to two main hospitals, the City and Princess Margaret Rose Orthopaedic Hospital. A decision had been made to build a new Royal Infirmary so the City Hospital became surplus to requirements. Its pharmacy was now a satellite of the Royal Infirmary. It was providing a service for fewer and fewer wards.

Mr Hunter's staff had increased from seven in 1973, when he was appointed, to 13 in 1992, two years before he retired. Originally, besides himself, there was a pharmacist, technician, two pharmacy assistants, one storeman and one secretary. By 1992, besides himself, there were at the City Hospital four pharmacists, one storekeeper and one storekeeper/clerk, two pharmacy assistants and four technicians, now called medical technical officers. At the Royal Hospital for Sick Children and Liberton Hospital, there were five extra staff under his jurisdiction.

Mr Hunter's department had given excellent service for many years, and his sadness at the hospital's closure echoed the sentiments of many other members of the hospital staff.

Department of Physiotherapy

The exact date when physiotherapists joined the staff of the City Hospital is unclear. In the early days many of their duties would have been carried out by the nursing staff, however improper that may seem to modern physiotherapists. These duties would have included the encouragement of sputum expectoration by tuberculous patients, the mobilisation of paralysed victims of poliomyelitis and of patients rendered weak after prolonged bed rest.

The original Physiotherapy Department occupied one of the open-sided tuberculosis wards converted into a single-storey, white painted, weatherboarded, pavilion-style building situated at the end of an uncovered concrete slab path to the south of Pavilion 5. Access was difficult for disabled or wheelchair-bound patients especially in bad weather. When the Geriatric Medicine Department started, most of the ward patients were treated there. About 1978–79, the new Physiotherapy Department with much improved facilities opened in the central block, adjacent to the lecture theatre. Shortly afterwards the uninhabited, white pavilion building was used as a bedding store. It was destroyed by fire, possibly as a result of arson, which was also responsible for the loss of the cricket pavilion and other easily vandalised structures in the hospital grounds.

Mrs Angela Lindsay, Superintendent of the department since 1992, has kindly supplied much of the following information including a list of her immediate predecessors as follows:

Dillys Williams	–1962
Elizabeth Ross	1962–1980
John Barber	1980–1984
Kirsten Dalkier	1985–1992
Angela Lindsay	1992–

Before the 1970s when the Care of the Elderly Unit demanded an increase in physiotherapy staff, there had simply been one Superintendent and three Basic Grade Physiotherapists. About 1974 a Senior II Grade was appointed to cover the Thoracic Surgical Unit but there was no overall increase in staff which then consisted of one Superintendent, one Senior II and two Basic Grade Physiotherapists. The team approach advocated by Professor Williamson, and the requirement of home visits, increased the workload. In time three part-time physiotherapists joined the staff. The first Senior I Grade Physiotherapist was to cover the Geriatric Unit and the day hospital.

Towards the end of her long career Miss Elizabeth Ross was actively planning the present Physiotherapy Department and physiotherapy services for the Assessment Unit and day hospital. Mrs Dalkier, appointed Superintendent in 1985, felt the department was being underused and she started up the out-patient area raising money through donations, raffles and cake and jumble sales. In 1988 a new Senior I Grade post was created to serve both the new out-patient area and the RIDU with especial emphasis on HIV-infected patients. The out-patient work began gradually with five new referrals per month from general practitioners who were given open access to the service.

When Angela Lindsay was appointed in March 1992, the staff consisted of 14 physiotherapists, including herself, nine of whom were full-time and five part-time. There were no physiotherapy helpers, only limited secretarial help and no computers. She developed an Outpatient Waiting List Initiative in June 1992 and saw the number of referrals grow rapidly to an average of 40 or 50 per month. This required an additional 0.5 whole time equivalent (WTE) Senior II staff post. Extension of the Waiting List Initiative in 1994 meant this post was extended to full-time and later 1.25 WTEs with additional secretarial hours. From 1993 to 1995 contracts were agreed with general practitioner fundholders so that, by 1995, this work accounted for 40 per cent of the out-patient department activity. By 1995–96 about 120 new patients were referred each month and a further 1 WTE senior grade post was approved.

In 1992 the first helper was appointed to assist with the increasing number of requests to obtain induced sputum samples from HIV-infected patients at risk of pneumocystis pneumonia. A hyperventilation service had been started in 1989 but this went to the Royal Infirmary in December 1993 when the Respiratory Medicine Unit moved there from the City Hospital. When still in action at the City Hospital, the 19-bedded Stroke Rehabilitation Unit was staffed by 2.6 WTE physiotherapists who came from the respiratory medicine wards. In the Care of the Elderly Unit in 1995, staffing ratios were changed as physiotherapists left, by converting part-time hours to helper hours to improve the 'skillmix'. After Mrs Lindsay was upgraded to Superintendent II because of the staffing increases and her enlarging role as manager, her complement of staff in 1995 was 10 full-time, 11 part-time physiotherapists, 3 part-time physiotherapy helpers and 1.70 WTE secretaries. Computerisation had arrived and a patient information management system was coping with contracts and billing.

From its tiny staff in the early 1970s, the department had therefore grown to provide an excellent service and create funds of its own through GP contracts. It remained devoted to the hospital's overall caring role in addition to its purely service commitments. Miss Elizabeth Ross continued to support the hospital's League of Friends long after she retired and many of the staff helped in various ways to raise funds for patients' comforts.

The traditional Wednesday tea and cake afternoons, which continued for 22 years, perhaps epitomise best the friendliness and cohesion of this department. As Mrs Lindsay explains, each member of staff took it in turn to supply a cake, ideally home baked, which was eaten at this weekly afternoon tea party get-together for all the staff. One hopes that when the Physiotherapy Department moves to the new Royal Infirmary, such informal but highly important staff meetings will not become diluted and lost in the context of a bigger organisation.

Occupational Therapy

Mrs Nola Meikle has been associated with the City Hospital on and off since the 1960s. She has kindly supplied much of the following information about the Occupational Therapy (OT) Department.

The earliest in a long line of occupational therapists at the hospital that she can recall is Avril Gardiner, a red haired lady who was larger than life. She had apparently not qualified as an occupational therapist but had previously worked in the armed forces where she provided diversionary therapy for wounded and sick troops. She was followed by Liz Davis who came to the hospital in the 1960s and was succeeded in turn by Marjorie Helm who was in charge of the OT Department from about 1974 until 1984 when she left to go to the Astley Ainslie Hospital. The next head of department was Rosemary (Romy) Crewe whose two and a half years' locum post was dogged by ill health which forced her to resign.

In 1986 Nola Meikle was appointed to the post of Head. She started work at the City Hospital in September 1986 at the same time as Professor MacLennan took up the Chair of Geriatric Medicine.

Mrs Meikle qualified in 1965 and worked with Dr Lowther and Dr (later Professor) Williamson in the day hospital at the Royal Victoria Hospital, thereafter having duties also at the City and Loanhead Hospitals. From 1967 to 1968 she acted as a nanny in Durban to the three children of Mr Carl Beckerling, a South African thoracic surgeon who was once registrar to Mr Andrew Logan, formerly of the City Hospital in Edinburgh but who had continued to work in Durban after retiring from the NHS in 1972. In the later 1960s Mrs Meikle held posts in King's College Hospital and Putney Hospital in London before moving back to Edinburgh where she provided OT services in the Eastern, Western and Northern General Hospitals.

In 1966 Mrs Meikle's work at the City Hospital was part-time, mostly single-handed, diversionary therapy. She often covered more than one area – the City and Royal Victoria Hospitals – still usually single-handed, but occasionally with another occupational therapist, Lettie Morrison.

In 1978 Mrs Meikle carried out a locum post at the City Hospital. She shared accommodation with the Physiotherapy Department and the medical social workers in the wooden building behind Pavilion 5. Without a creche at work or the back up at home that there often would be nowadays, she and the other para-medical workers took their babies to the hospital in carrycots. Shortly after, all the occupational therapists and physiotherapists moved to better accommodation, in the newly created department in the central block on the west side of the lecture theatre.

In 1986 the OT staff consisted of 5.5 trained occupational therapists and two assistants. In addition to her administrative and managerial duties the head of the department worked partly in the Respiratory Medicine Unit and partly in the RIDU. One Senior, one Basic Grade and one Assistant covered the Geriatric Assessment Unit; there was a full-time trained occupational therapist later a Senior, in the day hospital and another Senior in Respiratory Medicine.

The staff was later expanded with extra helpers especially in the day hospital and in the RIDU where Marjorie Helm had been particularly active looking after the hepatitis patients and intravenous drug misusers. There developed a need for a Senior I Grade and a Basic Grade occupational therapist to assist with the growing number of HIV-infected patients.

Mrs Meikle was anxious that frail elderly patients, often pitchforked into the RIDU by frustrated or overworked general practitioners with the flimsy diagnosis of 'diarrhoea and vomiting – ? infectious', should also receive appropriate OT input. Without even a basic minimum of diversionary therapy to stimulate them, old people would often settle into a hospital bed and become totally dependent. She always insisted, therefore, in having the clothes of elderly patients easily available on the ward so that they could 'learn' to dress themselves and get about the ward as soon as they were physically able.

Mrs Meikle appreciated that the full range of OT skills should be applied and that, where appropriate, the sometimes despised diversionary therapy — weaving baskets and making teddy bears — could be incredibly valuable. Overall functional assessment became increasingly important to predict, for instance, what a stroke victim could or could not do in his or her own home after hospital discharge. This often meant overcoming the resistance of some older consultants who seemed unaware of the sophisticated training undergone by modern occupational therapists especially in neurology, physiology and psychology. One senior occupational therapist so impressed a consultant, by diagnosing a brain tumour in its correct anatomical position, that he used this episode later in his lectures to illustrate the value of functional assessment by occupational therapists.

In the ENT Department occupational therapists helped with the physical and psychological rehabilitation of laryngectomees in a team effort with the physiotherapists and the speech and language therapist. Occupational therapy had therefore progressed rapidly from post-Second World War diversionary therapy to provide highly advanced services such as functional assessment and the appropriate aids to make it possible for disabled people to live at home. Provided that consultants appreciate their potential, occupational therapists and others in the professions allied to medicine will continue to make an inestimable contribution to the team effort.

Speech and Language Therapy Department

Up until July 1976 when Ms Sandra J. Anderson was appointed to a senior speech and language therapy post, there had been no formal service for the City Hospital. Previously a part-time therapist at Liberton Hospital would, if requested, attend the very few stroke patients with speech and language problems. The therapist from the Royal Infirmary visited post-laryngectomy patients and followed them up at the Royal Infirmary afterwards.

When Professor Williamson returned from Liverpool to the first Chair of Geriatric Medicine in Edinburgh in 1976, speech and language therapy was needed in his new Care of Elderly Unit. At the same time a growing need was identified in the ENT Department. A senior post in speech and language therapy was therefore created and Ms Anderson was appointed on 12 July 1976. She has continued ever since to work in an innovative, cheerful and enthusiastic manner much to the benefit of her patients. She has kindly provided the following information about her department.

Initially she was based at Liberton Hospital and managed single-handed to provide a service for Liberton, Longmore, Southfield, Bruntsfield, Loanhead and the Deaconess Hospitals as well as the City Hospital. To cope with the huge workload, extra resources were needed. On 3 March

1979 Ms Anderson was therefore transferred to the City Hospital from where she provided a service for only the City and Deaconess Hospitals until the latter closed in 1985.

For more than 20 years Ms Anderson has developed expertise in speech and language therapy in the ENT Department. She became acutely aware of the psychological and physical devastation that can follow major head and neck surgery and established a support group for laryngectomees. In 1980 the Lothian Laryngectomy Club was affiliated to the National Association of Laryngectomy Clubs – a branch of Macmillan Cancer Relief. At its inception the Lothian Laryngectomy Club was mirrored only by one similar club in Glasgow, but now there are several throughout Scotland. By 1995 the Lothian Club was raising about £1,500 every year to fund medical equipment, textbooks and staff courses all pertaining to head and neck surgery. In addition, items such as swimming aids are bought and the club's social events subsidised. In 1994 television and video-sets were provided for the four single laryngectomy rooms.

In 1981 Ms Anderson set up the first Scottish swimming group for laryngectomees which has a small but enthusiastic group of swimmers from Edinburgh and beyond. Of six such groups in the UK, Ms Anderson's is the only one in Scotland. In addition she has organised conferences, seminars and study days on aspects of laryngectomy for health care workers and patients.

In December 1993 when the Stroke Unit opened in the Care of the Elderly Unit, Ms Anderson had a colleague working with her for the first time:, Ms Emma Reymbaut, a part-time speech and language therapist. In May 1994, Ms Elma O'Donnell joined her as an assistant. Two months previously Ms Anderson moved from her unsatisfactory 'single office cum treatment room cum storeroom into a lovely new suite of rooms'.[5]

Specialist treatment was then given not only to head and neck surgery patients but to those with strokes and disorders of swallowing. Open access was offered to patients every morning and a monthly laryngectomy clinic was held with the medical staff. A stroke group was also flourishing until the Care of the Elderly Unit closed.

Ms Anderson pays generous tribute to all those doctors, surgeons, nurses and para-medical staff with whom she came in contact when she was working solo. Over those years she 'experienced nothing but kindness, support and offers of help'. She asks 'Will that same camaraderie and fellowship go with us when the City eventually closes?'. In its turn the hospital is indebted to Ms Anderson for her pioneering spirit and devotion to her patients.

Dietetic Service

Up to the early 1970s there was no regular dietetic service for the City Hospital. Despite her busy schedule, Miss Elizabeth Wilson, of the Diabetic and Dietetic Outpatient Clinic at the Royal Infirmary, was good enough to give advice for specific patients when requested. I and others on the Medical Staff Committee at the City Hospital, however, pressed for the hospital to have its own dietetic service and eventually it came.

Ms Enid Henery has kindly supplied the following information. By 1977 there was one Chief IV (full-time) and one Basic Grade Dietitian working at the City Hospital but also covering four other hospitals – Princess Margaret Rose Orthopaedic Hospital (PMROH), Liberton, Longmore and Bruntsfield Hospitals – as well as supervising a Basic Grade Dietitian at Astley Ainslie Hospital whose duties also extended to the Deaconess Hospital. During 1977 the Basic Grade Dietitian post was regraded to a Senior II post and a Basic Grade Dietitian was appointed to the medical wards, so allowing the Chief Dietitian time to manage the service and provide a senior post in the Care of the Elderly Unit. Temporary cover was arranged for Astley Ainslie Hospital and PMROH, weekly visits to Longmore and Bruntsfield Hospitals, and five or six sessions weekly at the Deaconess Hospital. When the City Hospital's day hospital opened in December 1977, the volume of work increased and a further recommendation was made for more dietetic staff.

The early members of the dietetic service included Jane Calder (Dietetic Manager), Carol Drabble, Alison Hendry and June Benson. From 1983 to 1987 Alison (Parker) Thompson was Dietetic Manager with Moyra Burns, Fiona Bell, Amy Fortune, Clare Keenan and Jan Clark. Alison Parker (Thompson) acted as Chief Dietitian for the ENT Unit and PMROH, Enid Henery held the Senior Grade II post in the Care of the Elderly Unit and Carol Drabble was the Basic Grade Dietitian for the medical corridor. They then covered the City, PMROH, Southfield Day Hospital and Hospital, Liberton and Loanhead Hospitals and the Currie Medical Centre.

By 1987 Enid Henery was Chief of service, Anne Lamb, the Senior II in the Care of the Elderly Unit, Caroline Penman held a senior post in the HIV/AIDS Unit, Fiona Bayne was responsible for nutrition education and Clare Keenan looked after the medical and respiratory medicine units. A 9-hour weekly secretarial post was included. In 1996, the staff consisted of Enid Henery, Anne Lamb, Fiona Bayne, Caroline Penman and Tracey Wilson.

Changes in staff and attachments to different hospitals and individual units within them resulted from the frequent organisational changes and regroupings of hospitals. The City Hospital belonged sequentially to the South Lothian District, the United Hospitals Unit and finally the RIE NHS Trust. After 1993–4, the dietitians at the City Hospital covered the City Hospital and PMROH only.

Enid Henery also recounts the changes in work required of dietitians over the past 20 years and the different locations in which dietitians worked because of the regroupings of hospitals. From the City Hospital having no dietitians at all in the early 1970s, the staff numbers grew although there were never enough for the demand. Dietetic practice became increasing sophisticated. Different types of expertise were needed as new medical and surgical techniques developed and new diseases such as HIV infection appeared. From simple referrals for overweight and diabetic patients, most of the work became devoted to nutritional support. From the 'home made' enteral feeds delivered by naso-gastric or oesophageal tubes in the 1970s, there are now also gastrostomy and jejunostomy feeds to prepare. Many proprietary preparations can be delivered by carefully controlled pumps rather than old gravity drip methods. Patients now continue enteral feeding at home so freeing hospital beds and reuniting patients with their families. The nutritional care of AIDS patients contributes greatly to their survival. The devotion of a Senior I Grade Dietitian to this service became increasingly important in the 1980s.

Research studies in the Care of the Elderly Unit involved the use of zinc in long-term care patients and a study of Vitamin D in the housebound elderly. Health promotion for both staff and patients was emphasised with sensible eating regimens. Sophisticated anthropometric measurement techniques in nutritional assessment were developed. Although the labour intensive home visiting had to be severely curtailed, good links with general practitioners were fostered. Student dietitians were seconded from the Royal Infirmary for a week's training and experience at the City Hospital. Computers were introduced in the 1980s for word processing, spreadsheets and forming databases.

Enid Henery is determined to transfer to the Royal Infirmary the enthusiasm, motivation, friendliness and expertise her staff have built up during 20 years of service at the City Hospital. In 1996 she wrote of the City Hospital:

> This hospital has been well known for its friendly staff and service to patients for a long time and I am pleased and feel privileged to have been part of that for the last 13 years or so.

Social Work Department

In mediaeval times an almoner literally distributed alms. In the late nineteenth century the word almoner came to mean a hospital official whose duties also involved the social condition of patients. With the burgeoning of the welfare state, hospital almoners became concerned as much with the welfare of patients in the broadest sense, as with their pecuniary condition alone. They now provide an invaluable bridge between the medical and nursing staff, the professions allied to medicine, the patients and their families. They must have a thorough knowledge of medical conditions, social environments, housing and nursing home facilities, interpersonal and family relations and the increasing complexity of modern systems of benefit.

Mrs Elizabeth Dunbar has kindly supplied much of the following information and has traced social work back to her early experiences with tuberculous patients and their families in the 1950s. In the Royal Victoria Dispensary (see Chapter 19) there was then a small social work department whose members made regular visits to the tuberculosis wards in the City and Royal Victoria Hospitals. Before Professor Crofton's triple drug therapy regimen of the 1950s, tuberculosis could remain open and highly infectious for months or years. Treatment was prolonged and arduous. It affected especially the very young, the old and the malnourished. In the overcrowded slums the finding of even one open case could pose a huge problem.

Parents and toddlers often shared one room or a 'single end' consisting of a room and kitchen. Controlling the spread of infection in such circumstances demanded close cooperation between physicians, health visitors, social workers and the MOH. The best solution was to rehouse the patient if at all possible and to provide individual bed and bedding, adequate clothing and an increased allowance for food and heating above the usual Sickness Benefit rates. The National Association for the Prevention of Tuberculosis and other voluntary organisations also contributed towards providing the necessities for such disadvantaged families. Medical social workers (MSWs) also tried to help families through difficult times. Often the prolonged hospitalisation of a breadwinner led to financial problems, strained marital relationships and caused the split up of families or engaged couples. Men and women in lodging houses often failed to cooperate with treatment. Typically ill-educated, alcoholic, with a history of psychiatric illness and no family ties, they might simply disappear not notifying a change of address when sent to prison or leaving the city altogether.

Tuberculosis was no respecter of social status. Mrs Dunbar recalls the sad case of one young lawyer called to the Bar in the 1950s. He and another young colleague contracted tuberculosis from a clerk who had a persistent 'winter cough'. One of these lawyers survived after extensive lung surgery and long convalescence; the other died.

Mrs Dunbar writes so vividly about the activities of her department that the following is quoted almost verbatim:

> Those patients with tuberculosis who were admitted to hospital were encouraged to take part in various educational and rehabilitation programmes, to relieve boredom and to make good use of time in an extended stay. In addition to the occupational therapy provided, one such attempt should be recorded. Mrs Sinclair Shaw, a talented French lady, came weekly to the City Hospital to conduct art therapy classes, the Chest, Heart and Stroke Association paying for all the art materials required. One or two of the most hardened 'Grassmarketeers' were surprised to find they had a talent which they never suspected and were very proud of their efforts. Perhaps for the first time in their lives being treated with courtesy by physicians, nursing staff and everyone else concerned, they felt they were of worth. Many responded to this.
>
> Throughout this time the head social worker was Miss Peggy Wood. Superficially, Peggy appeared to be the epitome of the old fashioned lady almoner, but her appearance belied her understanding and compassion. She devoted her life to work with TB patients and tribute should be paid to her hard work and dedication.
>
> In 1962 the senior social worker, who had worked so closely and effectively with Miss Wood in the Royal Victoria Dispensary, left to work in London. It was a sign of the rapid decline in the incidence of TB that Miss Shiells was replaced by a social worker in the City Hospital. By the time that Miss Wood retired in the late 1960s most of the specialties now existing in the City Hospital had been established and there were by then two full-time and one part-time social workers in addition to Miss Wood's successor. So over the years the emphasis gradually changed from an outpatient-based department with a small colony in the hospital, to a hospital-based department. From this time social work records were kept in the City Hospital and secretarial help was available. Each ward in the hospital had its designated social worker and an effort was made to meet the aptitudes and interests of the worker concerned. For example, one young MSW helped to run a support group for laryngectomy patients, which some other young people might have found difficult. Another worked in the last two remaining TB wards in the hospital. She enjoyed the challenges presented by the few remaining 'hard liners' and, as she came to the task from work

in Soweto, she had plenty of experience of difficult human situations to help her.

In the old days at the City Hospital many more of the staff lived in, including the Matron. One such lady, who retired many years ago, never went to bed without walking up the infectious diseases corridor to say good night to a young girl on a ventilator who had been stricken by polio. Such humanity was not at all uncommon, and the chief recollection is of the compassion, patience and understanding shown by all disciplines in the hospital. The social workers particularly appreciated the support and encouragement of senior physicians in the two main respiratory teaching units, who each in his own way made opportunities to discuss patients' medical and social needs. Other specialties in the hospital developed their own lines of communication. On a more frivolous level, the staff room in the old physiotherapy department down in the 'huts' provided much more than morning coffee for the OTs, PTs and MSWs based in that part of the hospital. Many fruitful exchanges of ideas and information took place.

Lastly, the members of the department enjoyed a very close and helpful relationship with various members of staff in the MOH's department in Johnston Terrace. The close working together was never better illustrated than by the case of a young Hong Kong Chinese boy who was admitted suffering from typhoid. He had just arrived in Edinburgh to live with an extended family and to work in a Chinese restaurant. Clearly, this was impossible. The MSW concerned had to support him for months in this bewildering situation. Eventually, an understanding landlady was found to take him in on discharge from hospital, educational classes for him were sought, particularly so that he could obtain fluency in English, and financial help was found to support him and pay for his classes.

Some considerable time later the MOH concerned was invited to lunch in a well-known Chinese restaurant when to his great consternation, the young Chinese boy whom he had banned from ever cooking and serving in a restaurant appeared through a bead curtain, dressed in an immaculate white jacket. Hasty enquiry was made, and the explanation was simple – the boy was working in a Chinese laundry and had been delivering clean table cloths!

In the late 1960s and early 1970s it proved difficult to provide continuity of service to the hospital. In addition to emigration and what the old Institute of Almoners used to call 'wastage through marriage', young social workers with good qualifications and perhaps two years' hospital experience found it easy to get jobs with good promotion prospects in the new local authority Social Work Departments. There are clear recollections of trying to provide a service to the entire hospital and the Royal Victoria Dispensary throughout one summer aided only by three students. At a time when job sharing was not so common as it is today, it was decided to recruit two older part-time MSWs to one job. These MSWs had settled homes in Edinburgh and family commitments, and it is gratifying to relate that one MSW in the City Hospital worked until retirement, and the other MSW was still in post in 1995.

It was also felt that it would be helpful to have a social work assistant to attend to more practical matters in patient care. Such an appointment was made, at the sacrifice of one part-time social worker. This meant that by the end of 1974 there were one full-time MSW and two part-timers in post, a full-time SW assistant and a full time secretary, with a newly appointed Principal MSW taking over the department in 1975.

From 1975, Mrs Kim Shandley, head of the department until 1982, takes up the story. Early in 1975 there were three part-time MSWs, one full-time MSW assistant and a full-time secretary and one newly appointed Senior MSW. Mrs Shandley's account follows, almost verbatim:

In April 1975 responsibility for hospital social work was transferred from Lothian Health Board to Lothian Regional Council Department of Social Work. Thereafter considerable reorganisation and consolidation took place within all hospitals in Lothian Region, under the guiding hand of the Director of Social Work, Mr Roger Kent.

The City Hospital became the co-ordinating centre for seven other hospitals – Princess Margaret Rose Orthopaedic, Astley Ainslie, Bruntsfield, Longmore, Liberton, Southfield, and Loanhead Hospitals. This grouping gradually strengthened the individual units, enabling exchange of ideas and experience over a wide range of clinical and social needs. A supportive, professional line management was established. Well-argued requests for staff increases enabled the assignment of a designated social worker to every ward or department, so that social work support to patients and their relatives could be organised most effectively, taking account of the needs of various clinical specialties.

As social work input developed, so did multi-disciplinary cooperation. Each discipline, medical and surgical, nursing, occupational and physiotherapy, out-patient (particularly the city centre TB Clinic in Spittal Street) administration and medical secretarial, domestic, catering, all co-operated and learned from each other, for the ultimate benefit of patients. One of the porters, a leading light in AA, was a most valuable consultant to the department and counsellor to several alcoholic patients in need. This cooperation was very rewarding for social workers during these years.

The well established professorial Department of Respiratory Medicine (Professor Sir John Crofton) followed in 1977 by the professorial Department of Geriatric Medicine (Professor J. Williamson) enabled social workers to obtain and develop knowledge and skills in centres of excellence to add to those acquired in communicable diseases, thoracic and ENT surgery. Social workers also contributed to teaching medical, nursing and social work students.

Patient care was always the uppermost priority throughout the hospital. Social workers were able to help patients and their relatives in many ways: welfare and financial information (requiring close cooperation with various offices of the Department of Health & Social Security), counselling in adjustment to ill health and bereavement, practical help with special needs such as change of house or employment and any arcane item which did not fit easily into any known clinical category! For example the marriage of a terminally ill patient and his partner of 12 years was a cooperative effort between staff of the ward, social work, catering and the Church of Scotland and was, against the odds, a memorably happy occasion.

The admission of a group of Vietnamese boat people provided an interesting insight into support systems of a different culture. Despite their comparatively destitute state, apart from polite responses in conversation and the heart-warming trust of the lovely children, they seemed to need little social support outside that provided within the family structure. The grandfather of one Vietnamese family could speak no English. To occupy his time while he was being investigated for an abdominal complaint he was given a stool to make by the OT. He finished weaving the cord top in record time, sitting cross legged on his bed with the twine tied to his big toe. The social worker concerned discovered that he had been a fisherman and this was how he mended his nets. He did not realise it was usual to pay for the materials and made several in quick succession to give to his family before the OT had the courage to stem the flow!

Another patient from afar off was a little girl from a nomad family in North Yemen who could speak no English on her admission but was communicating well by the time she was transferred to Princess Margaret Rose Orthopaedic Hospital for hand surgery. She was then fostered while continuing her treatment and is now living in the USA with relations of a Yemeni doctor who had taken an interest in her.

The geographic location of the Social Work Department in the gatehouse afforded many opportunities for casual, non-clinical encounters such as weary housemen in need of restorative cups of coffee. One such enthusiast found it an ideal place for bringing on his tomato plants, having previously been banished from growing them in the wards and residency! Life was often exhaustingly busy but never dull.

Hopefully the well established traditions of multi-disciplinary co-operation for the benefit of patients will be successfully transferred to pastures new when the hospital relocates.

Mrs Shandley was followed by Mr David Taylor MBE who had worked in Leith. Mr Taylor was much involved with the social needs of HIV-infected patients and their families when the explosion of intravenous heroin misuse and its consequences hit Edinburgh and Dr Brettle was building up the HIV/AIDS service. Mr Taylor became the AIDS Co-ordinator for Lothian Region on leaving the City Hospital. During this time the City Hospital Social Work Department came under the management of the Royal Infirmary. Mr Malcolm McEwan was in charge from 1986 to 1990. His title changed from Senior Principal Social Worker to Practice Manager of Social Workers. Mr Mike Stokes took over in 1990 and the next year saw further changes to the structure of the Social Work Department under the 1991 Community Care Act. All reference to medical social workers had been dropped over the years in favour of simply social workers.

Mrs Pam Leaver kindly contributed much of the information in the preceding paragraph. She came to the City Hospital in 1974 as a medical social worker and initially worked with Dr N. W. Horne's Chest Unit patients in Wards 5 and 5A and also in the ENT Department. In the Chest Unit she recalls the few remaining difficult-to-treat 'Grassmarke-teers' with tuberculosis and the patients undergoing chemotherapy for lung cancer. In 1975 the Social Work Department was taken over from Lothian Health Board to become the responsibility of the local authority, then the Lothian Regional Council. The complement of social workers by the later 1970s was approximately six, including a social work assistant.

In 1986 Mrs Leaver transferred to the RIDU after Mrs Marta Harley left. There was plenty of work for 1.5 WTE of social workers there when the impact of HIV infection was being felt. Another social worker who left her mark on the RIDU over a number of years was the understanding and often humorous Mrs Mae Baird who retired about the time Mrs Leaver came to the RIDU. The contribution of the almoners and (medical) social workers over the decades is acknowledged with much gratitude.

CHAPTER THIRTY-TWO

Records and Secretarial Services; Catering, Laundry, Area Sterilising Service; Domestic and Portering Services; Buildings, Grounds and Gardens

Records Office and Secretarial Staff
Late in the nineteenth century the brief notes recorded by nurses and doctors on temperature charts were often all that was kept to document a patient's admission, diagnosis, treatment, progress, and discharge or death. Because so many infections ran a similar course, records were often almost identical for patients suffering from conditions such as scarlet fever, unless complications set in or an unusual intervention or treatment was given. In a leather bound ledger the clinical observations on patients in the second City Hospital are noted in copperplate handwriting with a neatness and clarity that would shame modern medical and nursing calligraphers.[1] (See also the illustration on page 71.)

A legacy of this system was the simple double-sided sheet used in the infectious diseases wards well into the 1960s. Line drawings of the chest and abdomen were used to record abnormalities such as the distribution of rashes and, rather than a long personal and family history, boxes were available for ticking the relevant information. The top corners of the front page had boxes labelled *Head clean/dirty* and *Body clean/dirty* referring respectively to the absence or presence of hair and body lice.

Perhaps in the interests of research and the need to keep more detailed information in the event of litigation, much fuller case notes were next introduced and kept for a specified number of years along with the X-rays. This move coincided with the expansion of out-patient departments and services and the rapid increase in the number and sophistication of investigations. From then on the results of all manner of body fluid tests, ECGs, scans, X-rays and function tests increased the girth of the case note folders creating a storage problem for records departments. Putting case notes on microfiche only partly solved the difficulty, being expensive and not very user friendly. Similarly 'thinning' of X-rays and notes by medical staff was unpopular being both arbitrary and time consuming. Placing a finite limit on the time old case notes are kept before destruction has provided one answer and is the most commonly used method of providing space for current and future records.

Many of the former City Hospital staff remember with affection Jimmy Wilson at the records office. He had been a porter before taking up the post about 1948 at the start of the NHS. It seems amazing today that he coped with this task almost single-handed. His neat handwriting and the ruled margins of the admission books were meticulous. The secret of his beautiful tenor singing, sometimes heard in the hospital as well as in his local church choir, was to lubricate his voice beforehand with a teaspoonful of blackcurrant jam. He was much missed when he retired about 1974.

In the meantime, about 1966, Jimmy Knowles had become the City Hospital Records Officer and later the Group Records Officer. He was always an approachable man. Searching for missing records was never too much trouble, even though, as was often the case, a clinician who had instituted the search would apologetically find the mislaid case notes in his own possession. Jimmy Knowles left in the late 1970s to go to the Western General Hospital from where he left Edinburgh altogether for the mission field in Southern Africa. His son has carried on his tradition, being in charge of records at the Royal Infirmary.

When tuberculosis was still rife, the City Hospital and Royal Victoria Dispensary had close links and this also applied to the patients' records. Alyson Malone, formerly at the Royal Victoria Hospital, became the City Hospital's Records Officer and Information Manager and now works at the Lothian Health Board. Freda Coulter, formerly Office Manager for radiology in the Royal Infirmary, was appointed in charge of the City Hospital records office in March 1997.

When Jimmy Knowles left in the late 1970s his post was not filled, but fortunately, someone with much background experience became head of the department. This was Mrs Sheila Black who had worked variously as a cashier at the City Hospital, then in Princess Margaret Rose Orthopaedic Hospital and with the Scottish Special Housing Association until she returned to the City Hospital in the late 1970s. Outside the office her great interest was the group Queen with Freddie Mercury. Sadly, she was a heavy smoker who suffered from ill health, retired prematurely after her husband had died, and shortly after passed away herself.

Records officers, like Sheila Black, also had other duties, one of which was to recruit and supervise the hospital secretaries. A warm tribute must be accorded to all these ladies for their often unstinting and devoted work. Most consultants were privileged to have their own personal secretary or one was shared between two or three senior members of the NHS or academic staff. Many of these ladies were great characters. For instance in 1960 Dr Murdoch inherited Mrs Lilias Robertson who had been Dr Joe's secretary. She was an efficient and methodical person who was said to have been involved in deciphering ENIGMA during the Second World War. She always had *The Scotsman* crossword puzzle completed before mid-morning coffee and could type faster and more accurately on her mechanical typewriter than many modern typists can achieve on a word-processor. She struck fear and alarm into senior house officers and even consultants who dared to be late in signing 'her' letters, so missing the last posting time of the day. Among many other secretaries who gave long and dedicated service were Marjory Drummond in Respiratory Medicine, Joyce Holywell, Dr Horne's secretary, Mrs Burt who was for many years in the Care of the Elderly Unit and others too numerous to list here.

About 1991 the new HOMER system for tracing case notes was introduced and later PAS, Patient Administration System. Someone who can remember back to 1971 is the last Deputy Records Manager at the City Hospital, Ernie Whiteoak, who kindly provided much of the preceding information. He had worked in stores, pay and accounts department and then the records department and sadly had his present job terminated in March 1998 when the records office finally closed. Like Jimmy Wilson, Ernie has a fine tenor voice, and also plays the guitar, writes songs and sings in a small group.

Not all the City Hospital's records, however, were stored in the main records office. In the early 1960s when the Pyelonephritis Unit was established in Pavilion 14, the number of case notes rapidly multiplied. Patients were regularly followed up at the clinic and problems arose transporting their case notes between Ward 14 and the records office. For this reason, and for ease of access by research doctors, the case notes were transferred to Ward 14 where they were carefully looked after by the secretary, Mrs Alice Northwood, and her successors. They were moved to Ward 17 when the RIDU Out-patient Clinic moved there in the 1980s. To preserve strict confidentiality, Dr Brettle ordered fireproof and tamper-proof safes to house the case notes of HIV-infected patients. Being very heavy they had to be placed at intervals over the supporting beams throughout Pavilion 17. More secure accommodation became available later when a records store was built behind the new reception area in Ward 17.

The main records department was housed for many years opposite the medical library on the west side of the first floor of the New Medical Block. Because of the weight of case notes and X-rays, the floor underneath had to be strengthened. With the development of the City Hospital site by Morrison Homes, the New Medical Block is to be demolished. The X-ray Department, medical out-patients department and the offices of respiratory medicine, thoracic surgery and geriatric medicine, the medical library and the records office will then be no more.

Catering

When Robert Morham designed the hospital in 1896, ample provision was made for kitchens, sculleries, and food stores for the needs of patients and staff. A complex in the central block held these and the nurses' and servants' dining rooms. Dining space for medical staff was in the administrative buildings facing the main gate. Behind the kitchens were a vegetable store and vegetable scullery and, in the days before refrigeration, a room for fish and ice, a milk pantry, poultry larder, and finally fresh meat and cold meat larders. Being totally separate, these rooms would certainly have pleased today's food hygienists. Across the open courtyard was a covered area for storing food trolleys. Food was probably kept hot on pre-heated metal rings or in water jackets so as to reach the wards at least warm. The ward kitchens would only be used for some reheating of food and for simple preparations such as boiled eggs, hot drinks and toast.

Mr Tom Ferguson was the hospital's Catering Manager, and later Group Catering Manager, from his appointment in 1971 until 1985 when he transferred as Support Services Manager to the Royal Infirmary. He took over from Ms Eileen Wilson who subsequently worked in the Royal Edinburgh Hospital until her retirement. When he was Group Catering Manager, Mr Ferguson had responsibility for the City, PMROH, Bruntsfield, Deaconess and Elsie Inglis Memorial Maternity Hospitals. He was in charge at the City Hospital of 10–12 cooks, 2–3 trainees and 20–30 mainly part-time kitchen and dining room maids whose main tasks were clearing, washing up and cleaning.

The new hospital kitchen and self-service dining room for all grades of staff had been open for about seven months when Mr Ferguson took over in 1971. Up to this time the consultants had had a private dining room upstairs in the central block. The beautiful wooden floor of the main staff dining room was carpeted to reduce noise level and make cleaning easier. During Mr Ferguson's time, a new contract dishwasher centre was instituted. A major advance he introduced in 1972 was to change the ward trolleys from bulk service to a patient tray service. This required new trolleys in which individual dishes were kept hot with heavy metal rings below the plates. A sophisticated menu-card was introduced from which patients could chose the next day's meals.

Other changes which took place were, sadly, the gradual erosion of the resident doctors' privilege of dining separately. First the lunch service in the residency was withdrawn, next the evening meal and finally breakfast despite the support given to the junior doctors by the Physician Superintendent (see Chapter 27). Although not the direct responsibility of the catering management, the milk kitchen opposite Ward 15 also closed during this time. It had previously provided infant feeds for the children's wards but, as stricter food hygiene regulations were introduced, it was abandoned in favour of commercial, prepacked, individual feeds issued direct to the wards.

Mr Martin Henry succeeded Mr Ferguson and became Unit Catering Manager, initially responsible to Mr Jack Burton for the whole of the United Hospitals Unit (UHU). He worked at the City Hospital from December 1985 to September 1994 and took over some faithful, long-serving staff such as the ex-army Head Chef, Mr John Hastie, in the kitchen and Mrs Margaret Wishart in the dining room servery. Early changes made by Mr Henry included 'self-clear' in the dining room in 1986 which reduced the number of waitresses needed. Following a management efficiency work study, a popular incentive scheme was introduced which encouraged catering staff to aim for a 15 per cent bonus of gross earnings.

After a food poisoning scare in 1989, vacuum-packed pasteurised chicken was introduced, none of the consumers apparently being aware of any change in taste or quality. About 1989 also, competitive tendering for hospital services was introduced. Mr Henry laboured long over the specification of staff, wages equipment and service required, and won the in-house contract in April 1990 against fierce outside competition. The sense of achievement and the knowledge that 200 catering jobs in the UHU were secure for three years still brings a smile to his face.

For the next round of competitive tendering in 1993–94, Mr Henry was asked to cover the catering only for the City Hospital and PMROH, but this time the remit also included domestic services, sewing, personal laundry and the gardens. Seven companies competed. Mr Henry found he could provide 21 good quality meals each week for £11.49 per patient at 1993 prices. Once again, after months of hard work he won the tender for the City Hospital staff. By this time food for PMROH was cooked at the City Hospital and then transported. Mrs Mary Kelly then took over the domestic and portering services and the sewing room. Mr Henry subcontracted the care of the gardens and three full-time gardeners were employed. Their work included winter time snow clearing and road gritting in addition to forestry and gardening.

Mr Henry introduced several important changes. About April 1986 the night cooking service for staff ceased for economic reasons and was replaced by a vending service at the east side of the dining room. A new £35,000 MICO German dishwasher was installed and working in 24 hours during which obsolete equipment was also removed. A new dining room carpet was laid about 1992–93. To generate income, a popular service selling freshly baked bread and cakes for hospital staff became available on Fridays.

Mr Henry and his catering staff also offered healthy low-lipid and weight-reducing diets. Amusing, illustrated posters advertised enticing menus for festivals such as Christmas, New Year and other anniversaries. For example, hospital staff found it difficult to choose from a Burns' Day luncheon menu offering 'Cullen Skink, Fence Loupin' Haggis, Poached Dunoon Trout Fillet, Roast Rib of Scotch Beef, Vension in Red Wine and Port Served with a Crouton, Broccoli in Lockerbie Cheese Sauce, Lamb Athol Brose cooked in Elderberry Wine, Diced Neeps, Sliced Carrot, Mashed Tatties and Boiled Chips, followed by Cloutie Dumpling, Custard and Raspberry Crannichan [sic]'.

When Hong Kong was handed over to China in 1997, there was a truly Chinese menu starting with chicken and sweetcorn noodle soup with wafer paper prawns and ending with pineapple and banana fritters with lemon sauce, or lychees with ice cream. Mr Henry also successfully catered for conferences and other functions in the hospital.

Patients' menus were often innovative too. In 1992 a questionnaire was circulated of patients' expectations and satisfaction taking into account their age, length of time in hospital, special diets and vegetarian requirements. The response was remarkably good with evidence of overall satisfaction.

Another important contribution by Mr Henry was to emphasise cleanliness and food hygiene. In May 1992 he was runner-up for the Highfield Award at the annual conference in Inverness of the Royal Environment Health Institute of Scotland (REHIS) achieving the second highest marks in the Advanced Food Hygiene Diploma in Scotland within the previous 12 months. Mr Henry together with the Control of Infection Sister, Audrey McKenzie, were part of the successful training team. Over 150 catering and 25 domestic staff in the United Hospitals Unit gained certificates from REHIS.[2]

Sadly, as the City Hospital closes, so too do its kitchens, which have long provided morale boosting sustenance to staff and patients.

The Laundry

Although the hospital laundry was originally designed to cope only with its own linen, staff uniforms, and personal washing, it ultimately grew to be very large and provided a central service for many hospitals.

The wash-house and laundry buildings were tucked away in the south east corner of the hospital site. From the start there were separate facilities for the laundry of staff and patients. With the boiler house adjacent it was reassuring that there was:

> sufficient steam power ... provided for machinery and fittings of the most approved description for wash-house, laundry, disinfector, culinary purposes, electric lighting, and general heating of the entire premises, and for the sterilising of infected matters from drainage before entering the main outlet.[3]

The main entrance on the west of the laundry was a double-storey block with twin, mock-Tudor eaves. The rest was single-storey, but with high, ventilated, glass roofs, in functional, red brick surmounted by a tall, cylindrical chimney.[4]

In the mid-1950s central pooling of linen issues was decided upon.[5] By August 1956 all the laundering for the Group and Southfield Sanatorium came to the City Hospital. By the next year Rosslynlee, Longmore, Liberton and the Northern General Hospitals were all using the central service. The weekly output of items rapidly increased from 40,000 to 50,000 and by 1958 to 50,000–60,000[6] and then 65,000 weekly after an injection of £14,500 had been made for new machinery. Costs per item also fell, making the system economic. During Dr Horne's Superintendentship (1960–74) the output rose even further to 80,000 items weekly and there were worries that ageing equipment requiring replacement or repair could jeopardise the whole laundry service for the many hospitals the City Hospital then served.

For about 25 years up till 1979 when he retired, Mr Bob Strang was the laundry manager. He was succeeded by Mr George Nixon who was manager from 1979 to 1984–85. He subsequently became service manager in Ninewells Hospital, Dundee. During this time the City Hospital carried out the laundering for the following hospitals: Princess Margaret Rose Orthopaedic Hospital, Edinburgh Royal Infirmary, Southfield, Astley Ainslie, Royal Hospital for Sick Children, City, Deaconess, Elsie Inglis Memorial Maternity and Longmore Hospitals, to which were added Gogarburn, Rosslynlee and the Royal Edinburgh Hospitals about 1986.

In the year 1982–83 the City Hospital laundry coped with 38,523,000 pieces (averaging over 74,000 per week) at a unit cost of 13.33p.[7]

Although based at the Western General Hospital, Mr Gordon Rawson supervised the City Hospital laundry's final years from 1985 until 1987 when it closed. There were then 45 staff most of whom found re-employment at the Western General Hospital. Much of the workload, which had by then grown to 85,000 pieces weekly, was taken over by the Western General Hospital laundry and the rest by St John's Hospital at Howden.[8]

Area Sterilising Centre

The Area Sterilising Centre has been based at the City Hospital since 1985. Both Mr Mark Lavery[9] and Mr Ian Robertson[10] have provided information about its work.

The concept of a centralised sterilising service developed for two separate reasons. Firstly, the Second World War showed that prepacked sterile units could be used successfully in field hospitals close to the front. Secondly, studies in the UK in the 1950s showed the inadequacy of autoclaves in operating theatres. Until about 1955 each surgical unit had been responsible for its own sterilising procedures. Dr John H. Bowie, a Senior Lecturer in bacteriology at the University of Edinburgh and Jimmy Dick, his Senior Chief Technician, showed that sterilisation was unsatisfactory in more than 90 per cent of the hospital autoclaves they examined. The autoclaves either failed to sterilise their contents or caused heat damage to perishable items. Dr Bowie, therefore, soon promoted new systems such as downward displacement and automatically controlled, pre-vacuum autoclaves.

National studies carried out by the fledgling NHS confirmed Dr Bowie's findings and centralisation of sterilising services was recommended. Musgrave Park Hospital in Belfast was one of the first to adopt this system. In Edinburgh Sheila Scott, a Royal Infirmary theatre sister, conceived the idea in 1962 of preset trolley-top trays containing all the items required for defined surgical procedures. By 1969 this system included all the theatres, departments, wards and clinics in the Royal Infirmary and later supplied the needs of the Western General Hospital as well. The Royal Hospital for Sick Children had developed a similar, smaller, system for their own theatres and also supplied PMROH. Sheila Scott became an authority on sterilising services and an adviser to the Department of Health in London.

In the late 1970s the demand for sterilisation increased dramatically and the two units outgrew their premises. By October 1985 the central sterile supply services of the Royal Infirmary and Royal Hospital for Sick Children had amalgamated and moved to purpose-built premises at the eastern side of the City Hospital. This provided the first area-wide service in the UK.

One faithful member of the Area Sterilising Centre was Mr Ian Robertson. He had started as an apprentice machine man at 16, and then, aged 18, did his National Service in the RAMC. This simulated his interest in health care. Nurses' wages were very low, so he decided instead of a nursing career to be a hospital porter. By 1950, however, he had become an assistant to Dr Bowie and then started at the Theatre Service Centre in the Royal Infirmary.

Mr Robertson's later career advanced from Chargehand to Supervisor, Assistant Manager and finally Deputy Manager of the Area Sterilising Centre at the City Hospital from which post he retired in 1990 aged 62. He worked with Dr Bowie for 25 years contributing to all the developments that took place. He recalls the early experiments in the Royal Infirmary in 1958 when the first rectangular vacuum steam steriliser arrived from the USA. Thereafter he followed through the improved Drayton Castle machines Marks I and II which became increasingly sophisticated and automatic. Ultimately over 400 types of prepacked operation trays were available in addition to which certain surgeons demanded their favourite instruments packed and sterilised separately. Mr Robertson missed working in the Royal Infirmary when he moved to the City Hospital but commented favourably on the happy service which he helped to run there and the excellence of industrial relations throughout.[11]

Mrs Margaret Alexander, who had been theatre sister to Mr J. D. R. Cameron in Wards 15 and 16 in the Royal Infirmary had joined the Theatre Sterilising Centre in the early 1960s and became its manager, until the move to the City Hospital in 1985. When she resigned, Mr Robertson, her deputy, was already 59 and did not apply for the manager's post. Miss Rose Fleming who had been a Theatre Superintendent at the Royal Infirmary and Northern Group of Hospitals successfully applied for the manager's post in 1986. As she had had little experience with sterilising techniques, Mr Robertson became her teacher as well as deputy.[12]

When Miss Fleming retired about six years later, Mr Mark Lavery from Leeds succeeded her.[13] By this time the Centre had become very busy. It supplied all the hospitals in Lothian except for St John's Hospital in Howden which had its own service while the Western General had its own Central Sterile Supply Department (CSSD) for smaller packs. All the theatre trays for surgical operations in the Western General Hospital (except in the Department of Clinical Neurosciences) were, however, set and sterilised at the City Hospital. Should one of the larger sterilising centres fail, reciprocal services were agreed between the other major units in Scotland for appropriate back-up in such an emergency.

Mr Lavery has a staff of 90 (68 WTE) and his own transport system with drivers for collection and delivery from the hospitals he serves in Edinburgh and at Roodlands Hospital at Haddington. Everyone takes great pride in the work and morale is high. The service is open 24 hours daily seven days weekly except for 4 hours on Saturday and Sunday evenings. Although instruments arrive dirty, linen comes in clean but unsterile from the laundry. In the year 1996–97 the Area Sterilsing Centre supplied 75,000 theatre trays, each taking up to an hour to process, 121,401 supplementary instrument and ward packs and 63,509 surgical gown and linen packs.[14]

Maintenance of standards has top priority. In 1997 the quality control ISO 9002 was achieved and in the summer of 1998 Mr Lavery hopes the CE mark of the European Community will be on all his sterile products. This mark denotes not only the quality of the product itself but the safety and healthiness of the environment in which that product is made. Other guidelines to which standards must adhere are those of Good Manufacturing Practice (1989) about to be upgraded in the summer of 1998.

Discussions are taking place throughout Scotland about the future of central sterilising services particularly in view of the requirements of hospitals such as the new Royal Infirmary. It is hoped that in-house tendering for contracts will continue to be successful and commercial firms will not take over.

Support Services: Domestic Workers, Portering, Buildings, Grounds and Gardens

Patients and relatives inevitably notice the care provided by doctors, nurses and those in the professions allied to medicine. The staff in less glamorous posts also influence patient care even though their contributions go largely unrecognised. Indeed administrators, managers, supervisors and their staff are often first to be criticised. Yet patients and their families will remember the kind domestic giving them a much needed cup of tea, the porter who chats with an anxious patient being wheeled to the operating theatre, the cheering effect of a freshly painted ward or a well tended rose garden in the grounds. This chapter briefly pays tribute to the loyalty of some of these staff whilst recognising that basic grade domestic workers, porters and gardeners in 1998 were paid a mere £3.80 per hour.[15]

Mrs Mary Kelly, currently Deputy Support Service Manager for the RIE NHS Trust, became responsible to the City Hospital, then part of the United Hospitals Unit (UHU) in 1989. She already had a catering qualification but later worked with the Social Work Department in Glasgow and then in the Lothians at the Eastern General, Leith and

Edenhall Hospitals. She became Deputy Contract Manager for the City Hospital responsible for domestic services and portering, the latter previously run by Mr Jim Smith. An early task, set her by Mr Purves and Miss M. Buchanan, was the overhaul of cleaning in the Thoracic Surgery Unit following an outbreak of methicillin resistant *Staphylococcus aureus* (MRSA).[16]

Staff were difficult to recruit but, under the United Services Department, domestic and portering services were integrated. Mrs Kelly could therefore insist that porters took over some cleaning duties which they had not been asked to do before. When the UHU disbanded, Mrs Kelly became responsible for PMROH and the City Hospital alone. In 1994 when Mr Martin Henry left, Mrs Kelly also took over catering.

Mrs Kelly understands that the earlier domestic managers, like Mrs Shanks, were appointed directly by the Matron. Mrs Kelly's immediate predecessor was Mrs Mary Jeffrey, now a lecturer at Telford College. Domestic supervisors she can recall include Andrea Whiteheart, a Polish lady known as 'Yana' and then Mrs Wylis. Before competitive tendering was introduced, there were 80 whole time equivalents (WTEs) of domestic staff. This figure was regularly whittled away as departments in the hospital closed, running down to 24 WTEs when the only clinical units left were ENT, Maxillofacial Surgery and the RIDU. Latterly the ENT Department alone commanded a mere 11 WTE domestic staff.[17]

Similar staff reductions took place in portering from 26 WTEs in 1990 to 19.5 in 1994 and even fewer as more wards closed. Up to 1989, Mr Bob Devlin was Head Porter and subsequently Messrs Charlie Williamson (26 years' service at the City Hospital), John Cunningham, Al Robertson and Nigel Terry were portering supervisors. Affectionately remembered are the genial porter 'Stan' and the post-man Jimmy Gordon. Cleaning duties were added to those of portering about 1990. Until then a minimum of two porters covered night shifts.

Industrial relations at the City Hospital were normally good, grievances being sorted out expeditiously by diplomats like Dr Norman Horne and his successors before serious problems arose. About 1988, however, when a new incinerator was installed, some of the porters objected to the former boilerhouse attendant, who would otherwise lose his job, being put in charge. Conflict arose because the porters wanted the post for themselves. During the ensuing strike, rubbish piled up in the empty, old laundry and, only after the porters gave their permission, were Mr Jack Burton and Mr Jim Smith allowed to shift it. Next the medical, nursing and other staff formed a rota for dinner trolley runs. Unfortunately for the militant porters, but fortunately for the hospital, picketing of the Area Sterilising Service met with limited success only. Next the domestic workers refused to join the strike which then fizzled out after three weeks.[18]

The introduction of competitive tendering and the desire by all hospital workers to secure in-house contacts, encouraged unions and management to work together. Sadly, with Private Finance Initiative in future there will be no in-house bidding. Transfer of undertakings will apply but, when the City Hospital and PMROH are no more, job closures are inevitable. The new concepts of two-year employment contracts, migration planning and appropriate down-sizing are likely to be unpopular.

Mr David Pithie,[19] a former Hibs footballer who later played for Montrose and Leith Athletic, was a joiner to trade who rose to become General Foreman of the Royal Victoria and Associated Hospitals Group. He arrived in 1951 and retired in 1987. His staff at the City Hospital consisted of seven painters, three plumbers, three joiners, one blacksmith and one slater. He recalls the supervising engineers like Mr Ian MacDonald, Mr McIntosh and more recently Mr Ricky Barr now at PMROH and the late, always obliging Mr Tom Pearson, who was Clerk of Works and Senior Building Officer for the UHU. Another of the buildings officers was Mr Colin Waters.

An ethic strongly advocated by Mr Drummond, formerly on the hospital staff, was to emphasise maintenance, so that as much as possible was done by the hospital's own work force rather than by contracting out. Hence their conversion of the old, wooden TB wards into cricket pavilions and a temporary home for physiotherapists, occupational therapists and social workers. Similarly, about 1956–57 the hospital team moved the turntable TB isolation huts to the Royal Victoria and Southfield Hospitals. They later refurbished the visitors' room as the conference room. In Mr Tom Pearson's time they also fitted much of the new kitchens and dining room, the (David Flenley) Lecture Theatre and Regional Virus Laboratory.[20]

One major disappointment for Mr Pithie was to witness the vulnerability of the new shop built near the gatehouse and burgled despite having 9 in thick brick walls topped with concrete, iron bars on the windows, and the safe bolted to the floor. Despite all this, thieves drilled their way round the mortice lock and then wheeled away their takings in one of the hospital's cots.[21]

Mr Pithie was keen to promote promising staff, one of whom was Mr W. A. Maben, a red-bearded, cycling enthusiast. He came to the City Hospital as a plumber in 1974 and served as Estates Officer from 1989 to 1997, when he was transferred to the Royal Infirmary. He was responsible to Mr Pearson, Mr Peter White (for a short period only), Mr Colin Waters and then Mr Ricky Barr. By 1993 the estates management, buildings and engineering for PMROH and the City Hospital had combined for the purposes of competitive tendering, and are now the responsibility of Mr Phil Christie.[22]

Willie Maben's delight at the City Hospital was the trees. Until the UHU was disbanded, an area-wide forestry service had covered hospitals in Fife, the Borders and Lothians. Although the Royal Edinburgh Hospital won the contract for gardens in 1993, the City Hospital remained responsible for forestry until 1997. Originally there had been two foresters and 15 gardeners for the City Hospital alone. Fifty trees suffered with Dutch elm disease and were replaced. High winds counted for some of the pines most years. After essential thinning, some timber was sold for the benefit of the hospital every five years. Mr Maben had hoped to replace the losses with a mixture of broad-leaved trees and pines that would strengthen the woodland. The Coronation Wood near the west gate was of Scots pine, not the original Corsican pine, and was felled in the winter of 1988–89 to accommodate Milestone House.[23]

Mr Maben also looked after the greenhouses, walled garden and vegetable plots near the boiler house, which had originally supplied enough green foods for all the patients and staff. His other responsibilities included care of the cricket pitch and the two original football pitches.[24]

As a former plumber, Mr Maben was fascinated by the vast concrete-lined 100,000 gallon water cistern, 106 feet long, 86 feet broad and 12 feet deep, which lies in an elevated position above the hospital and is a feature of the fifth fairway of the Merchants' of Edinburgh Golf Course.[25] It had supplanted the originally projected water tower that was never built between the administrative buildings and the central block (see Chapter 15). This cistern supplied both tap water and the self-flushing system of the hospital's drains. At every routine inspection and cleaning, Mr Maben and his staff would marvel at the still excellent condition of this cistern's century-old concrete lining.

CHAPTER THIRTY-THREE

The Chaplains' Department, the Patients' Library and the League of Friends

The Hospital Chaplaincy

Despite the strict isolation policy designed to prevent the spread of infection in the hospital's early years, spiritual comfort was available, albeit in a haphazard way. For instance, a chaplain would have been allowed to visit a very sick or dying patient in the relative safety of a side room off the main ward. Despite Dr C. B. Ker's authoritarian rules forbidding contact with smallpox patients in the temporary wooden hospital, he did reluctantly permit visiting by such 'clergyman as will submit to the regulations, and relatives of absolutely hopeless cases' (see Chapter 17). Although routine clerical visits may have been discouraged depending on the type of infection in the ward, reference has already been made to the Sunday services conducted in the 1920s in the children's scarlet fever pavilions (see Chapter 18).

The Hospital Subcommittee of the Town Council's Public Health Committee from time to time set the fees for chaplains, who were from several different denominations, for attending the City Hospital and Polton Farm Colony.[1] These gratuities were increased in step with rising tram and cab fares; the Convener of the Church Committee received a free tram pass.[2]

By the 1930s when Dr Benson was Medical Superintendent the regulations about visiting had relaxed somewhat. The Minutes of the Church of Scotland's Presbytery of Edinburgh[3] suggest that Rev. John Bain of St Paul's Church served as Hospital Chaplain throughout the 1930s and probably until he died in 1942. The Presbytery's Convener of Hospital Services, or his local deputy, would regularly report on the work under their supervision. On 5 May 1931 Dr Burns, Convener of the City Hospital Services, reported that:

> The Chaplain, Mr Bain, had systematically visited the wards, infectious and otherwise, and had conducted services for the nurses. The convener had paid monthly visits to the hospital for conference. The services are greatly appreciated, and the expense is borne by the city. During the winter several

entertainments had also been arranged for. Acknowledgement was made of the willing assistance given to the committee by the Matron, Miss Pool.[4]

During the year ending April 1933, 148 visits were made to the hospital, 45 ward services conducted and 24 Sunday services for the nurses. Funeral arrangements were undertaken and all wards, infectious or otherwise, were regularly visited.[5] A similar record was made in a later report with the additional information that in November 1933 a communion service held in the 'Tubercular Wards' was so much appreciated that it was decided to repeat it quarterly in the future.[6] The report of 5 July 1938 recorded that over 40 patients in the 'tubercular wards' had partaken of the sacrament of the Lord's Supper, now held four times a year.[7] Besides 'The Chaplain is very grateful for gifts of Christian literature for distribution, and thanks are also well deserved by several city church choirs who give services of praise in the tubercular wards'.[8] Similar activities were recorded in 1941[9] and that the sacrament of Baptism had also been administered. It seems most likely that the spiritual needs of the long-stay patients with tuberculosis – and the staff – were being met with regular services but each report also mentions visits to *all* wards, infectious or otherwise.

The Jubilee Thanksgiving Commemorative Service in the nurses' recreation hall in 1953 was conducted by the 'Chaplain', Rev. George D. Monro, MA who was probably a hospital chaplain but not necessarily the City Hospital Chaplain at that time.[10] After this it is difficult to determine the succession of hospital chaplains until relatively recent times but the current and immediate past hospital chaplains are listed at the end of this chapter.

Rev. Dr. R. C. M. Mathers was the City Hospital's Chaplain from 1979 to 1994. He had held the charge of St Matthew's Church in Morningside for 32 years until his retirement in 1974. Afterwards St Matthew's amalgamated with South Morningside Church to become Cluny Parish Church. For the next five years Dr Mathers served as associate minister of St Andrew's and St George's Parish Church and as chaplain to staff in the stores of Princes Street.

When he left these posts to become the City Hospital's Chaplain in 1979, Dr Mathers quickly became aware of the need for pastoral care, not only of patients and their relatives, but of the clinical staff as well. Sister Ingram of Ward 6 approached him regarding the pre- and post-operative anxieties of patients undergoing major thoracic surgical operations, often for lung cancer. Dr Mathers therefore attended many of these worried people usually with a talk to calm them down and then he would give a blessing. When the HIV epidemic began, many

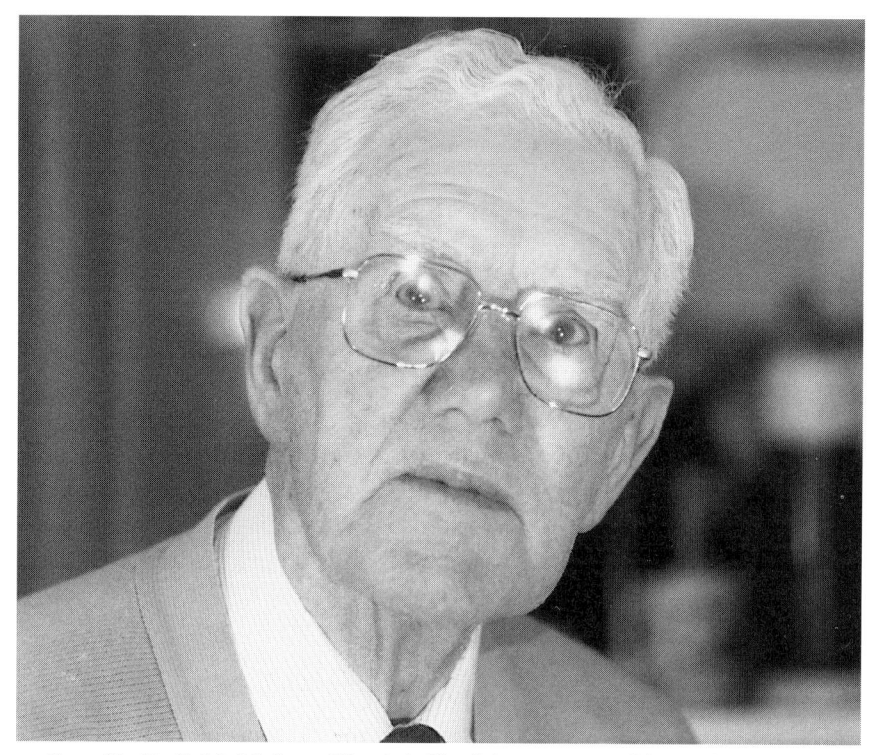

Rev. Dr R. C. M. Mathers, Hospital Chaplain, 1979–94. (Photo: By courtesy of Dr Kevin I. Wheeler)

infected people received solace from Dr Mathers who was tireless in his pastoral care and got to know many of them and their families very well. He found that a couplet of verse by John Greenleaf Whittier (1807–92) often provided comfort to those frightenend of dying:

> I know not where His islands lift their fronded palms in air,
> I only know I cannot drift beyond His love and care.

Dr Mathers found no difficulty in providing spiritual help for patients with AIDS irrespective of the route by which their infection had been acquired. He would say 'I may not condone what they do, but they are all God's children and deserve our love.'

Dr Mathers shared the emotional support of such patients with the nursing and medical staff. He regularly attended Dr Brettle's Friday afternoon meetings when AIDS patients were discussed in a confidential, multi-disciplinary forum. He willingly carried out funerals, baptisms, confirmations and even marriages as appropriate, often within the confidential atmosphere of the hospital chapel. He left Bible readings for those worried about their after-life. His contribution to the in-service training of the other chaplains and health care workers was much appreciated. Always approachable, gentle and courteous, Bob Mathers' soft, comforting voice and his serene face topped by white hair are now sadly missed. He died in 1999.

Dr Mathers' successor was Rev. Harry Telfer, minister to the Duncan Street Baptist Church.[11] From the London Bible College to charges in Westray in the Orkney Islands and Alloa in Clackmannanshire, he had also worked in Carluke where he was associated with Law Hospital before he came to Edinburgh in 1988. He took up the post of Chaplain in February 1990. He was therefore already familiar with the type of work involved, especially with AIDS patients, before Dr Mathers retired.

In 1995 his fellow Chaplains were Rev. Charlotte Henderson, who looked after what remained on the respiratory medicine corridor and thoracic surgery wards as well as the Care of the Elderly Wards 19A and B and the day hospital. Miss Norma Ronald cared for patients in the ENT and maxillofacial wards and the remainder of the Care of the Elderly, Wards 18A and B, 20 and 21. Both of these ladies had previous experience as prison chaplains. Continuing Dr Mathers' good work, Mr Telfer looked after patients in the RIDU. The Episcopal Chaplain was Rev. Geoffrey Hart and the Roman Catholic Chaplain was Father A. Mitchell who followed Fathers Victor Reiderer SJ and John Lees. The Chaplains were also invited to assist in a much valued course on stress management for the staff.

In 1995, Mr Telfer provided a quarterly service of worship in the day room of Wards 20/21, which was furnished as a chapel for the occasion, and to which relatives and staff were welcome. A number of local churches gave informal Sunday evening services and visiting choirs sang there every month. Holy Communion was provided on request and either administered by one of the hospital chaplains or by the patient's own minister or priest. Baptisms and weddings took place in the chapel and there was a continual need for the chaplains to take funerals especially for AIDS patients. Christian literature and audio-tapes were made available. Hospital chaplains from all over Scotland attended courses about pastoral care for AIDS sufferers, their partners and relatives. These were run in conjunction with the staff of Milestone House and the RIDU. Information was also provided through the Chaplains' Office about the availability of spiritual and pastoral care for patients of other religions.

The care and devotion of all the hospital chaplains to the patients, families and hospital staff deserves the highest praise.

Chaplaincy, the Library and the League of Freinds   393

RECENT CITY HOSPITAL CHAPLAINS [12]

Rev. Alastair Symington	1.5.77–31.1.85
Rev. Dr Robert Mathers	1.10.79–31.7.94
Rev. Joseph Ritchie	10.1.81–30.4.83
Rev. Donald Harper	1.5.83–30.6.85
Rev. Hamish McIntosh	1.2.85–31.12.89
Rev. Robert Gemmill	1.7.85–31.8.87
Rev. Dr Stanley Heavenor	1.11.87–10.9.92
Rev. Harry Telfer	22.1.89 to date
Rev. Hugh Drummond	5.10.93–31.7.94
Rev. Charlotte Henderson	1.8.94–31.3.98
Miss Norma Ronald	1.8.94–31.3.98

Library Services for Patients

When the New Medical Block was opened in 1961, a small medical library and reading room for staff were provided on the first floor above the medical out-patient clinic adjacent to the records office. Separate arrangements were made for patients.

Mrs Christine Craig has kindly provided the following information about library services for patients. As early as 1946 the Edinburgh Town Council approved a proposal by Mr Butchart of the Edinburgh City Libraries for a library service for hospitals. Staffing and fitment costs were to be met by the Public Health Committee. This service was later provided on an agency basis, the NHS Trust providing the premises and paying a proportion of the salary of a librarian and assistant. The standard and large print books, story books and audio-tapes were provided by the library authorities.

The service was originally much used by long-stay patients with tuberculosis, and some of the shorter-stay patients in the infectious diseases wards. The books and the trolleys carrying them had to be kept separate and required disinfection. In the later 1950s when there were fewer tuberculosis patients, disinfection was practised less. Other wards, with non-infectious patients, seemed to have avid book readers as well. From 1962, with the help of Women's Royal Voluntary Service (WRVS) workers, more of the wards could be supplied with books. Although the patients' library has moved three times in its history, the most recent location in the central block near the porters' room just north of the lecture theatre was most suitable for patients and staff alike. At one time it was also close to the hospital shop which further encouraged its use.

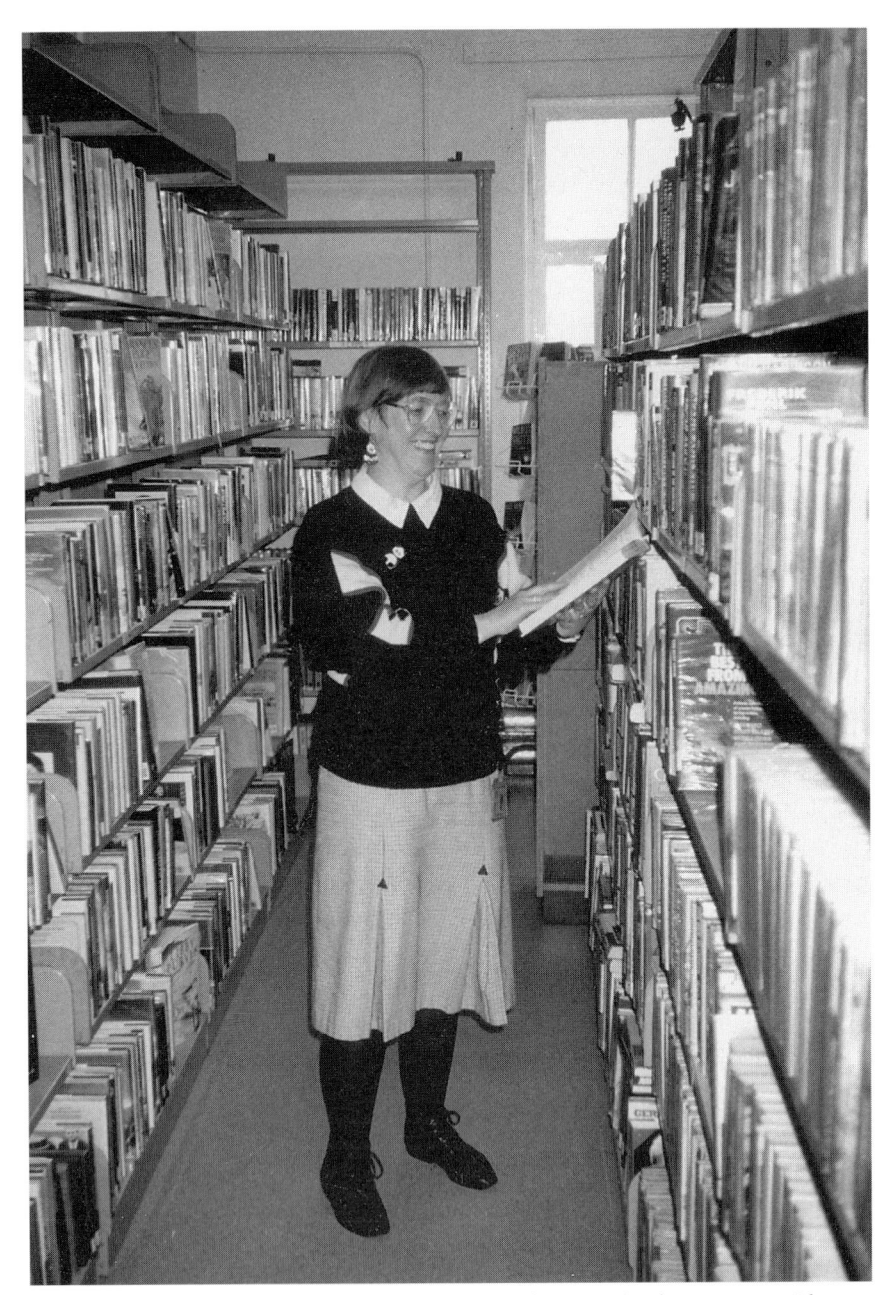

Mrs Christine Craig, Librarian of City Hospital Patients' Library, 1997. (Photo: J. A. Gray)

When the Care of the Elderly Unit was functioning, a library club for selected patients was formed. Patients with stroke disease made much use of it, as did the Occupational Therapy Department for diversionary work. Despite the imminent closure of the City Hospital, the patients' library services will continue to supply other Edinburgh hospitals.

Librarians at the City Hospital have been:

Mrs Lilias Tait, MBE	1946–75
Mrs Jane McDonagh	1975–82
Ms Gail McKinley	1982–84
Mrs Christine Craig	1984–present

The League of Friends of the City Hospital

In addition to the valuable service given by Greenbank Church volunteers in the hospital Tea Room from 1965 to 1997 (see Chapter 27), another voluntary body, the League of Friends also deserves recognition for the contribution it has made to the comfort and welfare of patients.

Mr Frank Snell, WS, an Edinburgh solicitor, now retired who later became the League's Honorary President, had been a patient in the City Hospital from August 1950 to September 1952. During that time he witnessed a dramatic improvement in the morale of staff and patients alike. The hospital was then witnessing the early development of thoracic surgery and, with the arrival of Professor Crofton, a vastly improved prognosis for patients with tuberculosis. Some measure of hope was at last being afforded to those previously 'incurable' patients with advanced, open tuberculosis whom Sir Robert Philip had sent to die in isolation at the City Hospital. A patient in the next bed to Mr Snell had already spent not just two but seven years in hospital. Years later Mr Snell was delighted to meet two Roman Catholic patients who had been so ill as to be given the last rites when he shared a ward with them. Both had since recovered.

Thirty years after being a patient himself, Mr Snell was visiting a badly disabled friend in the hospital and discovered that the patient's radio-headphone system had failed. As his friend had relied on this as his main source of entertainment, Mr Snell reported the failure to the hospital but was dismayed to find there were no funds available for repairing the system. This determined Mr Snell to set up a fund-raising body.[13]

With encouragement from Mr Geoffrey Redmond, the Hospital Secretary, and Miss A. E. Christie, Matron, Mr Snell organised a public meeting in Cluny Church Centre, Morningside, with the intention of starting up a League of Friends. The idea was endorsed enthusiastically. By 1985, with Mr Snell in the chair, the League's Committee was meeting monthly either in the conference room or the Tea Room of the hospital. Usually present were Miss Christie, and later Mr Robert Purves or Mrs Maureen Lees, Mr Michael Pearson, Sister Thomson of the Care of the Elderly Unit, Mr Geoffrey Redmond, Mr Ian Cunningham from the thoracic theatre, Mrs Marion Bowie of the day hospital (later Joint Secretary with Miss Sheila Finlay), Miss Mary Weir, Miss F. R. Fleming, Mrs and Miss Petzsch, Mr and Mrs Walter Naismith, Miss Elizabeth Ross, former Physiotherapy Superintendent, Dr Archie Milne and later myself together with Mrs Pat Macleod, the present Chairman. Mr Bill Watt became the Treasurer and later Mrs Bowie combined this post with that of Secretary.[14]

In addition to donations from ex-patients, their relations and friends, often in recognition of the care they had received at the hospital, the League held two major fund-raising events each year. The Summer Fair was held in the hospital grounds in June and a social event was held in November, originally in the recreation room of the nurses' home but, after the 1988 fire, in the staff dining room. At the Summer Fair there were stalls, competitions, games and a bouncy castle. Ice cream and teas were usually served in a marquee in case of inclement weather. The seventh Edinburgh Company of the Boys' Brigade under Captain Bill Shand wheeled patients round the stalls. Several bands enlivened the proceedings: Heriot's School Pipe Band, various army bands and in later years the Sunshine Band with toe-tapping and often nostalgic music much appreciated by the older generation. The November event was a wine and cheese party with a raffle, draw or silent auction to raise funds.

The League sponsored many projects including an expensive ventilator for the hospital's anaesthetists, a telephone trolley, library trolleys, transcutaneous electrical nerve stinulator (TENS) machines for relief of chronic pain, television sets, video and cassette players, headphones, paintings and framed posters for ward and waiting room walls, downies, a leaflet stand, art materials, an ejector seat and a camcorder. Day rooms and quiet rooms were refurbished, and assistance was given to wards for the provision of mural paintings and large plastic boxes of toys. At Christmas, money was made available to take patients from the Care of the Elderly Unit to the pantomime. Some funds each year were devoted to assisting nurses to attend further study courses. In many ways both patients and staff benefited from the activities of the League and tribute is due to the organisers of fund-raising events over the years. Much of the information about the League of Friends has been kindly been supplied by Mr Frank Snell and the present Chairman, Mrs Pat Macleod, who intends keeping the League going, at least until the last patients leave the hospital.

CHAPTER THIRTY-FOUR

The Future

There were probably many reasons why the City Hospital became unviable towards the end of the twentieth century. Some would say it had outlived its original purpose as a fever hospital. It had, however, provided more than adequate accommodation for several disciplines other than infectious diseases. From originally coping with fevers and tuberculosis only to providing a home for modern respiratory medicine, thoracic, ENT and maxillofacial surgery, and geriatric medicine, the City Hospital had adapted to encompass them all. There were also the laboratories to back them up: the Bacteriology and Scottish Mycobacterial Reference Laboratories, the Regional Clinical Virus Laboratory, the Respiratory Function Laboratory and the Rayne Laboratory. The X-ray and later the MRI scanning service, the professions allied to medicine and all the support services played their part.

There was, however, one very important facility missing, namely an intensive care unit. Whilst such a unit would have been unheard of in the first half century of the hospital's existence, it has since become an essential requirement for modern hospitals dealing with acute medicine and surgery. Although the surgical units had some high dependency areas within their own departments, the hospital had no central intensive care unit available to adults and children from the other disciplines.

Not unreasonably the Respiratory Medicine Unit felt this lack acutely and, with a desire also to be part of a large multi-disciplinary hospital such as the Royal Infirmary, Professor Haslett moved his unit there in 1993. It then became illogical for the thoracic surgeons to be so far separated from respiratory medicine physicians and, worse still for the surgical staff, to be on a split site, partly at the Royal Infirmary and partly at the City Hospital. They therefore moved to the Royal Infirmary in December 1997.

During this time the Care of the Elderly Unit was winding down after a policy decision to halve the number of continuing care beds in Lothian. As old people died in hospital or were sufficiently rehabilitated to go to their own homes or into nursing homes, their vacant beds were not reoccupied. The day hospital closed and the Stroke and Assessment Units were moved. It was sad for anyone who had known the hospital in previous years to see these once thriving centres of clinical excellence with their windows boarded up. With the loss of the Care of the Elderly Unit, the viability of the whole City Hospital was unlikely.

Throughout this time and for many years earlier, discussions had been taking place about the need for a new Royal Infirmary, its function, site, size and costing. Indeed at one stage a seriously considered option was to place the new Royal Infirmary at the City Hospital. This might have been feasible at one time on the grounds of space but the 131.5 acres originally bought at Colinton Mains Farm by the Town Council in 1895 had been nibbled away by Milestone House and the new Ambulance Head Quarters on Oxgangs Road North. In addition, if the University Medical School was to move from Teviot Place to be close to the new Royal Infirmary, there would certainly not have been enough room. It was also less convincingly argued that access roads to and from the City Hospital site would be inadequate for the traffic generated by a new Royal Infirmary and Medical School.

It is outwith the remit of this book to comment on the choice of Little France as the preferred location for the new Royal Infirmary. It is a green-field site on the south east fringes of Edinburgh and on the twisty Old Dalkeith Road. At the end of the nineteenth century, when Colinton Mains Farm was selected for the third City Hospital, it too was outside the city boundary. That choice also had raised questions about its distance from the city centre and the length of time it would take seriously ill patients with typhoid fever to reach the hospital with the transport then available (see Chapter 11).

The new Royal Infirmary at Little France is likely to cost more than £200 million. To pump-prime the project, both the Princess Margaret Rose Orthopaedic Hospital and the City Hospital will be sold off. The new Royal Infirmary will be a Private Finance Initiative. A consortium of BICC, the Royal Bank of Scotland and Morrison Construction are responsible for the development and building. Approval was given by the Secretary of State for Scotland in November 1994. The present Infirmary site will be developed by New Lauriston Ltd, a consortium of Edinburgh Development Investments and Morrison Construction.[1]

Unless space can be found in the meantime either at the present Royal Infirmary or elsewhere, it is likely that the ENT Surgery Unit and day care general surgery which has very recently come to the City Hospital will have to await the building of accommodation at Little France. Similarly the Regional Clinical Virus Laboratory and the Scottish Mycobacterial Reference Laboratory are likely to stay at the City Hospital until they go with the ENT Surgery Unit to be among the first occupants of the Little France site. The Maxillofacial Surgery Unit moved to St

John's Hospital at Howden, West Lothian, in June 1998. The adult part of the RIDU also moved in June 1998, so finally severing the near century-long responsibility of the City Hospital as the fever hospital for Edinburgh.

The RIDU now occupies a futuristic looking, modern construction (Wards 41–43) with a possible life span of 10 years. It is close to the west gate of the Western General Hospital to which it is connected by a steep corridor. The ground floor has office and out-patient accommodation and a large day room. Upstairs are 43 beds, mainly in single cubicles with negative pressure facilities, and one room adapted to take a patient with viral haemorrhagic fever should the need arise.

The paediatric component of the RIDU has been whittled down from the many *wards* originally occupied by children at the City Hospital to a mere six isolation *rooms* in child friendly but rather awkwardly shaped surroundings at the top of the Royal Hospital for Sick Children. To accommodate both infectious and immuno-compromised children in the same building, some of the rooms have a negative and positive pressure capability depending on the diseases to be isolated and treated.

What is to become of the City Hospital site? As a joint venture between Morrison Homes and Cala Homes it will be redeveloped as a £50 million housing complex, one of the largest in Edinburgh for some years.[2] Although the *Property Weekly* of *The Scotsman* suggested about 400 homes, a figure of 357–392 may be more realistic.[3] The site is a

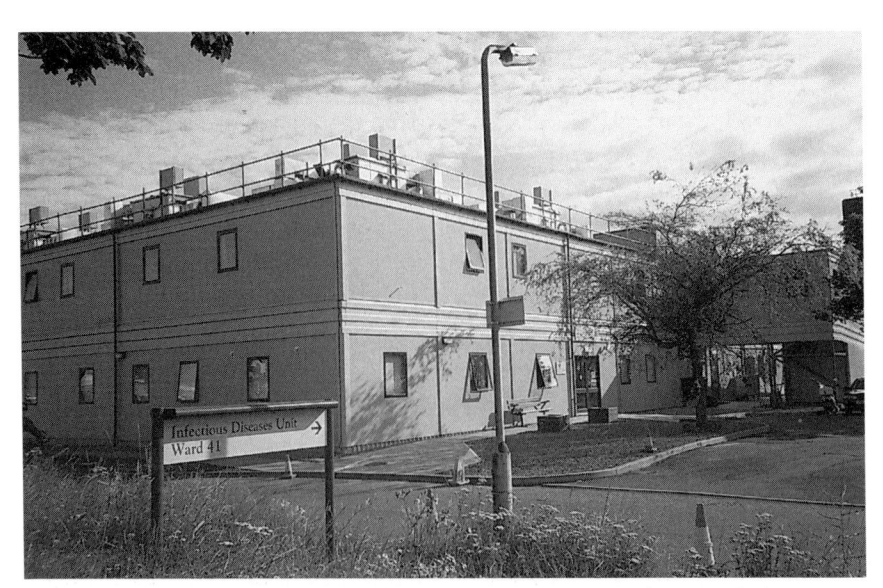

New home for the RIDU, Wards 41–43, Western General Hospital, from June 1998 (Photo: J. A. Gray)

conservation area but none of the old buildings is specifically listed. Early indications suggest the removal of most or all of the buff coloured brick buildings such as the 1965 medical residency, non-resident staff changing rooms, pharmacy, stores, dining room and kitchens and also the red brick buildings such as the central block, 'new' bacteriology laboratory, boiler house, wash-house and laundry.

Most of the red, Dumfriesshire sandstone buildings will remain except the New Medical Block (former servants' home), the day hospital (former typhus Ward 22) and Cottages 23 and 24 which will be pulled down. New four-storey flats will be built parallel to Greenbank Drive, north of the Pavilions 2–4 and 14–17 and five three-storey developments will occupy the grounds south of Pavilions 5–8 and 18–21. Three and four-storey flats will be built at the centre of the site south of the general offices. At the day hospital and in place of Cottages 23 and 24, new, mews-type dwellings will surround three sides of a central courtyard. On the east and south east of the site, detached and semi-detached houses will be built at a later stage.

An interesting feature will be a balancing pond south of Pavilions 5–7 which will take surface water off roofs and hard standings and prevent sudden flooding of the Braid Burn during heavy rain. Many of the original woodland features will be preserved. The Corsican pines and rough meadows are to provide recreational areas which will include the former cricket pitch. Many new trees are to be planted. One of the proposed names for the development, *Colinton Pines*, may therefore be appropriate.

The amount of traffic and vehicular pollution will probably not increase overall, although it will be greater during the morning and evening rush hour on weekdays. 'Rat-running' will stop as the west gate will be closed except for access by emergency services, cycles and pedestrians. The two main gates will be the original main gate and the north eastern entrance close to the ambulance depot, both opening onto Greenbank Drive.

Work started on the central and western parts of the site in the summer of 1998, initially excluding the day hospital, Cottages 23 and 24, Pavilion 17 and the MRI scanner building. The development of the eastern part of the site is not scheduled to start until the ENT Unit, the Regional Clinical Virus Laboratory and Scottish Mycobacterial Reference Laboratory, all situated in the north eastern corner, have gone to Little France.

Although the developers may find the style, shape and position of the buildings awkward, they may also bless the Town Council of the 1890s for choosing this attractive site with good elevation and drainage, and an open, gently southward sloping and therefore sunny position. A traditional corner shop, community centre and place of worship may yet be considered but in these days of two-car families, easily accessible shopping centres and widespread lack of interest in religious observance, they may not find a place.

Many former staff and patients will regret the passing of this fever hospital. It could be said that its working life is over because many of the diseases it was originally designed to accommodate have disappeared. Some illnesses like scarlet fever, which occupied 320 of the original 600 beds, have largely vanished or have become less virulent than they were when the hospital was built. Others like tuberculosis have been controlled in the West by surveillance, identification and modern chemotherapy. Immunisation has to a great extent defeated diphtheria, whooping cough, measles, rubella, mumps and poliomyelitis and it has totally eliminated smallpox. Antibiotics have revolutionised the management of many bacterial illnesses, and antiviral drugs are beginning to make a real impact in certain other infections. In time a vaccine will be developed to protect against HIV infection but already life expectancy in this disease is being prolonged by the judicious use of combinations of new, admittedly expensive, anti-retroviral agents.

Like a grand old lady, vivacious and vigorous in youth, the City Hospital is passing graciously into retirement, its job well done. By adapting and accommodating disciplines other than 'fevers', it has added greatly to its reputation. From the early days of mitral valve surgery to the later triumphs of minimal access thoracic surgery and from the gory days of almost indiscriminate tonsillectomies and adenoidectomies to the modern management of tinnitus, cochlear implants and the huge improvement in the results of major head and neck surgery with appropriate after care of laryngectomees in the ENT Unit, the surgeons at the City Hospital have made outstanding contributions. The introduction of artificial implants to reconstruct the face after trauma or malignancy is one of the triumphs of the maxillofacial surgeons. The rigorous pursuit and near conquering of the 'white death' at the City Hospital by Sir John Crofton, who introduced triple chemotherapy for tuberculosis, remains an achievement of global renown. Similarly the correct management of obstructive airways disease pioneered by the late Professor Flenley has benefited innumerable sufferers of emphysema. Before he went to the Royal Infirmary, Dr Andrew Douglas' work on sarcoidosis brought him and the City Hospital international recognition. Likewise Professor Haslett's cell function studies, Professor Neil Douglas' sleep apnoea research and Professor MacNee's studies on air pollution are all of major importance.

In geriatric medicine, Professor Williamson set the gold standard in the Care of the Elderly Unit. The Assessment, Stroke and Trauma Rehabilitation Units and studies in pressure sore care and prevention provided models for others to follow. In antibiotic therapy and the natural history of urinary tract infections the late Dr James Murdoch was a leader in the 1960s and 1970s. Dr Ray Brettle grasped the nettle of HIV infection and drug misuse, which no one else was willing to tackle in the 1980s, and so prevented Edinburgh's AIDS epidemic from escalating out of all proportion. The contributions of the Respiratory Function Laboratory and the Rayne Laboratory have been considerable. The siting of the Scottish Mycobacteria Reference Laboratory at the City Hospital was a major coup, stemming from the successive dedication of Drs Archie Wallace, Margaret Calder and Brian Watt. In the Regional Clinical Virus Laboratory the development of new techniques for detecting rotaviruses, hepatitis viruses, HIV and *Pneumocystis carinii* has also brought major benefits for patients.

All these disciplines have taken their part in medical education. The teaching of undergraduates, postgraduates, nurses and those in the professions allied to medicine has always been an important function of the hospital. Three successive Medical Superintendents, the Physician Superintendent Dr N. W. Horne and lay administrators have assisted in building up the hospital and in running it smoothly. Generations of nursing staff have come and gone. Some in the early days paid with their lives for their devotion to their patients after catching infections such as streptococcal sepsis, diphtheria, typhoid and tuberculosis. In more recent times, by caring for hepatitis and AIDS patients, some of whom were abusive and uncooperative drug misusers, the nursing staff have again selflessly risked their own health and safety. Happily this was recognised publicly on one occasion when Sister Margaret Kerr, was awarded the MBE for her leadership during the viral hepatitis outbreak of 1969–70. If the names of even a few of those, who have helped to make the City Hospital what it was and who contributed to the well being of their fellows, can be associated with the new housing projects, some measure of continuity will have been preserved. One hopes that, as the City Hospital closes, the staff will find new posts elsewhere and will take with them some of the spirit of this great hospital and happy memories of working there; similarly patients who survived their illnesses may be grateful for the services the hospital has provided. If this does happen, the City Hospital will have achieved its objective and may now slip quietly into well deserved retirement.

Abbreviated References and Selected Abbreviations

The following list contains short forms for references as used in the text and the Notes, with the full reference details given on the right. It also contains explanations for selected abbreviations, particularly those related to references.

Abercrombie MS and papers	Dr John Abercrombie, RCPEL, Box 4, Folder 31 (Cholera).
Alison MS and papers	Dr W. P. Alison, RCPEL, 1/6, 2/12 (Cholera).
Annual Report, MOH/PHD	The Annual Report of the Medical Officer of Health of the City of Edinburgh (for the appropriate year, usually published the following year). From 1908 these became the Annual Reports of the Public Health Department. Except for the amalgamation of several years during war time, they continue annually to 1974. Many enclose the Report by the Resident Physician, Colinton Mains Hospital and (later) by the Medical Superintendent of the City Hospital. ECL, YRA 244 and q YRA 244–24057.
Annual Statistical Report	Lothian Health Board Annual Statistical Report. LHSA, EUL, LHB 37/1/1–12.
An outbreak of typhus fever, 1899	An outbreak of typhus fever. Harvey Littlejohn (History) and Claude B. Ker (Clinical Features), *Transactions of the Medicochirurgical Society of Edinburgh*. 1899;162–184, ECL, YRA 649 (898) A 10058.

Abbreviated References and Selected Abbreviations 405

Bartholomew's Pentland Hills and Edinburgh District	Bartholomew's 1½ in map. Pentland Hills and Edinburgh District for pedestrians (undated). Edinburgh Geographical Institute.
Bartholomew's Pocket Plan of Edinburgh and Suburbs.	Bartholomew's Pocket Plan of Edinburgh and Suburbs: 3½ in to 1 mile (undated). Edinburgh Geographical Institute.
Boyd, *Leith Hospital*	D. H. A. Boyd, *Leith Hospital 1848–1988*. Edinburgh, Scottish Academic Press, 1990.
Brotherston, Early Public Health Movement	J. H. F. Brotherston, Observations on the Early Public Health Movement in Scotland. Memoir 8. London School of Hygiene and Tropical Medicine, 1952. London, H. K. Lewis & Co Ltd.
Building Specification, 15.4.1897	New City Hospital, Colinton Mains, Building Specification. City of Edinburgh Public Works Office, 15 April 1897. ECA.
Bunyan, Fairhurst, Mackie and McMillan, *Building Stones of Edinburgh*	I. T. Bunyan, J. A. Fairhurst, A. Mackie and A. A. McMillan, *Building Stones of Edinburgh*, ed. A. A. McMillan. Edinburgh, Edinburgh Geographical Society, 1987.
Chambers, *Traditions of Edinburgh*	R. Chambers, *Traditions of Edinburgh*. New Edition, 1868. Edinburgh and London, W. & R. Chambers Ltd, 1968.
City Hospital Extension, 9.12.1893	City Hospital Extension, I-Report by MOH and City Superintendent of Works, Edinburgh, 9 December 1893. Fly cover dated 10.5.1894. It also includes reports (and additional reports) by physicians, the City Superintendent of Works etc. and by the PHC. Only the page numbers of the total document

Clayson, Lecture to Joint Meeting, 1987	are referred to in the text. Plans are referred to separately. On 3.7.1987 to commemorate the opening of the Victoria Dispensary for Consumption in 1887, Dr Christopher Clayson, CBE, gave a lecture to a joint meeting of the Scottish Thoracic and the British Thoracic Societies and the Thoracic Society of Australia.
Clayson, Time was when youth grew pale ...	C. Clayson, Time was when youth grew pale, and spectre thin, and died. *Proceedings of the RCPE,* 1993;23:545–547.
Closed Record, Lord Provost *et al.* v. John Lownie and William Ormiston, 18.11.1902	Closed record in note of suspension and interdict for the Lord Provost ... of Edinburgh, – complainers; against John Lownie, Builder ... and William Ormiston, Surveyor ..., Respondents. First Division 18.11.1902. ECA, D16.
Colinton Hospital Report, 7.12.1895	Colinton Hospital. Report by MOH and Superintendent of Works on ... Proposed Buildings for Hospital at Colinton Mains. City Chambers 7.12.1895. ECL, C1/1.
Colinton Mains Hospital, Memorandum, 9.10.1903	Colinton Mains Hospital. Memorandum Accompanying Plans for the Information of the Local Government Board, prepared by R. Morham, Public Works Office, Edinburgh. 9.10.1903. SRO, HH 101/1359.
Collins, *The Influence of Scottish Medicine*	K. E. Collins, American Jewish Medical Students in Scotland, 1925–40, in *The Influence of Scottish Medicine,* ed. D. A. Dow. British Society for the History of Medicine and the Scottish Society

Abbreviated References and Selected Abbreviations 407

	of the History of Medicine, Carnforth, Parthenon Publishing Group, 1988.
Comrie, *History of Scottish Medicine*.	J. D. Comrie, *History of Scottish Medicine*, Vols I, II. 2nd edn. Wellcome Historical Medical Museum. London, Bailliere, Tindall & Cox, 1932.
Craig, *History of the RCPE*	W. S, Craig, *History of the Royal College of Physicians of Edinburgh*. Oxford, Blackwell Scientific Publications, 1976.
Crofton, Final Report on Tuberculosis Research 1952–65	Sir John Crofton, Final Report to the RVH Tuberculosis Trust. A review of research work supported by the Trust, 1952–65. Typescript in Vol. 4 of Minutes of RVH Tuberculosis Trust. LHSA, EUL.
Daiches, *Was – A Pastime from Time Past*	D. Daiches, *Was – A Pastime from Time Past*. Thames and Hudson, 1975.
DEG, SLHD	District Executive Group, South Lothian Health District, in Lothian Health Board. LHSA, EUL. LHB 28/1/1.
Description and Sketch Plan, 5.10.1896	Description and Sketch Plan of Proposed Hospital at Colinton Mains for the City of Edinburgh. Public Works Office, 5.10.1896. ECL, YRA 988c.
Deuchar, *The Prevalence of Epidemic Fever*	R. Deuchar, *Observations on the Prevalence of Epidemic Fever in Edinburgh and Glasgow and Means Suggested for Improving the Sanitary Condition of the Poor*. Glasgow, William Whyte & Co and William Collins, 1844. ECL, YRA 649–843.
Division of Medicine Minutes, SLHD Executive Committee	Division of Medicine Minutes, South Lothian Health District

	Executive Committee, LHSA, EUL, LHB 28/4/5
Eastwood and Jenkinson, *Western General Hospital*	M. Eastwood and A. Jenkinson, *A History of the Western General Hospital*. Edinburgh, John Donald Publishers Ltd, 1995.
ECA	Edinburgh City Archives, City Chambers.
ECL	Edinburgh Central Library, Edinburgh Room.
Edinburgh Evening News	*Edinburgh Evening News* (variously dated). ECL
Edinburgh Fever Hospital, 1903	*The Edinburgh Fever Hospital – Description with Plans and Photographs*. Edinburgh, George Stewart & Co, 1903. (With its foreword by Councillor W Lang Todd, this green, cloth-covered hardback copy may have been a presentation piece for the opening ceremony.) ECL. q. YRA 988c.
EML	Erskine Medical Library, University of Edinburgh.
Extracts from Mr Ballingall's letters	Typescript headed: Hospital. Town against Lownie. Extracts from Mr Ballingall's letters on the subject of delay. Filed with legal documents and Weekly Reports on Works in Progress. ECA, D16.
For consideration at Special Meeting of the Magistrates and Council, 26.2.1897	For consideration at Special Meeting of the Magistrates and Council to be held on Friday, 26.2.1897 ... New City Hospital, Colinton Mains. This contains reports by PHC *et al.* setting out past and present arguments for and against the move to Colinton and the number of beds needed. With TCM, ECA.
Fraser, *The Building of Old College*	A. G. Fraser, *The Building of Old College: Adam, Playfair & the*

	University of Edinburgh. Edinburgh University Press, 1989.
Gazetteer of Scotland	The Topographical, Statistical, and Historical Gazetteer of Scotland, Vols I,II. Glasgow, A. Fullerton & Co, 1843.
Gifford, McWilliam and Walker, Edinburgh	J. Gifford, C. McWilliam and D. Walker, The Buildings of Scotland, Edinburgh. Harmondsworth, Penguin Books, 1984.
Grant, Old and New Edinburgh	J. Grant, Cassell's Old and New Edinburgh: Its History, its People and its Places, Vols I–III. London, Cassell & Co. Ltd, 1883.
Gunn and Blanc, City Hospital, Bedford, George Heriot's Hospital, Edinburgh	C. B. Gunn and H. J. Blanc, City Hospital, Bedford, George Heriot's Hospital, Edinburgh. Edinburgh, E. & S. Livingstone. NMRSL.
Guthrie, The Royal Edinburgh Hospital for Sick Children	D. Guthrie, The Royal Edinburgh Hospital for Sick Children, 1860–1960. Edinburgh, E. & S. Livingstone, 1960.
Health in Lothian 1974–89	Health in Lothian 1974–89, LHSA, EUL, LHB 37/2/1.
Hendrie and Macleod, The Bangour Story	W. F. Hendrie and D. A. D. Macleod, The Bangour Story: A History of Bangour Village and General Hospitals. Aberdeen University Press, 1991; reprinted Edinburgh, Mercat Press, 1992.
Hospital Review, 1974	Hospital Review: Report on Hospitals in the SE Region Scotland (SERHB) Prepared by Iain J MacKenzie, Norman Nicol, ed. & des. by Ian D. Smith, Information Officer. March 1974. LHSA, EUL.
Hume and Boyd, Queensberry House Hospital	M. Hume and S. Boyd, Queensberry House Hospital: A History, ed. E. F. Catford.

Joint Minute in causa John Lownie against Lord Provost by James Walker	Edinburgh, Directors of Queensberry House Hospital, 1984. Joint Minute for the parties in causa John Lownie, ... Pursuer, against the Lord Provost ... of the City of Edinburgh, Defenders et e contra. Signed James Walker. ECA, D16.
Joint Print of Documents, Lord Provost *et al.* v. John Lownie and William Ormiston, 28.2.1903	Joint Print of Documents in note of suspension and interdict for the Lord Provost et al of the City of Edinburgh – Complainers and Respondents against John Lownie, ... and William Ormiston, ... Defenders. 28.2.1903. ECA, D16.
Judicial Reference	Judicial Reference – City of Edinburgh and John Lownie. ECA, D16.
Ker, *A Manual of Fevers*, 1911	C. B. Ker, *A Manual of Fevers*. London, Henry Froude, Oxford University Press and Hodder & Stoughton, 1911. LHSA, EUL, MAC, GD 1/46/5–5.
Ker's Infectious Diseases – A Practical Textbook, 1929	*Ker's Infectious Diseases – A Practical Textbook*, Revised by Claude Rundle, 3rd edn. London, Humphrey Milford, Oxford University Press, 1929.
Leitch, Two men and a bug ..., 1996	A. G. Leitch, Two men and a bug: One hundred years of tuberculosis in Edinburgh. *Proceedings of the RCPE*, 1996;26:295–308.
Letter to R. Morham from J. Murray & Sons, 30.3.1899	Letter to R. Morham Esq. from J. Murray & Sons, Corsehill Quarry, 30.3.1899, replying to Morham's of 28.3.1899, regarding the paucity of stone being supplied for Colinton Main's Hospital. Among Clerk of Work's

Abbreviated References and Selected Abbreviations 411

	Weekly Progress Reports, ECA, D16.
LHB Annual Report	Lothian Health Board Annual Report 1987–88. LHSA, EUL, LHB 37/1/13.
LHSA, EUL	Lothian Health Services Archive, Edinburgh University Library.
Littlejohn, *Sanitary Report*	H. D. Littlejohn. *Report on the Sanitary Condition of the City of Edinburgh*. Edinburgh, Colston & Son, 1865. ECL, YRA 490–43751.
M(A)C, SLHD	Medical (Advisory) Committee, South Lothian Health District (14.1.1975–11.5.1983) LHSA, EUL, LHB 28/4/1–2.
Mags. of Edinburgh v. John Lownie (1903) 5F. 711	Magistrates of Edinburgh v. John Lownie and William Ormiston. Court of Session (1903) 5F. 711–716.
Maitland, *History of Edinburgh*	W. Maitland, *The History of Edinburgh from its Foundation to the Present Time* ... Edinburgh, Hamilton, Balfour & Neil, 1753.
Memorandum by Bailie Pollard, 4.6.1896	Memorandum by Bailie Pollard, Chairman of the Health Committee, on Fever Hospitals on the Continent, with Reference to the New City Hospital about to be Erected at Colinton Mains, Edinburgh, 4.6.1896. ECA, C1/3.
Men of the Period	*Men of the Period, Scotland: The Records of a Great Country, Portraits and Pen Pictures of Leading Men*. Biographical Publishing Co. (ca. 1895) NLS:Biog. D. 5.1. M.
MOH	Medical Officer of Health
Minute of Agreement, 1913	Minute of Agreement between the Lord Provost and Council of the City of Edinburgh and the Parish Council of the City Parish

	of Edinburgh (Sir Thomas Hunter, WS.). 1913. ECA, D16.
Minutes of RIE Managers	Minutes of Meetings of the Managers of the Edinburgh Royal Infirmary. LHSA, EUL, LHB 1/1.
Minutes of Presbytery of Edinburgh	Minutes of the Church of Scotland's Presbytery of Edinburgh kindly supplied to Rev. Dr R. C. M. Mathers by Presbytery Clerk, Rev. W. Peter Graham.
Minutes of RV & AH BOM	Minutes of the Royal Victoria and Associated Hospitals Board of Management, 1948–74, which contain Reports of the BOM, Annual Reports for the City Hospital for Infectious Diseases (CH for ID) and Minutes of the General Purposes Committee (GP Committee), Finance Committee and the Medical & Allied Services Committee (M&AS Committee) LHSA, EUL, LHB 38/7/133–141 and 10/1/6–10/1/10.
Minutes of RVH Tuberculosis Trust	Minutes of the Royal Victoria Hospital Tuberculosis Trust, 1914–65. LHSA, EUL Minute Books Vols. (part of) 2, 3 and 4.
Minutes of Victoria Dispensary	Minutes of the Victoria Dispensary for Consumption and Diseases of the Chest, 1891–1905 followed by Minutes of the Royal Victoria Hospital for Consumption, 1905–1914. LHSA, EUL Minute Books, Vol. 1 and (part of) 2.
Murray, *Nuisances of Edinburgh*	A. Murray, *Nuisances of Edinburgh with Suggestions for the Removal Thereof Addressed to the Commissioner of Police*. Edinburgh, Adam & Charles Black, 1847. ECL YRA 490-B9909.

Abbreviated References and Selected Abbreviations 413

NLS	National Library of Scotland.
NMRSL	National Monuments Record of Scotland Library.
Obituary, Sir Robert William Philip	Anon. Obituary, Sir Robert William Philip. *Edinburgh Medical Journal*, 1939:46:180–182.
PHC	Pubic Health Committee.
PHC Minutes	Minutes of the Public Health Committee of Edinburgh Town Council (quoted by date of meeting). ECA.
PHD	Public Health Department.
PMROH	Princess Margaret Rose Orthopaedic Hospital (formerly PMRH for Crippled Children).
Pollard, *The Care of the Public Health*	J. Pollard, *The Care of the Public Health and the New Fever Hospital in Edinburgh*, 2nd edn. Edinburgh University Press, 1898. Pollard was assisted by Sir Henry Littlejohn, MOH, and Robert Morham, City Architect.
Post Office Plan of Edinburgh and Leith	Post Office Plans of Edinburgh and Leith, various dates. ECL.
PWO City Hospital Extension Plan, 9.12.1893	Public Works Office, City Chambers. City Hospital Extension, 9.12.1893. Sketch Block Plan from a Report by MOH and City Superintendent of Works. ECL. qYRA 988c–26342.
PWO City Hospital Extension Plan, March 1894	Public Works Office, City Chambers. City Hospital Extension. Alternative Plan (showing new wards on north-south axis). With reference to Report by Physicians. March 1894. ECL. qYRA 988c.
PWO City Hospital Extension Plan, 17.4.1894	Public Works Office, City Chambers. City Hospital Extension Sketch Block Plan, referred to in City Architect's

	report of 17.4.1894. ECL. q. YRA 988c.
RCPE	Royal College of Physicians of Edinburgh.
RCPEL	Royal College of Physicians of Edinburgh Library.
Reclaiming Note, 15.1.1903	Reclaiming Note for John Lownie against Lord Low's Interlocutor, 15.1.1903. This explores the suitability of William Ormiston as Arbiter. ECA. D16.
Report as to Smallpox Accommodation, 17.10.1910	Report by the MOH, Resident Physician at the City Hospital, and the City Superintendent of Works on the letter from the Assistant Secretary, Local Government Board as to Smallpox Accommodation. 17.10.1910. PHD, City Chambers. ECL. C3/12. By 1910 the MOH was Dr A. Maxwell Williamson, the Resident Physician still Dr C. B. Ker and City Superintendent, Mr J. A. Williamson.
Report as to the Treatment of Infectious Diseases, 1884	A Report by the Town Clerk and MOH as to the Present and Prospective Arrangements for the Treatment of Infectious Diseases in the City. 5.11.1884. ECL. qYRA 643.
Report by City Superintendent of Works as to Accommodation, 10.1.1891.	Report by City Superintendent of Works as to Accommodation for Staff at the City Hospital and other Matters. City Chambers, 10.1.1891. ECL. qYRA 988c B17867.
Report by the Committee of the College, 1894	Report by the Committee of the RCPE on the New City Hospital Site. MS in minutes of RCPE pp. 536–539 and printed in

	RCPEL and ECL. qYRA 988c, B17869.
Report by the Committee to the Managers of the Royal Infirmary, 18.2.1885	Report by the Committee Appointed to Deal with the Subject of the Fever Hospital Treatment of Infectious Diseases Reporting to the Managers of the Royal Infirmary, 18.2.1885. Minutes of the Managers, Vol. 33, pp. 263–273 LHSA, EUL. LHB 1/1.
Report on Colinton Mains Hospital, 19.5.1902	Report on Colinton Mains Hospital (in response to Public Health Committee's recommendations to supplement Mr Morham's report of 20.5.1901), 19.5.1902. ECA, 2/2.
Report on Probable Cost, 20.5.1901	New City Hospital, Colinton Mains. Report on Probable Cost. R. Morham, Public Works Office, City Chambers, Edinburgh. 20.5.1901. ECA, 2/1.
RIDU	Regional Infectious Diseases Unit.
RIE & AH Annual Report 1992–3	Royal Infirmary of Edinburgh and Associated Hospitals Annual Report 1992–3 (Copy from Mrs Ramage, secretary to Mr R. Purves, RIE).
RIE & AH Annual Report 1993–4	Royal Infirmary of Edinburgh and Associated Hospitals Annual Report 1993–4. LHSA, EUL. LHB 1/4/169.
RIE & AH Annual Report and Accounts 1994–5 (and 1995–6)	Royal Infirmary of Edinburgh and Associated Hospitals NHS Trust Annual Report and Accounts 1994–5 (and 1995–6). LHSA, EUL. LHB 1/4/170 (and LHB 1/4/171).
RIE & AH Report, 1974–88	Royal Infirmary of Edinburgh and Associated Hospitals Report, 1974–88. LHSA, EUL. LHB 1/4/164.

RVH	Royal Victoria Hospital
Samuel Papers	Papers, notes and certificates of Catherine B Samuel, who trained at the City Hospital qualifying as a Fever Nurse in September, 1920. LHSA, EUL. MAC GD 1/46/et seq.
SCD, EUL	Special Collections Department, Edinburgh University Library.
SLHD	South Lothian Health District.
Smith, *Edinburgh's Contribution to Medical Microbiology*	C. J. Smith, *Edinburgh's Contribution to Medical Microbiology*. Publication No. 7. University of Glasgow. Wellcome Unit for the History of Medicine, 1994.
Smith, *Historic South Edinburgh*, Vol. I	C. J. Smith, *Historic South Edinburgh*, Vol. I. Edinburgh, Charles Skilton Ltd, 1978.
Smith, *Historic South Edinburgh*, Vol. II	Vol. II, 1979.
Smith, *Historic South Edinburgh*, Vol. III	Vol. III, People, 1986.
Smith, *Historic South Edinburgh*, Vol. IV	Vol. IV, More People, 1988.
Smith, *Morningside*	C. J. Smith, *Morningside*. Edinburgh, John Donald Publishers Ltd, 1992.
Smout, *A Century of the Scottish People*	T. C. Smout, *A Century of the Scottish People 1830–1950*. Glasgow, William Collins Sons & Co Ltd, 1986. London, Fontana Press, imprint of Harper Collins, 1987.
Smout, *A History of the Scottish People*	T. C. Smout, *A History of the Scottish People 1560–1830*. Glasgow, William Collins Sons & Co Ltd, 1969. Edition quoted Fontana/Collins, 1977.
Special Meeting of the Town Council of Edinburgh, 26.2.1897	Special Meeting of the Town Council of Edinburgh, 26.2.1897. ECA. TCM 1896–7, pp. 217–225.
SRO	Scottish Records Office.

Stewart Smith, *The Grange of St Giles*	J. Stewart Smith, *The Grange of St Giles* ... Edinburgh, T. & A. Constable, 1898.
Sutherland, *Control and Eradication of Tuberculosis*	*The Control and Eradication of Tuberculosis: A series of international studies* ... ed. H. G. Sutherland. Edinburgh, William Green & Sons, 1911. RCPEL.
Tait, *A Doctor and Two Policemen*	H. P. Tait, *A Doctor and Two Policemen — The History of Edinburgh Public Health Department, 1862–1974*. Edinburgh District Council and Canongate Press, 1974.
Tait, Cholera Board of Health	H. P. Tait, The Cholera Board of Health, Edinburgh, 1831–34. *The Medical Officer.* 1957;98:235–237.
TCM	Edinburgh Town Council Minutes. ECA (under Town Council Records).
The Edinburgh Outbreak of Smallpox 1942	W. G. Clark, H. E. Seiler, A. Joe, J. L. Gammie, H. P. Tait and R. P. Jack, *The Edinburgh Outbreak of Smallpox 1942*. October 1944, Public Health Committee, City of Edinburgh PHD.
The Edinburgh Tuberculosis Scheme	Anon, The Edinburgh Tuberculosis Scheme. *Edinburgh Medical Journal*, 1937;44:285–297.
The Scotsman	*The Scotsman* (variously dated) ECL.
Turner, *Story of a Great Hospital*	A. L. Turner, *Story of A Great Hospital: the Royal Infirmary of Edinburgh, 1729–1929*. Edinburgh, Oliver & Boyd, 1937.
Weekly Report on Works in Progress	Weekly Report on Works in Progress in New City Hospital, Colinton Mains, the Property of the City of Edinburgh for the Week Ending ... These meticulously record the progress and problems encountered by Mr

George Ballingall, Clerk of Works, covering Contracts 1–3. They run consecutively from No. 1 (week ending 7.8.1897) to Nos. 343 and 236 (week ending 19.3.1904). ECA, D16.

Welsh, *A Practical Treatise on the Efficacy of Bloodletting* ...

B. Welsh, *A Practical Treatise on the Efficacy of Bloodletting in the Epidemic Fever in Edinburgh. Illustrated by Numerous Cases and Tables Extracted from the Journals of the Queensberry House Fever Hospital.* Edinburgh, printed by Bell & Bradfude and sold by Longman, Hurst, Rees et al., 1819. ECL, qYRA 649–818.

Notes and References

Full publication details for references given here in abbreviated form can be found in the list of Abbreviated References.

CHAPTER ONE

1. *Johnson's Journey to the Western Islands of Scotland and Boswell's Journal of a Tour to the Hebrides with Samuel Johnson, LL.D.* ed. R. W. Chapman, Oxford University Press, 1979, p. 173.
2. *Ibid*, p. 173.

CHAPTER TWO

1. Comrie, *History of Scottish Medicine*, Vol. I, Ch. 9, pp. 193–211. An authoritative account, quoted throughout this chapter, on the health regulations concerning leprosy, syphilis and plague.
2. M. Cant, *Villages of Edinburgh*, Edinburgh, Malcolm Cant, 1987, Vol. 2, p. 134.
3. J. Ritchie, Quarantine for plague in Scotland during the sixteenth and seventeenth centuries, *Edinburgh Medical Journal* 1948;55:691–701.
4. Maitland, *History of Edinburgh*, p. 32
5. J. G. Gray, *The South Side Story (An Anthology of the South Side of Edinburgh)*, Glasgow, W. F. Knox & Co Ltd. 1962, pp. 88–89. See also Stewart Smith, *The Grange of St Giles*, pp. 10–13; Grant, *Old and New Edinburgh*, Vol. III, pp. 47–49; C. Smith, *Between the Streamlet and the Town – A Brief History of the Astley Ainslie Hospital*, Polton Home Press, 1988.
6. Smith, *Historic South Edinburgh*, Vol. I, Ch. 11, p. 233.
7. *Ibid*., Chap. 1, pp. 8–12. See also Stewart Smith, *The Grange of St Giles*, pp. 13–20 which comments on the 10 different spellings of 'Sienna' in the Register of the Great Seal 1546–1580, No. 1980; and Grant, *Old and New Edinburgh*, Vol. III, pp. 51–54.
8. Smith, *Historic South Edingurgh*, Vol. I, Ch. 5, pp. 77–78.
9. Pollard, *The Care of the Public Health*, p. 8.
10. Maitland, *History of Edinburgh*, p. 85.
11. *Ibid*., p. 87.
12. Smout, *A History of the Scottish People*, Part Two Ch. 11 p. 253 Quoting the anonymous author of MS 316 in EUL, Folio 81, writing ca. 1760.
13. Tait, *A Doctor and Two Policemen*, p. 10.
14. Deuchar, *The Prevalence of Epidemic Fever*, p. 9.
15. *Ibid*., p. 6.
16. *Ibid*., p. 9.
17. Craig, *History of the RCPE*, p. 11.
18. Tait, Cholera Board of Health, pp. 235–237.

19. T. Latta, The treatment of cholera by the copious injection of aqueous and saline fluids into the veins, *Lancet* 1832;2:175–177.
20. Boyd, *Leith Hospital*, Ch. 1, pp. 6–8.
21. J. Abercrombie, *Suggestions Submitted to the Medical Practitioners of Edinburgh on the Characters and Treatment of the Malignant Cholera. Published for the Benefit of the Board of Health*, 7th edn, Edinburgh, Waugh & Innes, 1832, LHSA, EUL. Dr John Abercrombie (1780–1844) ran a proto-type *poliklinik* method of teaching. He was Lord Rector of Marischal College and, in 1828, Physician to the King in Scotland.
22. Abercrombie MS and Papers.
23. Tait, Cholera Board of Health, pp. 235–237.
24. Abercrombie MS and Papers.
25. Alison, MS and Papers. Dr Alison (1790–1859) was a great public health reformer. His *Observations on the Management of the Poor in Scotland and its Effect on the Health of the Great Towns* (1844) led to the Poor Law of Scotland, 1845. Among his papers are the daily cholera reports sent from local board secretaries to the Edinburgh Cholera Board of Health in the 1832 outbreak.
26. W. D. Adams, Statement of the Extra-professional services in connexion with Cholera in the Third Medical District of the City Parish, Edinburgh from 28 August to 30 November 1854. Prepared at the request of the Sanitary Committee of the Parochial Board. 1854 ECL, YRA 649–854 R501. The case histories make harrowing reading.
27. Ibid.

CHAPTER THREE

1. The Hon. Lord Cullen, *The Walls of Edinburgh – A Short Guide*, Edinburgh, The Cockburn Association, 1988. See also Pollard, *The Care of the Public Health*, p. 6.
2. Lord Cullen, *The Walls of Edinburgh*.
3. Tait, *A Doctor and Two Policemen*, p. 12.
4. W. Gilbert, *Edinburgh Life in the Eighteenth and Nineteenth Centuries*. Part 2 Edinburgh Life in the Nineteenth Century, Glasgow, Lang Syne Publishers Ltd, 1989, pp. 31–33. This edited reprint of Henry Grey Graham's account in *The Social Life of Scotland in the Eighteenth Century* provides a good description of the fires of 1824.
5. Littlejohn, *Sanitary Report*, p. 31.
6. Craig, *History of the RCPE*, p. 17. Quoting R. H. Campbell and J. B. A. Dow, *Source Book of Scottish Economic History*, Oxford, Blackwell, 1968, pp. 230–231.
7. Littlejohn, *Sanitary Report*, p. 38.
8. Chambers, *Traditions of Edinburgh*, p. 318.
9. Craig, *History of the RCPE*, p. 18.
10. Tait, *A Doctor and Two Policemen*, p. 14.
11. Smith, *Historic South Edinburgh*, Vol. II, Ch. 6, pp. 404–411. A very readable account of the development of Edinburgh's water supply. See also Pollard, *Care of the Public Health*, pp. 11–12.
12. Tait, *A Doctor and Two Policemen*, p. 14.
13. Littlejohn, *Sanitary Report*, p. 50.
14. Ibid., p. 51.
15. Murray, *Nuisances in Edinburgh*.
16. Ibid.

CHAPTER FOUR

1. Maitland, *History of Edinburgh*, p. 32.
2. *Ibid*, p. 33.
3. Deuchar, *The Prevalence of Epidemic Fever*, p. 8.
4. Tait, Cholera Board of Health, p. 235.
5. Brotherston, Early Public Health Movement, pp. 67–75.
6. *Ibid.*, p. 43.
7. Grant, *Old and New Edinburgh*, Vol. I, p. 240. Although Grant gives the date as 10 November, most sources quote 24 November, e.g. Tait, *A Doctor and Two Policemen*, p. 16 and J. Keay and J. Keay, *Collins Encyclopaedia of Scotland*, London, Harper Collins, 1994, p. 310.
8. Grant, *Old and New Edinburgh*, Vol. I, p. 203.
9. H. P. Tait, Sir Henry Duncan Littlejohn: Great Scottish Sanitarian and Medical Jurist. *Medical Officer* 1962;108:183–190. F. A. E. Crew, Centenary of Appointment of the First Medical Officer of Health for the City of Edinburgh. *Scottish Medical Journal* 1963;8:53–62.
10. J. D. Marwick and H. D. Littlejohn, Suggestions as to a Vaccination Act for Scotland. Edinburgh City Chambers. Marwick was the City Clerk. ECL, YRM 784-B16944.
11. Littlejohn, *Sanitary Report*.
12. Report on the Sanitary Condition of Saint-Giles' Ward as Ascertained by a recent House-to-House Survey with Recommendations for Improvements by the Public Health Committee. October 1889. Edinburgh, H & J Pillans & Wilson. ECL, q YRA 490.
13. Tait, *A Doctor and Two Policemen*. Hence the title of Dr H. Tait's book.
14. *Ibid.*, p. 20.
15. Littlejohn, *Sanitary Report*, plan opposite p. 113.
16. Smout, *A Century of the Scottish People*, p. 44; H. Clark, Living in One or Two Rooms in the City, in *The Scottish Home*, ed. A Carruthers, Edinburgh, National Museums of Scotland, 1996, pp. 62–63. Glasgow's City Improvement Act introduced the idea of ticketing in the 1860s and a similar enactment came into Edinburgh under the Municipal & Police Act, 1879 (42&43 VICT., 21.7.1879, in Ch. 132, pp. 80–82, ECA), although ticketing does not seem to have been enforced until 1899 when the four newly appointed inspectors managed to measure 2,000 houses in the first year. It is estimated that not all houses would have been visited until at least 1901. Annual Report of the Chief Sanitary and Market Inspector, 1899, p. 15 and 1900, pp. 5–6. ECA, SL 140/1/1.
17. H. D. Littlejohn, Report to the Town Council: On the Compulsory Intimation of Infectious Diseases 1875–76. ECL, YRA 643-B18057.
18. *Ibid*.
19. H. D. Littlejohn, What are the Advantages of a System of Notification of Infectious Diseases ...? A paper read at the Nottingham Congress of the National Association for the Promotion of Social Science. September 1862. London, Spottiswoode & Co ... ECL YRA 643-20204.
20. Annual Report, MOH, 1902, p. 29.
21. Annual Report, MOH, 1900, pp. 17–20.
22. Annual Report, MOH, 1902, p. 37.
23. H. P. Tait, Sir Henry Duncan Littlejohn: Great Scottish Sanitarian and Medical Jurist. *Medical Officer* 1962;108:183–190. F. A. E. Crew, Centenary of Appoint-

ment of the First Medical Officer of Health for the City of Edinburgh. *Scottish Medical Journal* 1963;8:53–62.

CHAPTER FIVE

1. Pollard, *The Care of the Public Health,* p. 10.
2. Turner, *Story of a Great Hospital,* p. 52.
3. Ibid., p. 51.
4. Ibid., p. 49.
5. Ibid., p. 49.
6. Fraser, *The Building of Old College,* pp. 33, 41.
7. *Gazetteer of Scotland,* Vol. 1, p. 449.
8. By 1843, the operating theatre in the attic was no longer in use.
9. The Lock Hospital accomodated patients with sexually transmitted disease.
10. *Gazetteer of Scotland,* Vol. 1, p. 449.
11. Smout, *A History of the Scottish People,* p. 251.
12. Welsh, *A Practical Treatise on the Efficacy of Bloodletting,* pp. 16, 17.
13. Ibid., p. 51.
14. Ibid., p. 52.
15. Turner, *Story of a Great Hospital,* p. 157.

CHAPTER SIX

1. Turner, *Story of a Great Hospital,* p. 157.
2. Chambers, *Traditions of Edinburgh,* pp. 353–362.
3. Hume and Boyd, *Queensberry House Hospital,* pp. 61–79.
4. Ibid., p. 79.
5. Ibid., p. 86.
6. Gifford, McWilliam and Walker, *Edinburgh,* p. 217.
7. Welsh, *A Practical Treatise on the Efficacy of Blood Letting.* Quoted often in this chapter as he details the work of an early nineteenth century fever hospital.
8. Turner, *Story of a Great Hospital,* p. 158.
9. Ibid.
10. Welsh, *A Practical Treatise on the Efficacy of Blood Letting,* pp. 2–3.
11. Ibid.
12. Ibid., pp. 1–4.
13. Ibid., pp. 5–7.
14. Ibid., p. 8. As in the old Royal Infirmary, the wide staircase in Queensberry House would have allowed patients, transported from home in chairs or on stretchers, to be carried easily to the upper wards.
15. Ibid., p. 7.
16. Ibid., p. 9.
17. Ibid., p. 10.
18. Ibid.
19. Ibid.
20. Ibid.
21. Ibid., p. 11.
22. Ibid.
23. Ibid., pp. 44–45.
24. Ibid., p. 46.
25. Ibid., pp. 44–45.

26. Turner, *Story of a Great Hospital*, p. 158.
27. Ibid.
28. Ibid.
29. Ibid., p. 160.
30. Tait, Cholera Board of Health, p. 235.
31. Turner, *Story of a Great Hospital*, p. 160.
32. *Gazetteer of Scotland*, p. 449.
33. Eastwood and Jenkinson, *Western General Hospital*, p. 8.
34. Abercrombie, MS and Papers.
35. Ibid.
36. Turner, *Story of a Great Hospital*, p. 160.
37. See Chapter 2, notes 19, 20.
38. Turner, *Story of a Great Hospital*, p. 159.
39. Ibid.
40. Ibid.

CHAPTER SEVEN

1. Report as to the Treatment of Infectious Diseases, 1884, p. 1.
2. Guthrie, *The Royal Edinburgh Hospital for Sick Children*, p. 11.
3. Report as to the Treatment of Infectious Diseases, 1884, p. 1.
4. *Gazetteer of Scotland*, Vol. I, p. 449.
5. Johnston's Plan of Edinburgh and Leith, 1851, ECL.
6. Ibid.
7. Tait, *A Doctor and Two Policemen*, p. 31.
8. Report as to the Treatment of Infectious Diseases, 1884, p. 1.
9. *Gazetteer of Scotland*, Vol. I, p. 449.
10. Tait, *A Doctor and Two Policemen*, p. 31.
11. View from the walk on the top of the Calton Hill, looking to the south. Drawn in stone by W. Westall, ARA. Sketched by Miss (later Lady) Mary Stewart, August 1822. Printed by C. Hallmandel (a print seen in an Edinburgh art gallery).
12. Eastwood and Jenkinson, *Western General Hospital*, pp. 10–11.
13. Edinburgh Parochial Board 1845–1893, St Cuthbert's Parochial Board & Combination, ECA, SL11.
14. Report as to the Treatment of Infectious Diseases, 1884, p. 1.
15. Ibid.
16. A printed circular enclosed with the handwritten PHC Minutes, ECA.
17. PWO, City Hospital Extension Plan 9.12.1893, p. 5 and Minutes of RIE Managers, 27.2.1885, Vol. 33, p. 274.

CHAPTER EIGHT

1. Boyd, *Leith Hospital*, p. 32.
2. This controversy is documented in the Minutes of RIE Managers and the PHC Minutes. Summaries giving both sides of the argument are 1. Report by the Committee to the Managers of the Royal Infirmary, 18.2.1885 with following Appendix, and 2. Report as to the Treatment of Infectious Diseases, 1884.
3. Report as to the Treatment of Infectious Diseases, 1884, p. 2.
4. Ibid.
5. Ibid.

6. *Ibid.*
7. *Ibid.*, p. 3., Report by the Committee to the Managers of the Royal Infirmary, 18.2.1885 pp. 10, 19–23.
8. Report as to the Treatment of Infectious Diseases, 1884, p. 3.
9. *Ibid.*, p. 3, and Report by the Committee to the Managers of the Royal Infirmary, 18.2.1885, p. 24.
10. Report by the Committee to the Managers of the Royal Infirmary, 18.2.1885, pp 24–25.
11. Report as to the Treatment of Infectious Diseases, 1884, p. 4.
12. *Ibid.*, pp. 5,6.
13. *Ibid.*, p. 5.
14. Report by the Committee to the Managers of the Royal Infirmary, 18.2.1885, pp. 7–8.
15. *Ibid.*, pp. 10, 14.
16. *Ibid.*, p. 14.
17. *Ibid.*, p. 15.
18. Minutes of RIE Managers, Vol. 33, p. 274.
19. *Ibid.*, Vol. 33, pp. 262, 277. The Lord Provost and Bailie Turnbull were *ex officio* representatives of the Town Council at the meetings of the Managers.
20. *Ibid.*, Vol. 33, p. 277.
21. Tait, *A Doctor and Two Policemen*, pp. 31–32.
22. Public Health Committee Draft Provisional Estimates, 1894–95, ECL and City Hospital Extension, 9.12.1893, p. 4.
23. Minutes of RIE Managers, Vol. 33, pp. 399–400.
24. *Ibid.*, Vol. 33, p. 429.
25. *Ibid.*, Vol. 33, p. 472.
26. See Chapter 30.
27. Tait, *A Doctor and Two Policemen*, p. 32.
28. Turner, *Story of a Great Hospital*, pp. 192–193.
29. Tait, *A Doctor and Two Policemen*, p. 32.

CHAPTER NINE

1. Pollard, *The Care of the Public Health*, p. 15.
2. Public Health Committee Draft Provisional Estimates, 1894–95, ECL.
3. Personal communication from an elderly Musselburgh resident, formerly a pupil at Campie House School.
4. PHC Minutes, numerous references in the 1890s.
5. Public Health Committee Draft Provisional Estimates, 1894–95, ECL.
6. PHC Minutes, 19.6.1891.
7. *Ibid.*, 19.6.1894.
8. Tait, *A Doctor and Two Policemen*, p. 35.
9. *Ibid.*, p. 35.
10. Turner, *Story of a Great Hospital*, pp. 192–193 and PWO City Hospital Extension Plan, 9.12.1893.
11. Gifford, McWilliam and Walker, *Edinburgh*, p. 187.
12. Public Health Committee Draft Provisional Estimates, 1894–95, ECL.
13. Report by City Superintendent of Works as to Accommodation, 10.1.1891, pp. 1–2.
14. PWO City Hospital Extension Plan 9.12.1893.

Notes for Chapter 9

15. TCM, 1893, pp. 230–231.
16. PHC Minutes, 28.2.1893.
17. PWO City Hospital Extension Plan 9.12.1893, p. 1.
18. Turner, *Story of a Great Hospital*, pp. 224–238.
19. W. Cowan, The Site of the Black Friars Monastery from the Reformation to the Present Day, Dec. 1913, *Book of the Old Edinburgh Club;* V, 67–93.
20. PHC Minutes, 11.4.1893.
21. Memorandam by Bailie Pollard, 4.6.1896.
22. PWO City Hospital Extension Plan, 9.12.1893, p. 1 .
23. *Ibid.*, p. 4.
24. *Ibid.*
25. *Ibid.*
26. *Ibid.*, p. 5.
27. PWO City Hospital Extension Plan, March 1894.
28. *Ibid.*
29. PWO City Hospital Extension Plan, 9.12.1893, p. 2.
30. *Ibid.*
31. *Ibid.*, p. 3.
32. PHC Minutes, 6.6.1893 and 20.6.1893.
33. PWO City Hospital Extension Plan, 9.12.1893, p. 3.
34. PHC Minutes, 14.6.1892.
35. PWO City Hospital Extension Plan, 9.12.1893, p. 3.
36. *Ibid.*
37. *Ibid.*, pp. 5–7.
38. *Ibid.*
39. *Ibid* p. 8.
40. *Ibid.*
41. TCM 21.2.1893 (Minute 33, p. 230).
42. PWO City Hospital Extension Plan, 9.12.1893, p. 7.
43. PHC Minutes, 25.9.1893.
44. Gifford, McWilliam and Walker, *Edinburgh*, p. 186.
45. *Ibid.*
46. PHC Minutes, 25.9.1893.
47. *Ibid.*, 27.2.1894.
48. *Ibid.*, 11.9.1894.
49. *Ibid.*, 27.11.1894.
50. *Ibid.*, 19.9.1893.
51. *Ibid.*, 28.5.1895.
52. Public Health Committee Draft Provisional Estimates, 1894–95, ECL.
53. PHC Minutes, 24.11.1891.
54. *Ibid.*, 1.9.1896.
55. *Ibid.*, 2.6.1896.
56. *Ibid.*, 14.1.1896.
57. *Ibid.*, 16.10.1895.
58. *Ibid.*, 18.7.1893.
59. *Ibid.*, 10.4.1894.
60. *Ibid.*, 16.1.1894.
61. *Ibid.*, 13.2.1894.
62. *Ibid.*, 3.7.1894.

CHAPTER TEN

1. Annual Report, MOH, 1898.
2. *Ibid.*, 1889–1895.
3. Boyd, *Leith Hospital*, p. 37.
4. *Ibid.*
5. PHC Minutes, 10.4.1894.
6. *Ibid.*, 8.5.1894.
7. *Ibid.*
8. *Ibid.*, 26.2.1895.
9. *Ibid.*, 5.6.1894.
10. *Ibid.*, 19.6.1894, 9.8.1894.
11. *Ibid.*, 11.9.1894.
12. *Ibid.*
13. *Ibid.*, 9.8.1894.
14. *Ibid.*
15. *Ibid.*, 11.9.1894.
16. *Ibid.*, 25.9.1894.
17. *Ibid.*, 17.6.1895, 21.6.1895.
18. *Ibid.*, 26.11.1895.
19. TCM, 8.9.1896, p. 601.
20. *Ibid.*
21. PHC Minutes, 1.9.1896.
22. *Ibid.*
23. *Ibid.*, 5.1.1897.
24. *Ibid.*, 4.5.1897.
25. *Ibid.*, 19.6.1894.
26. *Ibid.*, 3.7.1894.
27. *Ibid.*
28. *Ibid.*, 24.10.1894.
29. *Ibid.*, 17.7.1894.
30. *Ibid.*, 24.10.1894.
31. *Ibid.*, 19.6.1894.
32. *Ibid.*, 25.9.1894.
33. *Ibid.*
34. TCM, 1893–94, p. 518.
35. PHC Minutes, 27.11.1894.
36. *Ibid.*, 11.12.1894.
37. *Ibid.*
38. *Ibid.*, 2.1.1895, 15.1.1895, 29.1.1895.
39. *Ibid.*, 26.11.1895.
40. *Ibid.*, 14.5.1895.
41. *Ibid.*, 28.5.1895.
42. *Ibid.*, 27.8.1895.
43. *Ibid.*, 1.10.1895.
44. *Ibid.*, 26.11.1895.
45. *Ibid.*, 1.10.1895.
46. *Ibid.*, 26.11.1895.

CHAPTER ELEVEN

1. Pollard, *The Care of the Public Health*, p. 16.
2. Ibid., p. 18.
3. Ibid., p. 16.
4. Ibid., p. 18 and Chapter 10.
5. Minute of Extraordinary Meeting of the RCPE within their Hall on Monday, 28.5.1894. Bailie Pollard's letter is given in full. Minutes of RCPE, pp. 518–520. RCPEL.
6. Ibid.
7. Report by the Committee of the College, 1894.
8. Ibid., p. 539.
9. TCM, 21.5.1895, p. 457.
10. See ECA, SL 10/11.
11. TCM, 18.6.1895, p. 514.
12. Ibid., 17.9.1895, pp. 734–738 containing Reports by the MOH, pp. 734–735, Superintendent of Works, pp. 735–737, and Burgh Engineer, pp. 737–738.
13. Ibid.
14. Ibid. Report by the MOH, pp. 734–735.
15. Ibid. Report by Superintendent of Works, pp. 735–737.
16. Ibid. Report of the Burgh Egineer, pp. 737–738.
17. Ibid., p. 738.
18. Ibid.
19. Ibid.

CHAPTER TWELVE

1. *Men of the Period*, p. 81: Smith, *Historic South Edinburgh*, Vol. IV, pp. 269–270.
2. Gunn and Blanc, *City Hospital, Bedford, George Heriot's Hospital, Edinburgh*, p. 122.
3. Tait, *A Doctor and Two Policemen*, p. 35.
4. Smith, *Historic South Edinburgh*, Vol. IV, pp. 270–271.
5. Miss P. A. Morham, personal communication.
6. Building Specification, 15.4.1897.
7. *Men of the Period*, p. 87.
8. Hon. Judge Ralph Lownie, personal communication.
9. *Men of the Period*, p. 87.
10. Hon. Judge Ralph Lownie, personal communication.
11. *Men of the Period*, p. 87.
12. Smith, *Historic South Edinburgh*, Vol. II, p. 290.
13. Hon. Judge Ralph Lownie, personal communication.
14. *Men of the Period*, p. 87.
15. Hon. Judge Ralph Lownie, personal communication.

CHAPTER THIRTEEN

1. Colinton Hospital Report, 7.12.1895.
2. Ibid.
3. Description and Sketch Plan, 5.10.1896, p. 4 and View from SW. See also *Edinburgh Fever Hospital*, 1903, p. 17 and Chapter 32.
4. Memorandum by Bailie Pollard, 4.6.1896.

5. Robert Koch (1843–1910) a German bacteriologist after whom the tubercle bacillus was long known as Koch's bacillus. He developed new staining tests for bacteria and related some bacteria to the diseases they caused. In 1905 he won the Nobel Prize for work on tuberculin testing.
6. Memorandum by Bailie Pollard, 4.6.1896.
7. Ibid.
8. For consideration at special meeting of the Magistrates and Council, 26.2.1897.
9. Ibid.
10. Ibid.
11. Ibid.
12. Ibid.
13. Special Meeting of the Town Council of Edinburgh, 26.2.1897.
14. Building Specification, 15.4.1897.
15. Ibid.
16. Bunyan, Fairhurst, Mackie and McMillan, *Building Stones of Edinburgh*, pp. 30, 69, 70, 146.
17. Letter to R. Morham Esq. from J. Murray & Sons, 30.3.1899.
18. Building Specification, 15.4.1896.
19. Ibid.
20. TCM, 25.5.1897, p. 420.
21. TCM, 1897, p. 500.
22. Ibid., 1897, p. 502.
23. Ibid., 1897, pp. 501–502 and PHC Minutes, 20.7.1897.
24. PHC Minutes, 20.7.1897 and annotation and Minute, 23.7.1897.
25. Ibid., 31.8.1897.
26. Ibid.

CHAPTER FOURTEEN

1. *The Scotsman*, 15.5.1897.
2. Ibid.
3. Ibid.
4. Ibid.
5. Ibid.
6. Ibid.
7. Weekly Report on Works in Progress.
8. Ibid., Nos. 132, 10.2.1900–134, 24.2.1900.
9. Ibid., No. 1, 7.8.1897. Mr Lownie was also responsible for the access road.
10. Ibid., No. 8, 25.9.1897.
11. Mr Malcolm Cant, personal communication.
12. Ordance Survey Map, 'Slateford', 1895, Edinburgh Sheet 3.14. Reprinted courtesy of Trustees of the NLS, Edition by Alan Godfrey, Dunston, Gateshead, 1996. See also Post Office Plans, Edinburgh, Leith, Portobello, 1911–12, ECL.
13. *Colin Macandrew and Partners Limited 1882–1995: A Story of Achievement*. Edinburgh and Glasgow, produced by John Menzies for Colin Macandrew and Partners Limited, 1995. ECL, q YTH451 (c22906).
14. Weekly Report on Works in Progress, 13.11.1897.
15. Judicial Reference, enclosing letters of 11.12.1897 and 10.3.1898.
16. Extracts from Mr Ballingall's letters.
17. Ibid.

18. Judicial Reference, enclosing letters of 25.3.1898 and 18.8.1898.
19. *Ibid.*, letter of 7.1.1899.
20. *Ibid.*, letter of 17.2.1899.
21. *Ibid.*, letter of 10.5.1899.
22. *Ibid.*, letter of 25.3.1902.
23. *Ibid.*, letter of 29.3.1902.
24. *Ibid.*, letter of 1.4.1902.
25. *Ibid.*, letter of 9.11.1898.
26. Building Specification, 15.4.1897.
27. Closed Record, Lord Provost *et al.* v. John Lownie and William Ormiston, 18.11.1902.
28. Joint Print of Documents, Lord Provost et al v John Lownie and William Ormiston, 28.2.1903.
29. *Ibid.*
30. Mags. of Edinburgh v. John Lownie (1903) 5F. 711. The Hon. Lord Gill has kindly taken the trouble to unravel and explain these complex and prolonged legal actions.
31. Weekly Report on Works in Progress, No. 164, 22.9.1900.
32. *Ibid.*, No. 199, 25.5.1901.
33. Report on Probable Cost, 20.5.1901.
34. Report on Colinton Mains Hospital, 19.5.1902.
35. Joint Minute in causa John Lownie against Lord Provost.
36. Reclaiming Note, 15.1.1903; closed Record, Lord Provost *et al.* v. John Lownie, 1.3.1904.

CHAPTER FIFTEEN

1. Description and Sketch Plan, 5.10.1896.
2. Pollard, *The Care of the Public Health.*
3. *Edinburgh Fever Hospital*, 1903.
4. *Ibid.*, Prefatory note by Councillor W Lang Todd, Convener of the Public Health *Committee.*
5. Colinton Mains Hospital. Memorandum, 9.10.1903.
6. *Ibid.*, Supplementary Note pp. 14–15.
7. Building Specification, 15.4.1897.
8. Colinton Mains Hospital. Memorandum, 9.10.1903.
9. *Ibid.*
10. Mr Jim Smith, personal communication.
11. Mr Alec G. Welstead, personal communication.
12. Colinton Mains Hospital. Memorandum, 9.10.1903.
13. According to the Description and Sketch Plan, 5.10.1896. In the *Edinburgh Fever Hospital*, 1903, the number had increased from 320 to 329.
14. Description and Sketch Plan, 5.10.1896; Pollard, *The Care of the Public Health.*
15. Miss J. K. Taylor, personal communication.
16. Building Specification, 15.4.1897.
17. Mr Alec G. Welstead, personal communication.
18. Best described in Colinton Mains Hospital, Memorandum, 9.10.1903, pp. 7–10.
19. Weekly Report on Works in Progress, Nos. 343 and 326.
20. Mr Alec G. Welstead, personal communication.
21. Colinton Mains Hospital. Memorandum, 9.10.1903.

22. Colinton Mains Hospital, Memorandum, 9.10.1903, p. 11.
23. Professor Sir John Crofton and Dr N. W. Horne, personal communications.
24. Gifford, McWilliam and Walker, *Edinburgh*, p. 535.
25. Pollard, *The Care of the Public Health*, p. 44.

CHAPTER SIXTEEN

1. *The Scotsman*, 28.3.1903.
2. *Ibid.*, 14.5.1903.
3. *Edinburgh Evening News*, 13.5.1903.
4. *Ibid.*, 14.5.1903.
5. *The Scotsman*, 14.5.1903.
6. *Ibid.*
7. *Men of the Period*, p. 169.
8. *Ibid.*, p. 176.
9. *The Scotsman*, 14.5.1903.
10. *Ibid.*
11. Unfortunately Messrs Hamilton & Inches have no current record of the key made by them.
12. *Edinburgh Evening News*, 13.5.1903.
13. Smith, *Historic South Edinburgh*, Vol. IV, p. 272 and Smith, *Morningside*, p. 213.
14. The Lord Provost in some accounts was simply knighted by the King at the opening ceremony. The *Edinburgh Evening News* (13.5.1903), however, specifically refers to him being created a Baronet as Sir James Steel of Murieston, a name given to several streets in Dalry which he built. Mr Malcolm Cant, Personal communication, See also note 13.
15. Smith, *Historic South Edinburgh*, Vol. IV, pp. 271–273.
16. *Edinburgh Fever Hospital*, 1903 (Green, cloth-covered, hardback copy). See Chapter 15.
17. *The Scotsman*, 14.5.1903. A slightly different account of the planting of the King's elm tree is in *Edinburgh Evening News*, 14.5.1903.

CHAPTER SEVENTEEN

1. *Edinburgh Medical Journal*, 1925;23:265–269.
2. 'The General Treatment of Enteric Fever', MD thesis by C. B. Ker. SCD, EUL.
3. *Edinburgh Medical Journal*, 1925;23:265–269. The author's initials suggest Dr A. Logan Turner wrote Dr Ker's obituary.
4. An Outbreak of Typhus Fever, 1899.
5. Ker, *A Manual of Fevers*, 1911.
6. *Ker's Infectious Diseases – A Practical Textbook*, 1929.
7. Weekly Report on Works in Progress, No. 298, 9.5.1903.
8. See Chapter 16.
9. Weekly Report on Works in Progress, Nos. 317 and 210, 19.9.1903.
10. *Ibid.*, Nos. 322 and 215, 24.10.1903.
11. *Ibid.*, Nos. 337 and 230, 6.2.1904.
12. *Ibid.*, Nos. 343 and 236, 19.3.1904.
13. PHC Minutes, 26.11.1895.
14. Description and Sketch Plan, 5.10.1896.
15. Post Office Plans of Edinburgh and Leith, 1899–1900 and 1905–1906.
16. NMRSL, box file on City Hospital.

17. Bartholomew's Pentland Hills and Edinburgh District; Bartholomew's Pocket Plan of Edinburgh and Suburbs.
18. Annual Reports, MOH, 1892–1900.
19. *Ibid.*, 1900, p. 41.
20. *Ibid.*, 1904, pp. 38–40.
21. Weekly Report of Works in Progress, Nos. 339 and 232, 20.2.1904.
22. *Ibid.*, Nos. 340 and 233, 27.2.1904.
23. Annual Report, MOH, 1904, pp. 40–41.
24. *Ker's Infectious Diseases – A Practical Textbook*, 1929, p. 192.
25. *Ibid.*, p. 193.
26. *Ibid.*, p. 192.
27. *Ibid.*, p. 193.
28. *Ibid.*
29. Report as to Smallpox Accommodation, 17.10.1910.
30. *Ibid.*, p. 3.
31. *Ker's Infectious Diseases – A Practical Textbook*, 1929, p. 136.
32. *Ibid.*, p. 141.
33. Description and Sketch Plan, 5.10.1896 (Sheet 5).
34. See Chapter 18 for text of nursing regulations, 1905.
35. Annual Report, MOH, 1904, p. 45.
36. *Ker's Infectious Diseases – A Practical Textbook*, 1929, Plates 25 and 26.
37. *Ibid.*, p. 447.
38. Annual Report, MOH, 1904, pp. 45–47.
39. *Ibid.*, p. 46.
40. *Ibid.*, p. 51.
41. *Edinburgh Evening News*, 3.1.1912.
42. *Gazetteer of Scotland*, p. 449.
43. Comrie, *History of Scottish Medicine*, Vol. II, p. 644–645.
44. Tait, *A Doctor and Two Policemen*, p. 34.
45. PHC Minutes, 3.7.1894.
46. Tait, *A Doctor and Two Policemen*, p. 34.
47. Report by the Committee of the College, 1894.
48. Annual Report, PHD, 1909, pp. 54–55.
49. *Ibid.*, in Report by Dr Ker, p. 60.
50. *Ibid.*, pp. 54–55.
51. *Ibid.*, in Report by Dr Ker, p. 60.

CHAPTER EIGHTEEN

1. Miss J. K. Taylor, personal communication, and Chapter 17.
2. Nurses' Roll Call, January 1904, now in LHSA, EUL.
3. Staff Photograph, 1906, now in LHSA, EUL.
4. Staff Photograph, 1918, now in LHSA, EUL.
5. Miss J. K. Taylor, personal communication.
6. Annual Report, PHD, 1911, p. 54.
7. Samuel Papers, Lecture Notes, LHSA, EUL, MAC GD 1/46/4–3.
8. *Ker's Infectious Diseases – A Practical Textbook*, 1929, p. 145.
9. *Ibid.*, p. 140.
10. *Ibid.*, p. 139.
11. Samuel Papers, Lecture Notes, LHSA, EUL, MAC GD 1/46/4–3.

12. Daiches, *Was-A Pastime from Time Past*, pp. 64–67.
13. Samuel Papers, Lecture Notes, LHSA, EUL, MAC GD 1/46/4–3.
14. Annual Report, MOH, 1905, Dr Ker's Report, p. 45.
15. *Ibid.*, 1907, Dr Ker's Report, p. 46.
16. Annual Report, PHD, 1913, Dr Ker's Report, p. 58.
17. *Ibid.*, 1909. p. 49.
18. Annual Report, MOH, 1907, Dr Ker's Report, p. 54.
19. Intrathecally: into the cerebro-spinal fluid surrounding the spinal cord.
20. *Ker's Infectious Diseases – A Practical Textbook*, pp. 566–576.
21. Annual Report, PHD, 1914, Dr W.S.I. Robertson's Report, p. 51.
22. *Ibid.*, 1914, p. 52.
23. *Ibid.*, 1914, MOH's Report, pp. xiii–xiv.
24. Miss J.K. Taylor, personal communication.
25. Samuel Papers, Application Form, LHSA, EUL, MAC, GD 1/46/2–1.
26. PHC Minutes, 1917–19 Hospital Subcommittee Minutes, 3.6.1919 and 19.6.1919, ECA. See also Representation by MOH as to Nursing and Domestic Staff at the City Hospital, June 1919, ECA, C4/20.
27. *Ibid.*
28. *Ibid.*
29. *Ibid.*
30. *Ibid.*
31. Annual Report, PHD, 1919, Dr Ker's Report, p. 52.
32. *Ibid.*
33. *Ibid.*
34. Annual Report, PHD, 1920, Dr Ker's Report, p. 51.
35. *Ibid.*, 1920 pp. 43 and MOH, pp. x–xi.
36. *Ibid.*
37. *Ibid.*
38. *Ibid.*, 1921, Dr Ker's Report, p. 38 and MOH, pp. ix–x.
39. *Ibid.*, 1921, Dr Ker's Report, pp. 37, 38.
40. *Ibid.*, 1922, p. iii.
41. *Ibid.*, 1922, Dr Ker's Report, p. 40.
42. *Ibid.*, 1923, pp. iii–iv and 1924, p. v.
43. *Ibid.*, 1923, p. iv.
44. *Ibid.*, 1923, p. viii.
45. *Ibid.*, 1923, Dr Ker's Report, pp. 36, 37.
46. *Ibid.*, 1923, pp. v, vi.
47. *Ibid.*, 1923, pp. vi, viii.
48. *Ibid.*, 1924, p. iii.
49. *Ibid.*, 1924, p. iv.
50. *Ibid.*
51. *Ibid.*, 1924, Dr Joe's Report, pp. 47–49.
52. *Ibid.*, 1925, Dr Benson's Report, pp. 47–50.

CHAPTER NINETEEN

1. Minutes of Victoria Dispensary. Minutes of RVH Tuberculosis Trust. Sutherland, *Control and Eradication of Tuberculosis*. The Edinburgh Tuberculosis Scheme. Obituary, Sir Robert William Philip. Tait, *A Doctor and Two Policemen*, pp. 57–68. Clayson, Time was when youth grew pale ... Clayson, Lecture to Joint Meeting,

Notes for Chapter 19

1987. Crofton, Final Report on Tuberculosis Research, 1952–1965. Leitch, Two men and a bug ..., 1996.
2. Annual Report, MOH and Annual Report, PHD.
3. Leitch, Two men and a bug ..., 1996.
4. Tait, *A Doctor and Two Policemen*, p. 57.
5. Ibid., p. 57.
6. Annual Report, MOH, 1900, pp. 17–20.
7. Ibid., 1900, p. 18.
8. Ibid., 1900, pp. 17–20.
9. The Edinburgh Tuberculosis Scheme, p. 287.
10. The Edinburgh Tuberculosis Scheme, p. 289. Diagram shows the Dispensary with links to the Hospital for Advanced Cases (the City Hospital), the Sanatorium, Colonies and MOH.
11. Minutes of RVH Tuberculosis Trust, Vol. 3/4. p. 315.
12. Minute of Agreement, 1913.
13. Annual Report, PHD, 1921, pp. xii–xiii.
14. Ibid., 1924, p. 43.
15. Ibid., 1925, p. 42.
16. Ibid., 1921, p. xii.
17. Ibid., 1920, p. xvi.
18. Ibid., 1921, p. 38.
19. Minutes of RVH Tuberculosis Trust, 1905–1965, Vol. 1, p. 183.
20. Annual Report, MOH, 1906, pp. 18–19.
21. Ibid., 1906, p. 51.
22. A. Maxwell Williamson in Sutherland, *Control and Eradication of Tuberculosis*, Ch. 12, pp. 159–160.
23. Ibid., p. 160.
24. Ibid., p. 161. Dr Maxwell Williamson's diagram and pie charts show the beneficial effects of hospital isolation.
25. Ibid.
26. Ibid., p. 162.
27. Annual Report, PHD, 1908, p. 47.
28. Ibid., 1909, pp. 41–42.
29. Ibid.
30. Ibid.
31. A Maxwell Williamson in Sutherland, *Control and Eradication of Tuberculosis*, Ch. 13, p. 164.
32. Ibid.
33. Ibid.
34. The Edinburgh Tuberculosis Scheme, p. 290.
35. Minutes of RVH Tuberculosis Trust, Vol. 3, p. 16.
36. Prof. J. Williamson, personal communication.
37. Numerous references in Minutes of RVH Tuberculosis Trust, 1905–1965, especially the early volumes, record these generous donations.
38. Prof. J. Williamson, personal communication.
39. Clayson, Lecture to Joint Meeting, 1987.
40. The Edinburgh Tuberculosis Scheme, 1937, p. 294.
41. Sir John Crofton, personal communication.
42. Leitch, Two men and a bug ..., 1996.

43. Prof. J. Williamson, personal communication.
44. Sir John Crofton and Dr N. W. Horne, personal communications.
45. Dr A. C. Douglas, personal communication.
46. Crofton, Final Report on Tuberculosis Research, 1952–1965.

CHAPTER TWENTY

1. W. T. Benson, MD thesis, 'Diphtheria Carriers and their Treatment', SCD, EUL.
2. Annual Report, PHD, 1924, pp. 50–53.
3. *Ibid,* 1925–36 (Dr Benson's Reports on the City Hospital).
4. *Ibid.*
5. *Ibid.,* 1925, p. 46.
6. *Ibid.,* 1925–36.
7. W. T. Benson, The Control of Diphtheria: A Plea for Active Immunisation of the Pre-School Child. *Edinburgh Medical Journal,* 1934;41:293–304.
8. Annual Report, PHD, 1912, p. viii. The MOH was then Dr A. Maxwell Williamson.
9. W. T. Benson, The Control of Diphtheria: see note 7.
10. *Ibid.*
11. W. T. Benson, Clinical Recollections and Reflections, XX. Some Observations on the Notifiable Streptococcal Infections. *Edinburgh Medical Journal,* 1938;45:24–35.
12. *Ibid.*
13. *Ibid.*
14. *Ibid.*
15. Annual Report PHD, 1935, p. 31.
16. *Ibid.,* 1936, p. 34.
17. *Ibid.,* 1935, p. 31.
18. *Ibid.,* 1936, p. 34.
19. *Ibid.,* 1935, p. 31.
20. *Ibid.,* 1931, p. vi.
21. *Ibid.,* 1925, p. 46.
22. *Ibid.,* 1935, pp. 30–39.
23. *Ibid.,* 1929, p. 47 (Table).
24. *Ibid.,* 1927, p. 56.
25. *Ibid.,* 1936, p. 38.
26. *Ibid.,* 1929, p. 46.
27. *Ibid.,* 1927, p. 50.
28. *Ibid.,* 1928, p. 38.
29. *Ibid.,* 1929, p. 41.
30. *Ibid.,* 1929, p. 41.
31. Annual Report of the City of Edinburgh Infectious Diseases Hospital for the Year 1930, W. T. Benson, p. 4. One of two, 1930 and 1931, found at City Hospital. LHSA,
32. Annual Report, PHD, 1929, p. 42.
33. *Ibid.,* 1930, p. 40.
34. *Ibid.,* 1934, p. 39.
35. *Ibid.,* 1935, pp. 30–39.
36. *Ibid.*
37. See note 32, 1930, p. 3.

38. Annual Report, PHD, 1936, p. 33.
39. See Ref. 20, 1931, p. 4.
40. Annual Report, PHD, 1930, p. 56.
41. *Ibid.*, 1936, p. vii.
42. *Ibid.*, p. 33.
43. Obituary of W. T. Benson, July 1984, RCPEL.

CHAPTER TWENTY-ONE

1. A. Joe, MD thesis, 'Scarlatinal Arthritis: A Clinical and Statistical Study'. SCD, EUL.
2. Annual Report, PHD, 1937, pp. 41–43.
3. *Ibid.*
4. *Ibid.*
5. *Ibid.*
6. *Ibid.*, 1937, Report by Medical Superintendent of the City Hospital.
7. *Ibid.*, 1937, p. 48.
8. A. Joe, The Treatment of Cerebrospinal Fever by Sulphapyridine, *Edinburgh Medical Journal*. 1942:49;628–642.
9. Annual Report, PHD, 1937, Report by Medical Superintendent of the City Hospital.
10. *Ibid.*
11. *Ibid.*
12. Annual Report, PHD, 1938, Report by Medical Superintendent of the City Hospital, p. 3.
13. *Ibid.*, p. 14.
14. *Ibid.*
15. See note 8, p. 629.
16. *Ibid.*, p. 628.
17. *Ibid.*, p. 631.
18. *Ibid.*, p. 642.

CHAPTER TWENTY-TWO

1. Annual Report, PHD, 1939, p. 4.
2. Hendrie and Macleod, *The Bangour Story*, pp. 47–67.
3. Annual Report, PHD, 1939, p. 5.
4. *Ibid.*
5. Annual Report, PHD, 1941.
6. *Ibid.*, 1941, p. 7.
7. *Ibid.*, 1941, p. 26.
8. Eastwood and Jenkinson, *Western General Hospital*, pp. 73–81.
9. Annual Report, PHD, 1942, p. 5.
10. *Ibid.*, 1942, pp. 9–19 and *The Edinburgh Outbreak of Smallpox 1942*. Both are quoted extensively in the following pages.
11. *Ibid.*
12. *Ibid.*
13. *The Edinburgh Outbreak of Smallpox 1942*, p. 24.
14. Annual Report, PHD, 1942, p. 18.
15. Annual Report, PHD, 1942, p. 17.
16. City Plan and Guide (no publisher quoted) ca. 1927.

17. Annual Report, PHD, 1942, p. 17.
18. *Ibid.*
19. *The Edinburgh Outbreak of Smallpox 1942*, p. 22.
20. Miss J. K. Taylor, personal communication.
21. *The Edinburgh Outbreak of Smallpox 1942*, p. 23.
22. Annual Report, PHD, 1942, p. 17.
23. *The Edinburgh Outbreak of Smallpox 1942*, p. 22.
24. *Ibid.*, p. 24.
25. Annual Report, PHD, 1942, p. 18.
26. *The Edinburgh Outbreak of Smallpox 1942*, p. 23.
27. Mr W. A. Maben, former Estates Officer, personal communication. Mr David Pithie, former General Foreman, recalls that the smallpox buildings were only burnt down after the removal from the staff quarters of valuable wood fittings some of which were subsequently used for cubicles, cupboards and filing cabinets in the basement of the RVD in Spittal Street.

CHAPTER TWENTY-THREE

1. Annual Report, PHD, 1943, p. 1
2. *Ibid.*, 1943, pp. 31–33.
3. *Ibid.*, 1943, p. 30.
4. City Hospital Nurses' Register, recovered at City Hospital, LHSA, EUL.
5. Daily Record Book, recovered at City Hospital, LHSA, EUL.
6. Servants' Record Book, recovered at City Hospital, LHSA, EUL.
7. Mrs Isobel Lorimer (née Cruikshank), personal communication.
8. Mrs Isobel Lorimer (née Cruikshank), Mrs Jean Day (née Smith) and Mrs Pat Hunter (née McWilliams), personal communications.
9. Miss J. K. Taylor, personal communication.
10. *Ibid.*
11. Mrs Jean Day, personal communication.
12. Mrs Jean Day, Mrs Isobel Lorimer, Mrs Pat Hunter personal communications.
13. Mrs Isobel McFarlane (née McWilliams), personal communication.
14. Mrs Pat Hunter, Mrs Isobel McFarlane, personal communications.
15. Mrs Jean Day, personal communication.
16. Annual Report, PHD, 1944.
17. *Ibid.*, 1944, p. 6.
18. *Ibid.*, 1944, p. 33.
19. *Ibid.*
20. *Ibid.*
21. Mrs Pat Hunter (née McWilliams), personal communication.
22. Annual Report, PHD, 1950, Fifty Years Review, 1901–1950, p. 40
23. Annual Report, PHD, 1944, facing p. 33.
24. *Ibid.*, 1945, pp. 4–5.
25. *Ibid.*, 1945, p. 9.
26. *Ibid.*, 1945, p. 43
27. *Ibid.*, 1946, p. 6.
28. *Ibid.*, 1946, p. 56.
29. *Ibid.*, 1946, p. 11.
30. *Ibid.*, 1947, p. 3.
31. *Ibid.*, 1947, p. 11.

32. *Ibid.*, 1947, p. 114.
33. Miss J. K. Taylor suggests Ward 2A was the newly cubiclised ward used for infantile gastroenteritis.
34. Annual Report, PHD, 1947, p. 115.

CHAPTER TWENTY-FOUR

1. Annual Report, PHD, 1948, p. 3.
2. *Ibid.*, 1948, p. 11.
3. *Ibid.*, 1948, p. 12.
4. Minutes of RV & AH BOM, Resumé of activities, 1948–51, LHB 38/7/141.
5. *Ibid.*
6. Annual Report, PHD, 1948, pp. 32–36.
7. Pollard, *The Care of the Public Health.*
8. Annual Report, PHD, 1948, pp. 121–124.
9. Minutes of RV & A H BOM, Annual Report CH for ID, 1948, pp. 1–3, LHB 38/7/133.
10. *Ibid.*, 1948, p. 4.
11. *Ibid.*, 1948, p. 15.
12. Annual Report, PHD, 1948 pp. 55–56.
13. Minutes of RV & AH BOM, Annual Report CH for ID, 1948, p. 26, LHB 38/7/133.
14. Smith, *Edinburgh's Contribution to Medical Microbiology*, pp. 157–158.
15. *Ibid.*, p. 160.
16. *Ibid.*, p. 266.
17. Annual Report, PHD, 1948, p. 124.
18. Annual Report PHD, 1949, p. 3.
19. *Ibid.*, 1949, p. 12.
20. *Ibid.*, 1949, pp. 38 *et seq.*
21. *Ibid.*, 1949, p. 39.
22. *Ibid.*, 1950, pp. 12–13.
23. *Ibid.*
24. *Ibid.*, 1950, p. 14.
25. *Ibid.*, 1950, p. 80.
26. *Ibid.*, 1950, p. 89.
27. *Ibid.*, 1950, p. 91.
28. *Ibid.*
29. *Ibid.*, 1951, p. 13.
30. *Ibid.*, 1951, p. 91.
31. Minutes of RV & AH BOM, Resumé of activities, 1948–51, LHB 38/7/141.
32. Annual Report, PHD, 1951, p. 91.
33. Minutes of RV & AH BOM, Annual Report CH for ID, 1951, pp. 11–13, LHB 38/7/133.
34. Annual Report, PHD, 1951, p. 91.
35. *Ibid.*, 1951, p. 40.
36. Minutes of RVD & AH BOM, Annual Report CH for ID, 1951 p. 4, LHB 38/7/133.
37. *Ibid.* 1951, pp. 24–25.
38. *Ibid.*, 1951, pp. 21–27.
39. Minutes of RV & AH BOM, Resumé of activities, 1948–51, LHB 38/7/141.

40. Mr Andrew Logan, personal communication.
41. See note 39.
42. *Ibid.*
43. *Ibid.*
44. Annual Report, PHD, 1952, pp. 1–7.
45. *Ibid.*, 1952, p. 33.
46. Minutes of RV & AH BOM, Annual Report CH for ID, 1952, p. 1, LHB 38/7/133.
47. *Ibid.*, 1952, p. 2.
48. *Ibid.*, 1952, pp. 3–4.
49. Mr Andrew Logan, personal communication.
50. Minutes of RV & AH BOM, Annual Report CH for ID, 1965 (19.5.1965), p. 3/127. LHB 10/1/8.
51. *Ibid.*, 1965 (1.9.1965), p. 14/302. LHB 10/1/8.
52. *Ibid.*, 1967 (20.9.1967), p. 4/245. LHB 10/1/8.
53. *Ibid.*, 1968 (18.9.1968), p. 2/227 and (16.10.1968) p. 1/271, LHB 10/1/8.
54. Minutes of RV & AH BOM, Annual Report CH for ID, 1952, pp. 3–4 LHB 38/7/133.
55. *Ibid.*, 1952, p. 6.
56. *Ibid.*, 1952, pp. 3–4.
57. *Ibid.*
58. *Ibid.*
59. *Ibid.*, 1952, p. 5.
60. *Ibid.*, 1952, pp. 24–25.
61. Annual Report, PHD, 1953, p. 13.
62. *Ibid.*, 1953, p. 31.
63. *Ibid.*
64. *Ibid.*, 1953, p. 13.
65. Minutes of RV & AH BOM, Annual Report CH for ID 1953, p. 1, LHB 38/7/135.
66. *Ibid.*, 1953, p. 2.
67. *Ibid.*
68. *Ibid.*
69. *Ibid.*, 1953, p. 13.
70. Annual Report, PHD, 1953, p. 13.
71. Minutes of RVH & AH BOM, Annual Report CH for ID, 1953, p. 5, LHB 38/7/135.
72. *Ibid.*
73. *Ibid.*, 1953, p. 4.
74. *Ibid.*, 1953, pp. 22–23.
75. *Ibid.*, 1952, (Outstanding Developments), pp. 2–3., LHB 38/7/141.
76. *Ibid.*, 1953, p. 4.
77. Miss J. K. Taylor, personal communication and see ECL, YRA 988C–15750.
78. Address by Medical Superintendent at Commemorative Service, 13 May 1953, and see LHSA, EUL.

CHAPTER TWENTY-FIVE

1. Annual Report, PHD, 1954, p. 3. See also Chapter 19.
2. *Ibid.*, 1954, p. 15.

Notes for Chapter 25

3. *Ibid.*, 1954, pp. 34–36.
4. *Ibid.*
5. *Ibid.*
6. *Ibid.*
7. Minutes of RV & AH BOM, Annual Report CH for ID, 1954, pp. 1–23, LHB 38/7/137.
8. *Ibid.*
9. *Ibid.*
10. *Ibid.*
11. *Ibid.*, Outstanding Developments, 1954, LHB 38/7/141.
12. Annual Report, PHD, 1955, p. 19.
13. *Ibid.*, 1955, p. 142.
14. Minutes of RV & AH BOM, Annual Report CH for ID, 1955, pp. 1–23, LHB 38/7/138.
15. *Ibid.*
16. *Ibid.*
17. *Ibid.*
18. Minutes of RV & AH BOM, 1955, Outstanding Developments, LHB 38/7/141.
19. Minutes of RV & AH BOM, Annual Report CH for ID, 1955, pp. 1–23, LHB 38/7/138.
20. *Ibid.*
21. *Ibid.*
22. Annual Report, PHD, 1956, pp. 1–18.
23. *Ibid.*
24. Minutes of RV & AH BOM, Annual Report CH for ID, 1956 pp. 1–21. LHB 38/7/138.
25. Annual Report, PHD, 1956, pp. 1–18.
26. Minutes of RV & AH BOM, Annual Report CH for ID, 1956 pp. 1–21. LHB 38/7/138.
27. *Ibid.*
28. *Ibid.*
29. *Ibid.*, Annual Report, BOM, 1956, LHB 38/7/141.
30. Annual Report PHD, 1957, p. 13.
31. *Ibid.*, 1957, p. 15.
32. *Ibid.*
33. *Ibid.*
34. Minutes of RV & AH BOM, Annual Report CH for ID, 1957, pp. 1–22, LHB 38/7/138.
35. Minutes of RV & AH BOM, Annual Report, BOM, 1957, LHB 38/7/141.
36. Minutes of RV & AH BOM, Annual Report, CH for ID, 1957, pp. 1–22, LHB 38/7/138.
37. *Ibid.*
38. Minutes of RV & AH BOM, Annual Report, BOM, 1957, LHB 38/7/141.
39. *Ibid.*
40. Annual Report, PHD, 1958, pp. 1–184.
41. *Ibid.*
42. Minutes of RV & AH BOM, Annual Report for CH of ID, 1958, pp. 1–21, LHB 38/7/138.
43. *Ibid.*

44. *Ibid.*
45. *Ibid.*
46. *Ibid.*
47. *Ibid.*
48. *Ibid.*
49. *Ibid.*
50. *Ibid.*, Annual Report, BOM, 1958, LHB 38/7/141.
51. *Ibid.*
52. Minutes of RV & AH BOM, G. P. Committee, 6.10.1958, p. 5/248, LHB 10/1/6.
53. *Ibid.*, BOM, 20.8.1958, p. 4/168, LHB 10/1/6.
54. *Ibid.*, BOM, 19.8.1959, p. 4/187, LHB 10/1/6.
55. Annual Report PHD, 1959, pp. 1–131.
56. Minutes of RV & AH BOM, Annual Report BOM, 1959, LHB 38/7/141.
57. *Ibid.*
58. *Ibid.*
59. *Ibid.*
60. *Ibid.*, GP Committee, 12.1.1959, p. 6/330, LHB 10/1/6.
61. Annual Report, PHD, 1960, pp. 1–134.
62. Minutes of RV & AH BOM, BOM, 18.3.1959, p. 3/428, LHB 10/1/6.
63. Anon., Obituary, Alexander Joe, *British Medical Journal*, 1962;2:1620.
64. Anon., Obituary, Alexander Joe, *Scottish Medical Journal,* 1963;8:38.
65. Anon., Obituary, Alexander Joe, *British Medical Journal*, 1962;2:1620.

CHAPTER TWENTY-SIX

1. Minutes of RV & AH BOM, BOM, 15.7.1959, p. 1/158, LHB 10/1/6.
2. *Ibid.*, BOM, 21.10.1959, p. 1/241, LHB 10/1/6.
3. *Ibid.*, BOM, 18.11.1959, p. 1/288, LHB 10/1/6.
4. *Ibid.*, BOM, 16.12.1959, p. 4/329, LHB 10/1/6.
5. *Ibid.*, BOM, 20.1.60, p. 1/369, LHB 10/1/6.
6. *Ibid.*, BOM, 16.3.1960, p. 1/447, LHB 10/1/6.
7. See Chapter 16.
8. Minutes of RV & AH BOM, 1960–1974, LHB 10/1/6–10.
9. Dr N. W. Horne, personal communication.
10. Mr A. G. Welstead and Mr David Pithie, personal communications.
11. Collins, *The Influence of Scottish Medicine*, p. 154.
12. Minutes of RV & AH BOM, G P Committee, 10.10.1960, p. 5/223, LHB 10/1/6.
13. *Ibid.*, BOM, 18.1.1967, p. 4/592, LHB 10/1/8.
14. *Ibid.*, BOM, 21.1. 1967, p. 3/154, LHB 10/1/8.
15. *Ibid.*, BOM, 18.5.1960, p. 2/104/1, LHB 10/1/6.
16. *Ibid.*, BOM, 20.7.1960, p. 5/163, LHB 10/1/6.
17. *Ibid.*, BOM, 21.6.1961, p. 6/143, LHB 10/1/6.
18. *Ibid.*, BOM, 16.1.1963, p. 2/427 and BOM 20.2.1963, p. 1/467, LHB 10/1/7.
19. *Ibid.*, BOM, 20.5.1970, p. 1/73, LHB 10/1/9.
20. *Ibid.*, BOM, 24.6.1970, p. 1/116 and BOM 15.7.1970, p. 3/172, LHB 10/1/9.
21. *Ibid.*, BOM, 21.10.1970, p. 3/324, LHB 10/1/9.
22. *Ibid.*, BOM, 17.1.1962, p. 5/406, LHB 10/1/6.
23. *Ibid.*, BOM, 21.2.1962, p. 2/438, LHB 10/1/6.

24. *Ibid.*, BOM, 21.3.1962, p. 2/476, LHB 10/1/6.
25. *Ibid.*, BOM, 18.4.1962, p. 4/38, LHB 10/1/7.
26. *Ibid.*, BOM, 4.7.1962, p. 9/133 and BOM 18.7.1962, p. 3/173, LHB 10/1/7.
27. *Ibid.*, BOM, 17.4.1963, p. 3/37, LHB 10/1/7.
28. *Ibid.*, BOM, 15.5.1963, p. 3/89 and GP Committee, 7.5.1963 p. 8/58, LHB 10/1/7.
29. *Ibid.*, GP Committee, 7.5.1963, p. 10/64, LHB 10/1/7.
30. *Ibid.*, GP Committee, 7.5.1963, p. 10/64, LHB 10/1/7.
31. *Scottish Medical Journal*, 1971;16:209–215.
32. The late Dr F J Wright, personal communication.
33. *Ibid.*
34. Minutes of RV & AH BOM, BOM, 17.4.1963, p. 5/53, LHB 10/1/7.
35. *Ibid.*, BOM 17.7.1963, p. 1.149, LHB, 10/1/7.
36. *The Scotsman*, 28.6.1963.

CHAPTER TWENTY-SEVEN

1. Minutes of RV & AH BOM, BOM, 21.2.1968, p. 1/473, LHB 10/1/8.
2. *Ibid.*, BOM, 21.7.1965, p. 1/227, LHB 10/1/8.
3. *Ibid.*, BOM, 21.8.1965, p. 1/256, LHB 10/1/8.
4. *Ibid.*, BOM, 20.10.1965, p. 2/411, LHB 10/1/8.
5. *Ibid.*, BOM, 21.2.1968, p. 1/474, LHB 10/1/8.
6. *Ibid.*, M & AS Committee, 7.9.1966, p. 10/337, LHB 10/1/8.
7. *Ibid.* BOM, 21.2.1968, p. 1/474, LHB 10/8.
8. *Ibid.*, M & AS Committee, 3.11.1965, p. 10/429, LHB 10/1/8.
9. *Ibid.*, BOM, 20.12.1967, p. 1/381, LHB 10/1/8.
10. *Ibid.*, M & AS Committee, 2.12.1970, p. 9/373, LHB 10/1/9.
11. *Ibid.*, M & AS Committee, 1.11.1972, p. 10/415, LHB 10/1/10.
12. *Ibid.*, BOM, 20.12.1972, p. 2/527, LHB 10/1/10.
13. Professor James Williamson, personal communication.
14. *Ibid.*
15. Smith, *Edinburgh's Contribution to Medical Microbiology*, pp. 152–168.
16. Minutes of RV & AH BOM, BOM, 18.1.1961, p. 3/383 and BOM, 15.3.1961 p. 1/477, both LHB 10/1/6.
17. Smith, *Edinburgh's Contribution to Medical Microbiology*, p. 164.
18. *Ibid.*
19. Minutes of RV & AH BOM, BOM, 17.2.1965, p. 5/518, LHB 10/1/8.
20. Dr G. J. R. McHardy, personal communication.
21. Minutes of RV & AH BOM, Finance Committee, 11.7.1960, p. 13/135, LHB 10/1/6.
22. *Ibid.*, BOM, 15.6.1960, p. 3/104, LHB 10/1/6.
23. *Ibid.*, BOM, 20.12.1961, p. 1/348, LHB 10/1/6.
24. *Ibid.*, BOM, 18.4.1962, p. 1/25, LHB 10/1/6.
25. *Ibid.*, BOM, 20.6.1962, p. 5/117, LHB 10/1/6.
26. *Ibid.*, GP Committee, 11.11.1963, p. 13/320, LHB 10/1/6.
27. *Ibid.*, BOM, 17.11.1965, p. 1/453, LHB 10/1/8.
28. *Ibid.*, BOM, 20.10.1965, p. 4/419, LHB 10/1/8.
29. *Ibid.*, BOM, 17.11.1965, p. 1/453, LHB 10/1/8.
30. *Ibid.*, BOM, 16.2.1966, p. 1/624, LHB 10/1/8.
31. *Ibid.*, BOM, 16.11.1966, p. 2/473, LHB 10/1/8.

32. *Ibid.*, BOM, 21.12.1966, p. 1/523, LHB 10/1/8.
33. *Ibid.*, M & AS Committee, 6.3.1968, p. 11/498, LHB 10/1/8.
34. The late Dr H. A. Raeburn, SAMO, SE Regional Hospital Board (Scotland), and his son, Professor J. A. Raeburn, were both looked after by Miss Miller when they were junior doctors at the City Hospital. Personal communication.
35. Minutes of RV & AH BOM, BOM 17.8.1960, p. 1/167, LHB 10/1/6.
36. *Ibid.*, BOM, 21.6.1961, p. 1/121, LHB 10/1/6.
37. *Ibid.*, GP Committee, 9.3.1964, p. 15/16, LHB 10/1/7 and BOM, 19.7.1967, p. 1/186, LHB 10/1/8.
38. *Ibid.*, GP Committee, 12.7.1965, p. 18/207, LHB 10/1/8.
39. *Ibid.*, BOM, 20.12.1961, p. 3/353, LHB 10/1/6.
40. *Ibid.*, M & AS Committee, 6.3.1963, p. 7/495, LHB 10/1/7.
41. *Ibid.*, BOM, 16.6.1965, p. 4/169, LHB 10/1/8.
42. *Ibid.*, GP Committee, 12.11.1962, p. 11/314, LHB 10/1/7 and BOM 18.12.1963, p. 3, LHB 10/1/7.
43. *Ibid.*, BOM, 20.9.1967, p. 1/226, LHB 10/1/8.
44. *Ibid.*, BOM, 18.10.1967, p. 1/284, LHB 10/1/8 and BOM, 15.11.1967, p. 1/325, LHB 10/1/8.
45. *Ibid.*, GP Committee, 7.11.1966, p. 17/449, LHB 10/1/8.
46. *Ibid.*, BOM, 18.11.1964, p. 5/359, LHB 10/1/7.
47. *Ibid.*, GP Committee, 11.1.1965, p. 10/429, LHB 10/1/7.
48. *Ibid.*, BOM, 21.7.1965, p. 3/236, LHB 10/1/8.
49. *Ibid.*, BOM, 20.11.1963, p. 1/337, LHB 10/1/7.
50. *Ibid.*, GP Committee, 9.1.1967, p. 13/556, LHB 10/1/8.
51. *Ibid.*, BOM, 20.6.1962, p. 2/104 and p. 7/128, LHB 10/1/7.
52. *Ibid.*, BOM, 18.5.1960, Table, LHB 10/1/6.
53. *Ibid.*, BOM, 18.3.1964, p. 2/534, LHB 10/1/7.
54. *Ibid.*, BOM, 15.12.1965, Table LHB 10/1/8.
55. *Ibid.*, BOM, 21.4.1971, Table, LHB 10/1/9.
56. *Ibid.*, BOM, 21.12.1960, p. 3/342, LHB 10/1/6.
57. *Ibid.*, BOM, 16.8.1961, p. 2/E. 34, LHB 10/1/6.
58. *Ibid.*, Nursing Committee, 1.11.1961, p. 5/289, LHB 10/1/7.
59. *Ibid.*, Nursing Committee, 6.6.1962, p. 1/67-p. 2/68, LHB 10/1/7.
60. *Ibid.*, BOM, 18.7.1962, p. 4/186, LHB 10/1/7.
61. *Ibid.*, BOM, 19.6.1963, p. 1/121, LHB 10/1/7.
62. *Ibid.*, BOM, 17.7.1963, p. 3/161, LHB 10/1/7.
63. *Ibid.*
64. *Ibid.*, BOM, 16.10.1963, p. 3/291, LHB 10/1/7.
65. *Ibid.*, Nursing Committee, 6.5.1964, p. 14/59, LHB 10/1/7.
66. *Ibid.*, BOM, 21.10.1964, p. 2/292, LHB 10/1/7.
67. *Ibid.*, Nursing Committee, 5.1.1966, p. 12/533, LHB 10/1/8.
68. *Ibid.*, M & A S Committee, 1.6.1966, p. 13/121, LHB 10/1/8.
69. *Ibid.*, Nursing Committee, 3.2.1965, p. 10/471–473, LHB 10/1/8.
70. *Ibid.*, Nursing Committee, 3.2.1965, p. 10/474, LHB 10/1/8.
71. *Ibid.* M & AS Committee, 1.6.1966, p. 13/121, LHB 10/1/8.
72. *Ibid.*, Nursing Committee, 7.4.1965, p. 10/12, LHB 10/1/8.
73. *Ibid.*, Nursing Committee, 1.9.1965, p. 18/318, LHB 10/1/8.
74. *Ibid.*, BOM, 21.4.1965, p. 4/42, LHB 10/1/8.
75. *Ibid.*, BOM, 16.6.1965, p. 10/199, LHB 10/1/8.

76. *Ibid.*, BOM, 16.6.1965, p. 9/192, LHB 10/1/8.
77. *Ibid.*, Nursing Committee, 2.6.1965, p. 10/149, LHB 10/1/8.
78. *Ibid.*, M & AS Committee, 1.6.1966, p. 10/114, LHB 10/1/8.
79. *Ibid.*
80. *Ibid.*, M & AS Committee, 1.6.1966, p. 12/117, LHB 10/1/8.
81. *Ibid.*, Nursing Committee, 5.1.1966, p. 12/532, LHB 10/1/8.
82. *Ibid.*, BOM, 20.4.1966, p. 3/26, LHB 10/1/8.
83. *Ibid.*, M & AS Committee, 6.7.1966, p. 13/176, LHB 10/1/8.
84. *Ibid.*, BOM, 21.7.1971, p. 3/226, LHB 10/1/9.
85. *Ibid.*, M & AS Committee, 3.9.1969, p. 11/231, LHB 10/1/9 and BOM 17.9.1969, p. 3/277, LHB 10/1/9.
86. *Ibid.*, BOM, 19.11.1969, p. 2/376, LHB 10/1/9.
87. *Ibid.*
88. *Ibid.*, BOM, 19.11.1969, p. 3/378, LHB 10/1/9.
89. *Ibid.*, M & A S Committee, 2.12.1970, p. 10/379, LHB 10/1/9.
90. *Ibid.*, M & A S Committee, 2.12.1970, p. 10/380, LHB 10/1/9.
91. *Ibid.*, M & A S Committee, 5.4.1972, p. 13/13(b), LHB 10/1/10.
92. *Ibid.*, BOM, 18.7.1973, p. 1/227, LHB, 10/1/10.
93. *Ibid.*, M & A S Committee, 5.9.1973, p. 11/261, LHB 10/1/10.
94. *Ibid.*, BOM, 18.5.1960, p. 2/68, LHB 10/1/6.
95. *Ibid.*, BOM, 20.7.1960, p. 3/150, LHB 10/1/6.
96. *Ibid.*, BOM, 17.8.1960, p. 5/182, LHB 10/1/6.
97. *Ibid.*, BOM, 19.12.1962, p. 5/402, LHB 10/1/7.
98. *Ibid.*, BOM, 20.2.1963, p. 2/469, LHB 10/1/7.
99. *Ibid.*, BOM, 20.11.1963, p. 6/358, LHB 10/1/7.
100. *Ibid.*, BOM, 16.6.1965, p. 2/162, LHB 10/1/8.
101. *Ibid.*, BOM, 15.9.1965, p. 4/418, LHB 10/1/8.
102. *Ibid.*, BOM, 15.12.1965, p. 4/514, LHB 10/1/8 and GP Committee, 6.6.1966, p. 17/125, LHB 10/1/8.
103. *Ibid.*, M & A S Committee, 7.6.1967, p. 12/113, LHB 10/1/8.
104. *Ibid.*, BOM, 19.7.1967, p. 4/204, LHB 10/1/8.
105. *Ibid.*, GP Committee, 11.9.1967, p. 12/208, LHB 10/1/8.
106. *Ibid.*, BOM, 17.4.1968, p. 3/29, LHB 10/1/9.
107. *Ibid.*, BOM, 22.5.1968, p. 3/74, LHB 10/1/9.
108. *Ibid.*, GP Committee, 10.6.1968, p. 15/101, LHB 10/1/9.
109. *Ibid.*, BOM, 17.12.1969, p. 4/438, LHB 10/1/9.
110. *Ibid.*, GP Committee, 12.1.1970, p. 17/470, LHB 10/1/9.
111. *Ibid.*, BOM, 24.6.1970, p. 2/123, LHB 10/1/9.
112. *Ibid.*, BOM, 15.7.1970, p. 2/168, LHB 10/1/9.
113. *Ibid.*, GP Committee, 10.5.1965, p. 18/97, LHB 10/1/8.
114. *Ibid.*, BOM, 19.5.1965, p. 5/137, LHB 10/1/8.
115. *Ibid.*, BOM, 18.9.1968, p. 5/239, LHB 10/1/9.
116. Mr A G Welstead, personal communication.
117. Minutes of RV & AH BOM, M & A S Committee, 7.11.1973, p. 10/376, LHB 10/1/10.
118. *Ibid.*, BOM, 21.11.1973, p. 3/434, LHB 10/1/10.
119. *Ibid.*
120. *Ibid.*, BOM, 21.11.1973, p. 3/434 *et seq*, LHB 10/1/10.
121. *Ibid.*, BOM, 19.12.1973, p. 1/470, LHB 10/1/10.

122. *Ibid.*, BOM, 28.3.1974, p. 1/631, LHB 10/1/10.

CHAPTER TWENTY-EIGHT

1. Mr W. J. Farquhar, OBE, formerly of Clinical Research Audit Group (CRAG) Secretariat, NHS Management Executive, The Scottish Office kindly helped to correct some of my misconceptions.
2. Dr Sheena Parker and Mr Don Nicolson, personal communications and RIE & AH Report 1974–1988, pp. 5–6.
3. DEG, SLHD, 10.1.1974, p. 1 and 30.7.1974, p. 74.
4. M(A)C, SLHD, 14.1.1975, p. 1.
5. Division of Medicine Minutes, SLHD Executive Committee, 27.9.1974.
6. RIE & AH Report 1974–88, pp. 5–6.
7. Mr Jack Burton, personal communication.
8. Dr Sheena Parker, personal communication.
9. Mr Jim Smith, personal communication.
10. Hospital Review 1974, p. 133.
11. *Ibid.*
12. *Ibid.*, pp. 134–5.
13. *Ibid.*, pp. 136–7.
14. *Ibid.*, pp. 134–135.
15. *Ibid.*
16. *Ibid.*, pp. 136–137.
17. *Ibid.*
18. *Ibid.*, pp. 134–135.
19. Annual Statistical Report, 1975, p. 9, LHB 37/1/1.
20. *Ibid.*, 1975, p. 9 LHB 37/1/1; 1982, p. iii, LHB, 37/1/8.
21. *Ibid.*, 1982, p. iii, LHB, 37/1/8.
22. *Ibid.*, 1975, p. 9, LHB 37/1/1.
23. *Ibid.*, 1979, p. 12, LHB, 37/1/5.
24. *Ibid.*, 1975, p. 9, LHB, 37/1/1.
25. *Ibid.*, 1981, p. 12, LHB, 37/1/7.
26. *Ibid.*, 1980, p. 12, LHB, 37/1/6.
27. *Ibid.*, 1975, p. 50, LHB, 37/1/1 and 1986, p. 78, LHB 37/1/12.
28. DEG, SLHD, 5.11.1974, p. 111 (14).
29. Division of Medicine Minutes, SLHD, Executive Committee, 28.3.1977, 342.00–342.04.
30. K. B. Hymes *et al.*, *Lancet* 1981;2:598–600.
31. Kaposi's sarcoma and *Pneumocystis carinii* pneumonia amongst homosexual men in New York and California, *Mortality and Morbidity Weekly Report (M & MWR)*, 1981;30:305; Update on Kaposi's Sarcoma and opportunistic infections in previously healthy persons – United States, *M&MWR*, 1982;31:294.
32. R. P. Brettle, MD thesis, 1994, SCD, EUL.
33. C. A. Ludlam *et al.*, *Lancet* 1985;2:233–236.
34. J. R. Robertson *et al.*, *British Medical Journal* 1986;292:527–529.
35. See also Ch. 27.
36. Health in Lothian 1974–89.
37. *Ibid.*, pp. 25–26.
38. *Ibid.*, p. 113.
39. R. P. Brettle, MD thesis, 1994, SCD, EUL.

40. Health in Lothian 1974–89, p. 113.
41. LHB, Annual Report, 1987–88, p. 5.
42. *Ibid.*, p. 7.
43. *Ibid.*, 1991–92, p. 12.
44. Mr B. Liston, Fire Officer, personal communication.
45. R. P. Brettle, MD thesis, 1994, SCD, EUL.
46. *Ibid.*
47. R. P. Brettle *et al.*, *British Medical Journal* 1987;295:421–424.
48. R. P. Brettle *et al., AIDS Care* 1990;2:171–181.

CHAPTER TWENTY-NINE

1. Mrs Hilary Flenley kindly gave me access to her late husband's papers.
2. D. C. Flenley, *Concise Medical Textbooks: Respiratory Medicine*, 1st edn, 1981, 2nd edn, 1990 London, Bailliére Tindall.
3. J. Rees, *British Medical Journal*, 1991;303:67.
4. Both Dr Patricia Warren and Miss Sylvia Merchant kindly provided details of the Respiratory Function and Rayne Laboratories.
5. Prof. N. J. Douglas, personal communication.
6. Prof. W. MacNee, personal communication.
7. Dr M. F. Sudlow, personal communication.
8. Mr E. W. Cameron, personal communication.
9. *Ibid.*
10. RIE & AH Annual Report & Accounts, 1994–5, p. 16.
11. *Ibid.*, 1995–6, p. 4.
12. Prof. A. G. D. Maran, personal communication.
13. RIE 7 AS Annual Report & Accounts, 1994–5, p. 16.
14. RIE & AH Annual Report, 1992–3.
15. *Ibid.*, p. 12.
16. *Ibid.*, 1993–4, pp. 11–12.
17. RIE 7 AH Annual Report & Accounts, 1994–5, p. 16.
18. Prof. A. G. D. Maran, personal communication.
19. Personal communication, Mr G. Lello.
20. Prof. A. G. D. Maran, personal communication.
21. RIE & AH Annual Report, 1993–4, p. 14.
22. RIE & AH Annual Report & Accounts, 1994–5, p. 16.
23. RIE &AH Annual Report, 1992–3, p. 32 and RIE & AH Annual Report & Accounts, 1995–6, p. 39.
24. RIE & AH Annual Report & Accounts, 1995–6, pp. 4,14.
25. RIE & AH Annual Report, 1993–4, p. 7.
26. *Ibid.*, 1993–4, p. 11.
27. *Ibid.*
28. RIE & AH Annual Report & Accounts, 1994–5, p. 16.
29. RIE & AH Annual Report & Accounts, 1995–6, pp. 4, 14.
30. Mr E. J. Rawlings, personal communication.

CHAPTER THIRTY

1. Annual Report, MOH, 1907, p. 46.
2. Miss J. K. Taylor kindly provided much information for this chapter with papers and photographs she kept of the hospital.

3. Miss A. E. Christie also kindly gave much oral information about her years at the hospital. See also notes 7 and 9.
4. Mr R. Purves' recollections about nursing and ancillary staff have been most valuable.
5. Mrs M. Lees provided information about the last few years of the hospital.
6. Papers of the Lorimer family, relations of the author's wife.
7. Miss A. E. Christie and Mr Ron Munro have examples of this medal struck by Messrs. Alex Kirkwood of Edinburgh, who still retain blanks. In a letter of 17.12.1890 to Dr Wood, Medical Superintendent of the second City Hospital, Sir Henry Littlejohn explained that the medals were the gift of Bailie Russell (later Lord Provost Sir James Alexander Russell) and were to remain the property of the City of Edinburgh. The Badges Book of the City Hospital (with Sir Henry's letter, now with LHSA, EUL) shows that Miss E. L. Sandford, Lady Superintendent of Nurses at the second City Hospital, returned her medal on 15.12.1903 and Miss I. Thomas, Matron at Colinton Mains, received hers (possibly the same one) on the next day. Later medals (Miss Christie's example is from 1914) had the name of the nurse and her dates of training inscribed on the reverse, so the rules may have been relaxed by then to allow nurses to retain their medals.
8. Mrs Pat Hunter (née McWilliam) kindly supplied the badge illustrated. She trained at the City Hospital from 1938 to 1941.
9. Miss A. E. Christie kindly supplied the badge illustrated.
10. Mrs Mina Begg, personal communication. See also Chapter 28.

CHAPTER THIRTY-ONE

1. Description and Sketch Plan, 5.10.1896, Sheet No. 5.
2. *Ibid.*
3. Annual Report, MOH, 1907, p. 46.
4. Annual Report, PHD, 1919, p. 53.
5. Ms Sandra Anderson, personal communication.

CHAPTER THIRTY-TWO

1. Clinical records ledgers from the second City Hospital are now at LHSA, EUL
2. *United Hospitals' Unit News,* Spring 1992.
3. Description and Sketch Plan, 5.10.1896, p. 3.
4. *Edinburgh Fever Hospital,* 1903 (photograph pp. 14–15).
5. Minutes of RV & AH BOM, Annual Report 1956.
6. *Ibid.,* 1957.
7. Mr George Nixon, personal communication.
8. Mr Gordon Rawson, personal communication.
9. Mr Mark Lavery, personal communication.
10. Mr Ian Robertson, personal communication.
11. *Ibid.*
12. *Ibid.*
13. Mr Mark Lavery, personal communication.
14. *Ibid.*
15. Mrs Mary Kelly, personal communication.
16. *Ibid.*
17. *Ibid.*

18. Mr Jim Smith, personal communication.
19. Mr David Pithie, personal communication.
20. *Ibid*.
21. *Ibid* and see Mr A. G. Welstead's account in Chapter 26.
22. Mr W. A. Maben, personal communication.
23. *Ibid*.
24. *Ibid*.
25. *Ibid*.

CHAPTER THIRTY-THREE

1. PHC Minutes 27.1.1920, item 63, p. 55 and 19.2.1918, item 21, p. 50.
2. *Ibid.*, 10.6.1919, item 10, p. 264.
3. Minutes of Presbytery of Edinburgh.
4. *Ibid.*, 5.5.1931, p. 233.
5. *Ibid.*, 4.7.1933, p. 620.
6. *Ibid.*, 3.7.1934, p. 155.
7. *Ibid.*, 5.7.1938, p. 155.
8. *Ibid*.
9. *Ibid* 22.7.41, p. 714.
10. Rev. Dr R. C. M. Mathers personal communication and see Chapter 24.
11. Rev. Harry Telfer, personal communication.
12. Mr John K. Thomson, Chaplaincies Administration, National Mission, The Church of Scotland kindly supplied this list.
13. Personal communication, Mr Frank Snell.
14. Mrs Pat Macleod, personal communication.

CHAPTER THIRTY-FOUR

1. Mr Alan A Ezzi, Project Manager, New Royal Infirmary of Edinburgh, personal communication.
2. Personal communication, Mr Derick Reid, Morrison Homes, who kindly supplied information on the development of the City Hospital site, as also Ms Gillian Gray, Cala Homes (Scotland) Ltd.
3. *The Scotsman Property Weekly*, 9.10.1997.

Index

Abercrombie, Dr John, on cholera 14, 16
Acquired Immuno-Deficiency Syndrome (AIDS) 320
Action for Children in Hospital 353
Adam, William
 architect 38
 Infirmary Street gates 70
Adams, Dr W.D., cholera doctor 17–18
Adams, Miss M.I., Matron 219, 225–6, 227, 228–9, 258, 302, 305, 351, 358
adult respiratory distress syndrome (ARDS) 335
AIDS
 15-bedded unit at City Hospital 325
 antibody 322
 counselling 322
 hospice 2
 infection rates 325
 nutritional care 369
AIDS-associated mycobacterial infections 294
airing grounds 67
Aitken, Professor Cairns, RIE NHS Trust Chairman 313
albendazole 285
Alexander, Mrs Margaret, Theatre Sterilising Centre Manager 384
Alison, Dr William Pultney (1790–1859) 24, 25–6
Alston, Dr Douglas M, Chairman of Board of Management 269, 271, 285, 298–9
ambulance
 horse-drawn 150
 motor 152–3; in 1930s 194
 stretcher 152
aminoglycosides 276
Anaesthetics Department 287–9
Anderson, Ms Sandra, Speech and Language Therapy Department 366–7
animal waste 22–3
animals, stray, slaughter 9, 10
Area Executive Group 311

Ashfield Nursing Home, Chamberlain Road, grave slab 11
Asiatic cholera outbreak 1831, 1848 46–7
Astley Ainslie Hospital 10
 carer respite 346
Astor Committee, tuberculosis recommendations 174–5

Baillie, Mrs Christine, radiographer 348
Bain, Miss, smallpox contact sister 209
Bain, Rev. John, chaplain 389
Baird, Mrs Mae, medical social worker 375
balconies 125, 188–9
 additional 201
Ballingall, Mr
 Clerk of Works 111–13, 117; Weekly Report on Works in Progress 117, 143–4, 146
Balm Well of St Katherine 7–8
Barber, John, Superintendent of Physiotherapy 362
Barclay, Dr Roger, District Medical Officer 311
Barr, Mr Ricky, supervising engineer 387
Bath, Dr George, AIDS Coordinator 326
Bath, Dr J.C.J.L. 293
Battle of the Sites 64
BCG vaccine 176
 use 242
Beatson, Dr George 150
bed pan, metal, cleansing 125
bed
 1893 65
 cost rise 163
Begg, Mrs Mina, RIDU out-patient sister 327, 356, 357–8
Bell, Fiona, dietician 368
Bell, Miss, Lady Dispenser 359
Benson, Dr Walter T.
 Medical Superintendent 163, 164, 165, 183–91; Diploma in Tropical Medicine and Hygiene 184;

retirement activities 194;
vaccination for seamen 184
Benson, June, dietician 368
Benton, Dr Claire, Consultant Dermatologist 323
Berlin, efficient infectious disease provision 99
Best, Professor J, HIV-dedicated MRI scanner 323
Biggam, Major General Sir Alexander 283
Bingham, Dr Jim 327
Binnie, Night Superintendent Sister 357–8
Binning, Nurse Alice, prizewinner 241
Birrell, Dr J.F., paediatric ENT Consultant 286
Bissett, Dr Kate 326
Black, Mrs Sheila, Group Records Officer 377
Black Death 9
Blood Transfusion Service 322
Boddie, Mrs Maureen 327
Boissard, Dr G 293
Bolas, Mr Gordon, dentist for AIDS patients 323
Bowie, Dr John, Senior Lecturer in bacteriology 383
Boyle, Sister Sheena, AIDS Unit 326
Brakenridge, Dr D.J., Convener, New City Hospital Site 86
Brayton, Miss, Regional Nursing Officer 280
Brettle, Dr Raymond
  HIV research team results 329–31
  HIV-dedicated MRI scanner 323
  'Human Immunodeficiency Virus, the Edinburgh Epidemic' MD thesis 320
  new out-patient clinic 326
  self-referral HIV screening clinic 321, 323
  Senior Registrar, part-time Reader 316–17, 318–19
  work on HIV infection 403
Brindle, Miss, pharmacist 359
British Tuberculosis Association 243
  Certificate 250
Broach, Miss Maggie, Assistant Matron 219

bronchopneumonia, influenzal 199
Brown, Dr A.A., Vice-chairman of South Lothian District Medical Committee 311
Brydon, Dr J.W., death from meningitis 193
bubonic plague 7, 9–10, 12
Buchanan, Miss Margaret 292
Buchanan, Miss Marion, Director of Nursing Services 352
Bucknall, Dr, report on drug misusers 321
Building Committee, 1901 cost report 118
Burgh Muir, infection isolation 10
Burns, Dr, Convener of City Hospital Services 389
Burns, Dr Sheila
  Consultant Virologist 293
  Regional Virus Laboratory Director 324
Burns, Moyra, dietician 368
Burt, Mrs, secretary to Care of the Elderly Unit 377
Burton, Mr Jack
  Lothian Health Board Unit Administrator 312
  United Hospitals Unit 380

Calder, Dr Margaret 403
  Director of Bacteriology Laboratory 178, 293–4
Calder, Jane, Dietetic Manager 368
Cameron, Dr Jennesse 327
Cameron, Mr Evan W, cardio-thoracic surgeon 339, 340
Cameron, Professor Charles 176–7
Cameron Hospital, Windygates 315
Campanella, Mr Ciro, Senior Lecturer in cardiac surgery 339
Campie House 92
  convalescent fever patients 61
  costs 62
campylobacter 316
canicola fever 255
Canongate (Poorhouse) Hospital (1st City Hospital) 48–52
  1890 smallpox patients 58
  1890 use 74–5, 77–8, 80

Index

1890s costs 61
smallpox or cholera patients 6
cardiac surgery 246, 248
  preparation 288
Carswell, Dr James, Tropical Diseases Unit 283–4
Carswell, Mr G. 349
Carter, Sir David, Professor of Surgery 340
case notes 376–7
Casualty Services 212
Caves, Mr Philip, Senior Lecturer in cardiac surgery 289, 338
cement delivery delays 112
Centers for Disease Control, Atlanta, Georgia 319–20
cephalosporins 276–7
Chalmers Street, Royal Victoria Dispensary 169
Chambers, Dr William, provost, improvement scheme 61
chapel 129–30
Chapman, Dr Brian J., Consultant Geriatrician 345
Charity Workhouse 49
Chase, Mr A.R., Clinical Instructor 301
chemotherapy, controlled trials 180–1
Chest, Heart, and Stroke Association 371
Chest Unit 2
chickenpox, single-storey blocks 122
children, slum 22
Chisholm, Mrs Anne, testing for HIV encephalopathy 326
chloramphenicol 243
chlorhydroxyquinolone 261
cholera
  epidemics 14
  notification 15, 16, 31
  outbreak 1866 48
'Cholera Board of Health Edinburgh, 1831–34' 14, 16–17, 25
Christie, Miss A.E, Deputy Matron, later Matron 303, 304, 351, [B]352[b]–3, 395
Christie, Mr Phil, Estates Management 388
Christison, Sir Robert, Professor of Materia Medica and Jurisprudence 42, 53–4

City Fever Hospital 1870 49 see Canongate (Poorhouse) Hospital
City Hospital (Third)
  access 121
  administrative buildings 127
  advanced tuberculosis patients 170
  (Alternative) Extension Plan 1894 66
  Area Sterilising Centre 383–5
  Assessment Unit 403; physiotherapy services 363
  Bacteriology Department 1904 149
  Bacteriology Laboratory 69, 178, 315, 398; Extension 294
  Bank of Scotland branch 271, 299
  bed provision costing 101–2
  beds, 600 capacity 122
  bird's-eye projected view 98
  building costs 1960s 297
  building delays 110
  building difficulties 108–19
  building inauguration party 108–9
  bus service 306–7
  Care of the Elderly Unit 2, 271, 289–92, 341, 345–7, 398; physiotherapy use 362–3; speech therapy requirement 366
  catering 379–81
  chaplaincy 389–93
  children's ward for non-pulmonary TB 177
  Christmas dance 186
  Department of Geriatric Medicine, social workers 374
  Department of Respiratory Medicine 2; social workers 374
  description 120–31
  Diamond Jubilee Celebrations 285
  Dietetic Service 368–9
  during 2nd World War 204–15
  Ear, Nose and Throat (ENT) Department 286–7
  ENT Department 271, 399; occupational therapy services 366; speech therapy requirement 367
  fauna in grounds 3
  foundation 1903 1
  gardens 121
  general medical admissions 300
  Geriatric Day Centre 271

Group Catering Officer 244
Hospital Secretary 269
Hospital Steward 194
industrial relations 386–7
Infectious Diseases Unit, fall in length of stay 316
joined Royal Infirmary NHS Trust 1994 2
Jubilee Thanksgiving Commemoration Service 251, 390
laundry 128–30, 315, 382–3; centralisation 260; system conversion 251
League of Friends 364
lecture theatre 130
library 298
Maxillofacial Department, move to St John's Hospital 1998 345
Medical Records Office 298
Medical Residency 295, 296–7
medical staff: 1928 185; 1954 254
Medical Superintent's house 127
MRI scanning service 398
New Medical Block 263, 270
non-pulmonary tuberculosis patients 1921 170
Occupational Therapy 364–6
open-sided TB ward 172
patients' library services 393, 394–5
pharmacy 263, 271, 315, 359–62
Physiotherapy Department 362–4
planning 97–107
portering 386–8
Pyelonephritis Unit 270, 277, 282
Records Office 376–9
redevelopment 400–2
Regional Infectious Diseases Unit *see* Regional Infectious Diseases Unit
Royal opening 1903 132–3, 134–8
screening clinic (CHSC) 322–3
secretarial staff 376–8
servants' home 128
shop 256
site choice 85–90
Social Work Department 370–5
Speech and Language Therapy Department 366–7
Stroke Rehabilitation Unit 346, 347, 363, 367, 398, 403
Sub-Post office 256, 299

Tea Room 304, 305–6
teaching rooms 1965 298
temporary smallpox hospital 144–5
Thoracic Surgery Unit 246, 289, 338–40; transfer to RIE 1997 338
Trauma Rehabilitation Unit 403
Tropical Diseases Unit 270, 282–5
water cistern 388
Western General Hospital laundry 270
X-ray Department 241, 244, 347–50
City Hospital Pharmacy Bulletins 360
City Hospital Welfare Association 256
City Infectious Hospital 55, 57
Clark, Dr W.G., MOH 204–7, 216, 224–5
  infant mortality fall 235
  on NHS transition 235
Clark, Jan, dietician 368
Clark, Professor Frank, Lothian Health Board General Manager 312
Clayson, Dr Christopher 176
coaches for patient transport 152
Colinton Mains
  smallpox hospital 210
  tuberculosis beds 237
Colinton Mains Farm, as site for fever hospital 87–9, 399
Colinton Mains Fever Hospital 52
'Colinton Mains Hospital – Memorandum Accompanying Plans for ... the Local Government Board' 120
Colledge, Dr Nicola, Consultant Geriatrician 345
College of Surgeons in Ireland 340
Colonial Office consultancy 283
Committee for Lighting and Cleaning 30
Committee for Streets and Buildings 30
Community Care Act 1991 375
Community Drugs Problem Service (CDPS) 325, 327
Community Drugs Project 326
Comrie, Dr John D. 7
Conn, Dr Nancy 292
Connery, Sean, at Milestone House 328
contagion measures 13
Contagious Diseases (Animals) Acts 32
Cooper, Mr, Burgh Engineer, on drainage 88–9

Copenhagen, efficient infectious disease provision 99–100
Coronation Wood 388
Corynebacterium diphtheriae 201
Cossar, Sister, outpatient clinic 327
cotrimoxazole 324
Coulter, Freda, Records Officer 377
covered ways 126–7
Cowan, Dr David L., paediatric ENT surgeon 342
Cowan, Miss, Assistant Matron 353
Cowgate, proposal for temporary hospital 77
Cowgate/Grassmarket Improvement Scheme 164
Craig, Mr Jimmie, Laboratory Assistant 238, 292
Craig, Mrs Christine, librarian 393–4
Craiglockhart Poorhouse 87
  smallpox in 163
Crewe, Rosemary, occupational therapist 364
cricket 307–8
Crofton, Sir John, Professor of Respiratory Medicine 81, 167, 177–9, 180–1
  1951 teaching commitments 244
  antimycobacterial therapy 14
  combination drug anti-TB therapy 179, 402
  joint author *Clinical Tuberculosis* 272
  move from Southfield to City Hospital 263
Crompton, Dr Graham K. 294, 308
cross-infection 45
Croughan, Mr Michael, Senior Chief Medical Laboratory Scientific Officer 294
Cruickshank, Dr Alistair 290
Cruickshank, Professor Robert 292
Cubie, Dr Heather 324
Cummack, Dr D. Hunter, Consultant Radiologist 239, 347
Cunningham, Mr John, portering supervisor 386
Currie, Dr Colin T., Senior Lecturer in Geriatric Medicine 291–2, 345
cycloserine 276–7
cystitis 277
cystoscopy 349

Daiches, Professor David, as patient 157–8
Dairies, Cowsheds and Milk-Shops Order 1885 32
Dale, Dr Bryan A.B., ENT unit 342
Dalkier, Mrs Kirsten, Superintendent of Physiotherapy 362, 363
Davidson, Dr Iain A., RIE Medical Director 313
Davidson, Mrs Sue 327
Davidson, Professor Sir Stanley 283
Davis, Liz, occupational therapist 364
Day, Mrs Jean 219–20, 221, 222–3
Department of Health & Social Security, cooperation with MSWs 374
Destitute Sick Society 13
Deuchar, Robert, Secretary to Edinburgh Fever Board 25
Devlin, Mr Bob, Head Porter 386
Dhillon, Dr Bal, Consultant Ophthalmologist 323
dialysis patients, hepatitis deaths 279
Diana, Princess of Wales, at Milestone House 327–8
Dick, Jimmy, Senior Chief Technician in bacteriology 383
dietary changes 369
dining rooms, plan 115
diphtheria
  1904 mortality 149
  1923 school outbreak 165
  1940 increase 204
  Dr Benson for child immunisation 186–7
  late nineteenth century 65
  notification 1879 31
  temperature and progress chart 71
  ward plan 124
Diploma of Public Health 163
  courses at City Hospital 185–6
Directorate for Psychiatry of Old Age 346
disease transmissibility 7
Dobson, Mr Ken, United Hospitals Group General Manager 313
Docherty, Mr Stuart, Unit Administrator assistant 312
Dodd, Dr Keith 287
Donald, Dr A.B. 201

Douglas, Dr Andrew C. 178, 179, 181–2, 337
  sarcoidosis 402
Douglas, Dr Graham, Senior Registrar 317
Douglas, Ms Pauline 326
Douglas, Neil J.
  Director of Scottish National Sleep Laboratory 336
  Professor of Respiratory and Sleep Medicine 335–6
  sleep apnoea research 402
Drabble, Carol, dietician 368
drainage, inadequate 23
Drinker respirator 190, 200, 231
drug misuse 319
  needle sharing 2
drug misusers, AIDS 322
Drummond, Marjorie, Respiratory Medicine secretary 378
Drummond, Provost George 25, 37–9
Drummond Street Cholera Hospital 14, 47
Dunbar, Mrs Elizabeth, almoner 370–1
Duncan, Dr A.H., District Medical Officer 311
Duncan, Miss, Lady Dispenser 359
Dundee, King's Cross Hospital 315
Dyer, Mrs, child play coordinators arrangement 353
dysentery
  1951 outbreak 243
  bacillary 198, 201; increase 202
  children 222
  decrease 316
  flexner 201

East Pilton Fever Hospital 74, 162–3
  later Pilton Hospital, advanced tuberculosis patients 170
  tuberculosis accommodation 164
Easterbrook, Dr C.C., Crichton Royal Mental Hospital 230
Eastern General Hospital, thoracic surgery 246
ECHO viral infection 259
E.coli 026 261
E.coli 0157 261
E.coli, urinary infections 277

Edinburgh City Hospital: A Noteworthy Enterprise of Fifty Years Ago 236
Edinburgh Fever Board 13, 25
Edinburgh Fever Hospital – Description with Plans and Photographs 1903 120
Edinburgh Health Care 345
Edinburgh Joint Stock Water Company 22
Edinburgh Medico-Chirurgical Society 69
Edinburgh Municipal and Police Act 1879 31
Edinburgh Outbreak of Smallpox 1942 211
Edinburgh Public Health Committee 1–2
Edinburgh Tuberculosis Scheme 163, 168, 171
Edmond, Dr Elizabeth, Laboratory Director 293
Egan, Mr Vince, testing for HIV encephalopathy 326
Elder, Dr Herbert C., Tuberculosis Officer 176–7, 192, 218
electric lighting 100
Emergency Hospital Scheme 204, 206, 225
Emmanuel, Dr Xavier 324
emphysema, Norman Salvesen Research Trust 335
encephalitis lethargica 198
ENT surgeons, golf prowess 342
ENT surgery 2, 340–44
'epidemic fever' 7, 13, 39–40
erysipelas
  30 bed provision 123
  late nineteenth century 65
  notification 32
  treatment by RIE 55
ethambutol 181
European Association of Cardio-Thoracic Surgeons 340
European Society of Pneumology 334
evacuee clinics
  Broomlee Camp 216
  Middleton House 216
Ewing, Nurse Jean, prizewinner 237
Ex-Far East Prisoners of War Association, memorial library 282–3

Fairley, Mr Robert, Deputy Secretary of Board and cricketer 308

Fairley, Nurse Anne, prizewinner 255
Farquhar, Mr W.J., District
    Administrator 311
Farquharson, Dr I.M., ENT Consultant
    286–7
Ferguson, Mr Tom, Catering Manager
    379
Fever Board 47
Fever Hospital Committee
    1893 remit 63
    1896 modified approval of Morham
        plans 101
Fever House, 1885 Town Council
    purchase 58
Fever Nurse Certificate 354
fever nurse training 58
fever patients, early care 7–18
Fever Register, abeyance 302
fevers, nineteenth century, hospital
    requirement 1
fire drill 72
fires 19, 21
    in nurses' home 328-[B]9[b]
Fital, Mr Tony, ECG technician 348
Flegg, Dr Peter J, Senior Registrar 317,
    327
Fleming, Miss Rose, Area Sterilising
    Centre Manager 384
Flenley, Dr David C., Professor of
    Respiratory Medicine 332, 333–4
    emphysema 402
    Rayne Laboratory 334
    Recent Advances Series 334
    Respiratory Medicine 334
Flexner and Jobling's antitoxin 160
Flodden Wall 20
food boxes 190
food, electric trolleys 232
Food Hygiene (Scotland) Regulations
    1959 263
food poisoning, increase 316
Ford, William, Professor of
    Experimental Pathology, Manchester
    278
forest laws 7
Fortune, Amy, dietician 368
Foster, Mr G. 349
France, Dr A.J., Senior Registrar 317
Fraser, Dr Andrew 38

Fraser, Professor Sir John, surgeon 170
fresh air as therapeutic agent 188
Friendly Conference 55, 57
Friends of the City Hospital 248
fumigation 52

Gallo, Dr Robert 320
gamma camera 349
gamma globulin protection 255
Gardiner, Avril, occupational therapist
    364
Gardiner, Dr W.T., consultant otologist
    163, 164, 191
gastroenteritis 1947 232
gastrointestinal infections 1894 75
Gay Switchboard 322
Geddes, Dr Alastair, Professor in
    Birmingham 278, 279
General Police and Improvement
    (Scotland) Act 1862 29
Genito-Urinary Medicine Unit, rotation
    scheme with RIDU 317
gentry in Old Town 21
George II, Royal Infirmary of
    Edinburgh Charter 1736 38
George Watson's Hospital 51, 53
Geriatric Medicine Unit 259
Gilloran, Dr J.L., MOH 180
Girvan, Mr, Head Porter 348
Glasgow
    1955 smallpox outbreak 242
    municipal responsibility for infectious
        disease 57
    smallpox outbreak 211–12
Gloucester, HRH the Duchess of 285
Gordon, Jimmy, postman 386
Gowans, James, Convener of Public
    Health Committee 1877 51
Grant, Dr Ian W.B. 178, 182, 294
Grant, Dr Robin, HIV neurological
    problems 323
Grant, Dr William E., rhinologist 342
Gray, Dr Chris, Professor of Geriatric
    Medicine 292
Gray, Dr James A., Consultant Physician
    282
    RIDU 316
Greenbank Church 304
Greening, Dr Andrew 335

Greenwood, Dr Judy OBE, Consultant Community Psychiatrist 325
Greig, Consultant Colonel 283
Grieve, Miss Agnes, Group Nursing Officer 351–2
Griffiths, Dr Harold W.C. 287
Griffiths Report 1985 312
Group Nursing Training Scheme 301
Gruer, Dr Rosamund, District Medical Officer 311
Guy, Dr John, Tuberculosis Officer 175–6

haemophiliacs, HIV–infected Factor VIII 321
Haemophilus influenzae type B vaccine 253
Hallam, Dr N. 324
Hamilton, Mr David, Professor of Cardiac Surgery 339
Hamilton, Ms Barbara 327
Hand, Nurse Denis, prizewinner 248
Hargreaves, Mr David 324
Hargreaves, Chief Medical Laboratory Scientific Officer 293
Harley, Mrs Marta, medical social worker 375
Harris, Dr Edward 294
Hart, Rev Geoffrey, Episcopal chaplain 392
Haslett, Dr Christopher, Professor of Respiratory Medicine 335–6
  cell function studies 402
Hastie, Mr John, Head Chef 380
Hayhurst, Dr Valerie 327
Helm, Marjorie, occupational therapist 364, 365
Henderson, Rev. Charlotte, chaplain 392
Hendry, Alison, dietician 368
Henery, Ms Enid, Care of Elderly Unit dietician, later Chief of service 368, 369
Henry, Mr Martin
  Highfield Award runner-up 1992 381
  Unit Catering Manager 380–1
Henryson, James, 1585 plague surgeon 11
hepatitis
  infectious 258–9
  non-A, non-B 279, 319
  serum 279–80
  type A 319
  type B 2; infection increase in 1980s 325
  type C 319
  viral 279–80; 1975 notification 315–16
heroin
  misuse 2
  misusers and HIV infection 321
Hetherington Committee, on salaries 205
High School Yards, reception building, costs 62
99–103 High Street
  official cleansing 9
  tenement collapse 1751 26
Hindmarsh, Mr J. 349
HIV
  counselling 329
  heroin-associated epidemic 319
  infection 2, 317, 318–27; funding 325
  patients 285
  patients' clinic 2
  patients' spiritual care 390–1
  research team results 329–31
  self-referral screening clinic 321
  testing 293
HIV-positive mothers, risk infection 323–4
Hodge, Vere, Consultant Col. 283
Holywell, Joyce, secretary to Dr Horne 378
HOMER system for tracing case notes 378
Horne, Dr Norman W., Physician Superintendent 178, 264, 270, 271, 272, 273–4, 311, 403
  joint author *Clinical Tuberculosis* 272
  Modern Drug Treatment of Tuberculosis 272
Hospital Review 1973 314–15
Houses of Reception and Quarantine 62, 77
housing
  overcrowding 26
  'ticketing' 30
housing defects 19, 21–3
housing improvement 30
Hughes, Dr P. 327

Index

Human T-cell lymphocytic Virus III (HTLV-III) *see* HIV
Hunter, Mr Andrew B.H., Principal Pharmacist 359, 360–2
hyperventilation service 363
hypothermia induction 287–288

identity card 226
Illingworth, Mr C.F.W., Consulting Surgeon 191
Inchkeith, syphilis colony 9
incinerator provision 76
infantile paralysis *see* poliomyelitis
Infantile Paralysis Fellowship 56, 245
infectious disease
  bed decrease 316
  beds, 1870 on 61
  clinical teaching 55
  early control 7–18
  figures in the 1890s 74
  intimation form [B]32[b]
  notification 31
Infectious Disease (Notification) Act 1889 31–2
infective jaundice 279
Infirmary, old site, reorganisation and expansion 61–73
Infirmary Buildings, old, fever hospital set up 1885 57–8
Infirmary of Edinburgh 1729 37
Infirmary Fever House 55–7
  established 58
  medical staff 59
Infirmary Street
  cost increase 85
  Extension Plans 1894 66
  Hydro Extractor and Disinfector 68
  lift installation 67
  nurses' home 67
  provisional cost estimates 1894–95 72
  servants' accommodation 68
Infirmary Street Baths, power supplied to hospital 68, 71
influenza
  pandemic 1918 162
  type A 259
Inglis, Dr J. (Hamish) M., Regional Virus Laboratory Director 293, 324
intravenous pyelography (IVP) 348

intubation for diphtheria 149
Irish building labourers 22, 26, 39
iron lung 231
isolation cottage 122, 124
isoniazid 179, 181, 251

James, Dr Alexander, Consultant Physician 161, 164, 192
James IV, and Chapel of St Roque 10
Jardine, Mr Frank, Consulting Surgeon 191
Jeffrey, Mrs Mary, domestic manager 386
Joe, Dr Alexander, Medical Superintendent 164, 193, 197–203, 205–7, 221–2
  achievements 264–5
  Jubilee address 252
  with Lord Provost and nurses 227, 228
  wartime teaching 227
Johnstone, Dr Frank, Consultant Obstetrician 323
Jones, Dr Gwyneth 327
Jones, Dr Michael 285, 327
  locum Consultant 328–9
Jones, Mr Trevor, Lothian Health Board General Manager 312

kanamycin 277
Kaposi's sarcoma 319–20
Kay, Dr A. Barry, later Professor of Allergy and Clinical Immunology, London 182, 348
  production of *A Midsummer-Night's Dream* 307
Keenan, Clare, dietician 368
Kelly, Mrs Mary, Deputy Support Service Manager 385–6
  domestic services and sewing room 380
Kent, Mr Roger, Director of Social Work 373
Ker, Dr Claude B., Medical Superintendent 141, 142–3, 146–7, 160
  600 bed support 103, 108
  lectures to nurses 161
  and nursing staff 155
  tuberculosis treatment 173
Kerr, Dr Alastair I.G., Director of ENT unit 341–2

Kerr, Sister Margaret 280–1 MBE 403
Kincairney, Lord, 1904 judgment 119
kitchens, plan 115
Knowles, Mr Jimmy, Group Records Officer 298, 377

Laing, Dr Robert 327
Laing, Miss M.S., District Nursing Officer 311
Lamb, Anne, Care of Elderly Unit dietician 368
Lamb, Dr David 182
laryngectomees, swimming group 367
Latta, Dr Thomas, of Leith 14, 47
Lavery, Mr Mark, Area Sterilising Centre Manager 384–5
Lawrie, Dr J.H.D. 193
League of Friends of the City Hospital 395–7
Learmonth, Nurse Janet, prizewinner 244
Leaver, Mrs Pam, medical social worker 375
Leen, Dr Clifford, Consultant Physician 319
Lees, Father John, RC chaplain 392
Lees, Mrs, Acting Principal Nurse, later Principal Nurse 313, 353, 354
Leitch, Dr A. Gordon 167, 337–8
Leith
  Port of, Medical Inspection Report 184
  smallpox epidemic 1893–94 74
Leith Hospital
  accommodation during epidemics 53
  HIV screening clinic 323
Leith Hospital 1848–1988 14
Leith Improvement Scheme 164
Lello, Mr Glenn, Senior Lecturer in maxillofacial surgery 344
leprosy hospital 1584 9
Liberton 7
lincosamines 276
Lindsay, Mrs Angela, Superintendent of Physiotherapy 362, 364
linen supply reorganisation 255
Lister Institute, meningococcal antitoxin 160

Littlejohn, Sir Henry Duncan MOH 28–33, 167–8
  approved new hospital 69
  Campie House fares requests 62
  Canongate Hospital concern 74–5
  and Morham, Robert, *City Hospital Extension* 63
  requests permanent infectious diseases hospital 49
  Rules for the Hospital 72
  scarlet fever bed shortage 75
  Town Council land sale upset 58
Livingstone, John, apothecary, d.1645 11
Lloyd, Dr E.L. 283, 284
Lock Hospital 47
lodging houses 21, 26
  inspection 30
Logan, Mr Andrew 178, 246–247, 339
Lothian Health Board 2, 308–9
Lothian Laryngectomy Club 367
Lownie, John, building contractor
  biography 94, 95–6
  tender acceptance 106
Lowther, Dr C.P. 290
LRC Department of Social Work, 1975 hospital social work responsibility 373
Lumsden, Dr R.B., ENT Consultant 286
Lusby, Mr John, Lothian Health Board General Manager 312
Lymphadenopathy Associated Virus (LAV) *see* HIV

Maben, Mr W.S., Estates Officer 387–8
MacCallum, Dr Linda 327
McCallum, Mr J.R., paediatric ENT Consultant 287
McCartney, Dr J.E. 238
McCormack, Mr Robert J.M. 178, 246, 248, 289
  thoracic surgery development 338–9
McDonald, Lady, wife of Provost 108
MacDonald, Mr Ian, supervising engineer 387
McDowall, Dr G.D., ENT Consultant 286–7
McEwan, Mr Malcolm, Practice Manager of Social Workers 375

Index 459

McHardy, Dr G.J.Ross, Consultant Respiratory Physiologist 295, 337
McHardy, Dr Sue 327
McIntosh, Mr, supervising engineer 387
McIntyre, Dr J. Clark, ENT anaesthetist 287, 341
McKenzie, Audrey, Control of Infection Sister 381
Mackenzie, Councillor M.R. 306
Mackie, Mr (C.) Larry, Group Nursing Officer 352, 353
Mackie, T.J., Professor of Bacteriology 237–8
McLay, Dr K., ENT Consultant 286–7
MacLennan, Dr W. (Bill) J, Professor of Geriatric Medicine 345
MacMichael, Dr Neil 290
Macnamara, Dr James, Senior Hospital Medical Officer 294
MacNee, Dr W. (Bill), Professor of Respiratory and Environmental Medicine 324, 335–7
air pollution studies 402
McNeill, Dr R.A., ENT Consultant 286–7
Macpherson, Bailie, Public Health Commmittee 68
McQueen, Dr Callum 287
MacQueen, Dr Malcolm D. 283, 284
Macrae, Dr Alistair D., Consultant Virologist 293
Macrae, Dr William R., ENT anaesthetist 287, 341
McWilliams, nurse Isobel 221–2
McWilliams, nurse Patricia 221
Main, Dr Margaret, Senior Medical Assistant 230, 231, 239
Mair, Dr John 180
Maitland, William, *History of Edinburgh 1753* 25
malaria 14
Malcolm-Smith, Dr N.A. 287
Malone, Alyson, Records Officer and Information Manager 377
Mankad, Mr Pankad, Consultant in cardiac surgery 339
Mansbridge, Councillor Mrs N. 307
Maran, Dr Arnold G.D. Professor of Otolaryngology 342, 343–4
City Hospital Head of Service 287, 313
President of Royal College of Surgeons 342
voice laboratory at RIE 342
Marshall, Mr James, charge nurse 357
Masonic Lodge, High School Yards, scarlet fever use 75
Mass Radiography Unit 235
Mathers, Rev. Dr R.C.M., Hospital Chaplain 326, 390, [B]391[b]–2
Matthews, Dr J.D., Vice-Chairman, Division of Medicine, South Lothian Region 311, 317
maxillofacial surgeons 341
face reconstruction 402
maxillofacial surgery 2, 344–5
Meadowside House children's infectious disease hospital 48
measles
80 bed provision 123
1940 increase 204
1944–5 outbreak 227–8
1956 epidemic 257
1975 rise 315
first-case notification 165
late 19th century 65
notification 1879 31
penicillin benefit 242
rise in 1890s 74
treatment by Canongate Poorhouse 55
Medical Officer of Health (MOH) 29
Medical Officer of Health (MOH) department, Johnston Terrace 371
medical social workers (MSWs) 370–5
Meikle, Dr J. Halley 149
Meikle, Mrs Nola, Head of Occupational Therapy 364, 365–6
meningitis
cerebro-spinal 190, 202
notification 160
Merchant, Miss Sylvia 334, 335
mercury vapour lamps 190
Microbiology Laboratories 292–4
Milestone House 327–8
nurse training 353
military personnel treatment 162
milk, tuberculosis infection danger 32

Miller, Dr Fred, joint author *Clinical Tuberculosis* 272
Miller, Lord Provost James 251
Miller, Miss Marion, residency maid 297
Milne, Dr Archie C., Consultant Anaesthetist 248, 287–8, 340, 341
Minimal Access Therapy Training Unit Scotland (MATTUS) 340
Mitchell, Father A., RC chaplain 392
Mitchell, Mr Roy, maxillofacial implants 344
MMR (measles, mumps and rubella) immunisation, introduction 315
Moffat, Dr Margaret, virologist 178–9, 292, 293
Mok, Dr Jacqueline, Consultant Community Paediatrician 323, 330
monasteries, early patient care 7–18
Monro, Rev. George D.
  chaplain 390
  Jubilee Service 251
Montagnier, Dr Luc 320
Morham, Robert, City Architect 62–3, 65
  arguments with John Lownie 114–17
  biography 92, 93–4
  Building Specification 1897 121
  Building Specification for Colinton Mains Hospital 94
  correspondence with Lownie 111–17
  in favour of Colinton Mains site 88
Morrison, Lettie, occupational therapist 365
mortality
  and overcrowding 29–30
  recording 31
Moussa, Dr Sami A., Consultant Radiologist, radiological diagnosis of AIDS 323, 349–50
MRC Streptomycin Trial 1948 178
Muir, Professor Alexander L. 337
Muirhead, Dr Claud, Consulting Physician 65, 67, 68, 69, 86
Municipal Fire Brigade 21
Murdoch, Dr James McC., Consultant Physician 264, 270, 282, 403
  biography 275–6, 278–9
  Pharmacy Committee chairman 360
  RIDU 316

Murie, Ms Ruth, later Mrs McCabe 327
Murray, Alexander, Inspector of Lighting and Cleansing 23
Murray, Dr J.A.M., Consultant, ENT unit 341

Napier University, Edinburgh Lung and Environment Group Institute 337
National Association for the Prevention of Tuberculosis 370
National Health Insurance Act 1911 237
National Health Service 233
National Insurance Act 1911 170
naval personnel treatment 162
needles
  exchange 326
  sharing and drug misusers 321, 322
neomycin 261
nephritis, post-streptococcal 187
New Surgical Hospital 47
New Town Dispensary 25
Newlands, Dr Bill, ENT unit 341
Newsam, Mr Jack E. 277, 349
newspapers, patient progress bulletin 149–50, 151
NHS Trust Control of Infection Committee 294
NHS Trusts formation 313
Nicolson, Mr D.G., District Finance Officer 311
nitrofurantoin 276
Nixon, Mr George, laundry manager 382
Northwood, Mrs Alice, secretary to Pyelonephritis Unit 378
Nuisances in Edinburgh 1847 23
nurses
  ambulance 155, 357
  badges 354, 355–6
  combined training programme with Royal Infirmary 259–60
  fall in numbers training 236
  fever certificate 155
  fever training 58
  grading revision 303
  High School Yards building 62–3
  immunisation 187, 188
  infectious diseases contracted 158, 160–63, 165, 187, 191, 193, 199, 200, 218

out-reach, for AIDS patients 323
pay 161–2
Prize Giving 1947 233
procedures 220
recruitment problems 242–3, 300–4
scarlet fever segregation 148–9
senior sisters' tug o' war (against doctors) 245
shortage 300–4
smallpox segregation 147
'student' 219
training and State Examination 186
treatment for tuberculosis 218
uniforms 302
nurses' home 101, 112, 128
  fire 328–9
  plan 115
Nurses' Roll Call 1904 154
Nursing Staff Regulations 158–60

O'Brien, Mr Jack 349
Observations on the Management of the Poor ... and its Effects on the Health of the Great Towns 26
O'Donnell, Ms Elma, speech and language therapist 367
Officer of Health provision 29
Old Tolbooth Wynd 50
On the Prevention of Tuberculosis 1900 32
Ormiston, William, surveyor, arbiter between client and builder 114, 116, 119
overcrowding 61
  reduction 30
Owens, Mr John J., RIE NHS Trust Chief Executive 313
oxygen tents 202

Paderewski Medical School 206, 217
para-aminosalicylic acid (PAS) 179, 181, 251
paratyphoid fever, type B outbreak 1962–3 279, 301
Parker, Dr Sheena, United Hospitals Group General Manager 312
Parker, Sister Shirley, AIDS Unit 326
Parrish's Syrup 226
PAS (Patient Administration System) 378

patient information management system 364
patients, transportation to hospital 150, 152–3
Paulit, Dr John, 1645 physician 11
paving and draining 30
Pearson, Dr R.C.M. 193, 201
Pearson, Mr, Business Manager 354
Pearson, Mr Mike, City Hospital Business Manager 313
Pearson, Mr Tom, UHU Clerk of Works 387
penicillin 237
  introduction 225
penicillins 276
Penman, Caroline, HIV/AIDS Unit dietician 368
pentamidine, inhaled 324
Pettit, Nurse Elner J.J., prizewinner 257
Philip, Sir Robert, Professor of Tuberculosis 14, 32, 167–8, 169, 175–6
  tuberculosis mortality fall 176
Phillips, Mr C.J., Chairman of Board of Management 271, 299
phthisis *see* tuberculosis, pulmonary
physiotherapy 244, 251
Pickens, Dr Sam, Senior Registrar 316
Pithie, Mr David, General Foreman of Royal Victoria and Associated Hospitals Group 387
plague
  isolation 10
  notification 9
  see also bubonic plague
Play in Scottish Hospitals 353
Pneumocystis carinii
  detection 293
  pneumonia 320, 324
Police Acts 1771 23
police inspection of dairies, meat markets, etc. 30
poliomyelitis 190, 198, 201, 206, 231–2
  vaccine limited 258
Pollard, Bailie James, Convener of Public Health Committee 61, 63, 90
  biography 91–2
  breaking ground party 108
  Care of the Public Health, etc. 120
  European fact-finding mission 64

for purchase of Colinton Mains estate 89
Polton Farm Colony 389
polymixin 237
Pool, Miss Mary, Matron 165, 191, 205, 217, 351
Poor Law Amendment Act 1845 26
population increase 26
porter's gatehouse lodge 102
Portobello, temporary hospital 77
Postgraduate Board for Medicine, clinical courses 298
Practical Treatise on the Efficacy of Bloodletting in the Epidemics of Fever in Edinburgh 43
prepacked sterile units 383
Pressure Sore Prevention and Care 346–7
Pringle, Nurse Margaret, prizewinner 243
private patients 58
Prontosil 188, 202
Proseptasine 188
Proseptinase 202
Public Health Committee 30
　cholera hospital accommodation 75
　Joint Subcommittee 69
　possible rebuilding of City Hospital 63
Public Health Department
　Annual Reports 167
　NHS hospitals under 236
public health movement 25–33
Public Health (Scotland) Act 1867 30, 51
Public Health (Scotland) Act 1867, Town Council responsibility for infectious disease 56
public health statistics, Littlejohn appointment centenary 33
Public Works Office
　1897 Building Specification for the New City Hospital at Colinton Mains 103–4
　block plan from Description and Sketch Plan 1896 101
puerperal fever
　increase 198–9
　notification 32
puerperal sepsis 190, 357
　reduction 242
Pullen, Dr Herbert, Consultant in Infectious Diseases in Leeds 278

Pulmonary Function Service 295
Purves, Mr Robert, City Hospital Manager 313, 353, 354
　RIE Director of Operations, Nursing and Quality 354
Pyelonephritis Unit 276–78, 348
pyrazinamide 181

quarantine 25
　High School Yards building 62
　regulations 9–10
Quarryhole Park, temporary hospital 75–6
Queen's Park, temporary hospital 77–8
Queensberry House Fever Hospital, 1818–35 41, 42–7
　bleeding 43
　nurses 43–4
　patient accommodation 43
quinolones 276

rabies provision in Budapest 98
radiography, mass miniature 14
radiology, mass miniature campaign 179
Raeburn, Dr Hugh A., Senior Administrative Medical Officer 280
Ragged School 49
railings at old Royal Infirmary 70
Railton, Miss Rosemary, Group Chief Pharmacist 359–60
Rankin, Dr A.L.K. 193, 238
rationing after the war 226
Rawlings, Mr E. Jimmy, Group Superintendent Radiographer 347, 348, 349
Rawson, Mr Gordon, laundry manager 383
Rayne Laboratory 398, 403
　cell biology 334
　exercise laboratory 335
　radiographers use 349
　sleep studies 335
Red Cross, Scottish Branch 245
Redmond, Mr Geoffrey, Hospital Secretary 271, 395
Regional Clinical Virus Laboratory 263, 315, 344, 398, 399, 403
Regional Infectious Diseases Unit (RIDU) 315–18

Index 463

case notes 378
children's ward 341
move to Western General Hospital [B]400[b]
occupational therapy services 365
Registered Nurse Training Committee 301
Reid, Dr Kenneth, Royal Victoria Dispensary 181
Reid, Mr Kenneth, Senior Lecturer in cardiac surgery 339
Reiderer, Father Victor S.J., RC chaplain 392
Reorganisation of the NHS in Scotland 1974 314
Report on the Sanitary Condition of the City of Edinburgh 1865 29–31
Report on the Sanitary Condition of Saint-Giles' Ward 1889 30
Respiratory Diseases 1969 181
Respiratory Function Laboratory 294–5, 398, 403
Respiratory Medicine Unit, transfer to RIE 1993 338, 398
Respiratory Physiology Laboratory 315
retrograde pyelography 349
Reymbaut, Ms Emma, speech and language therapist 367
Rhind, Dr George 335
Richardson, Dr Alison, Clinical Psychologist 323
rifampicin 181
Rist, Dr Edouard, writing on Philip 168
Ritchie, Dr John 149
Robertson, Dr Roy, West Granton Medical Group and drug misusers 321
Robertson, Dr William S.I., MOH 160, 164
Robertson, Mr A.I., portering supervisor 386
Robertson, Mr Ian, Area Sterilising Centre Deputy Manager 384
Robertson, Mr Walter W., Surveyor, HM Board of Works 104, 114, 116
Robertson, Mrs Lilias, secretary to Dr Joe and Dr Murdoch 378
Robertson, Professor J.D., Chairman of South Lothian District Medical Committee 311
Robson, Dr James, Professor of Medicine 337

Ronald, Miss Norma, chaplain 392
Rooyen, Dr C.E. van 193–4
Ross, Dr J.D. (Ian) 178, 182, 272
Ross, Dr Jonathan 317
Ross, Miss Elizabeth, Superintendent of Physiotherapy 362, 363, 364
Rosslynlee Mental Hospital 258
Royal Blind Asylum, mattress order 75
Royal College of Physicians 13
  1900 laboratory analysis of infectious specimens 168
  and cholera 16
  Crofton as President 1973 181
  laboratory, sputum analysis 32
  Report on the New City Hospital Site 1894 86
  research laboratory 14
Royal Commission 1976–9 311
Royal Commission on the Poor Laws of Scotland, 1844 26
Royal Environment Health Institute of Scotland (REHIS) 381
Royal Hospital for Sick Children, refusal to admit infectious patients 48
Royal Infirmary 37–40
  1879 move to Lauriston 64
  building 1738 38–9
  fever wards admission check 30
  move to Lauriston Place 53; pavilion for infectious diseases 53
  new 399
  rebuilding 2
  thoracic surgery 246
Royal Infirmary Convalescent Home 208–9, 210
Royal Victoria and Associated Hospitals Board of Management 236
Royal Victoria Dispensary 254
  case notes 377
  Lauriston Place 169
  social work department 370, 371, 373
  X-ray cover by City Hospital 347
Royal Victoria Hospital 236
  X-ray cover by City Hospital 347
Royal Victoria Hospital Tuberculosis Trust 175, 179, 180
rubella, 1979 outbreak 315
Russell, Dr J.A., provost, improvement scheme 61

Sabin poliomyelitis vaccine 232
St Andrew's Ambulance Association 50
St Catherine of Sienna, Convent of 10
St Cuthbert's and Canongate Combination 51
St Cuthbert's Charity Workhouse 46
St John Ambulance Association 150
St Patrick's Roman Catholic School 58
St Roque (Roche), Chapel of 10–11
salaries 1894–95 72
Salk poliomyelitis vaccine 232
Salmon Report 303
salmonella 316
salmonella food poisoning 260
Salmonella typhimurium food poisoning 253
salmonellosis 256
salvage chemotherapy 179
Sanderson, Dr Robert, head and neck surgeon 342
Sandford, Miss E.L., Lady Superintendent of Nurses 154, 351
Sang, Mr Chris, cardio-thoracic surgeon 339
Sangster, Dr George, Consultant Physician 239–40, 261, 278, 316, 317
Sanitary Districts 29–30
sanitation
  defects 26
  New Town 22
  Old Town 21
Sanocrysin 179, 192
Saughton prison, HIV screening clinic 323
scabies, High School Yards building 62
scarlatina, notification 1879 31
scarlet fever
  1933 epidemic 188
  immunisation 186–7
  late nineteenth century 65
  milk-borne 164, 165
  mortality decline 187
  notification 1879 31
  patient numbers 65
  pavilions 101
  penicillin benefit 242
  penicillin intramuscular injections 357
  regimen 156
  reinfection and complications prevention 188
  rise in 1890s 74–5
  treatment by RIE 55
  ward plan 124
Schick testing 164
  1924 campaign 165
Schultz-Charlton diagnostic skin test 187
Scott, Dr Charles E., Aural Surgeon 191
Scott, Mrs Anne 327
Scott, Sheila, RIE theatre sister 383
Scott Forrest, Dr 206, 227, 230
Scottish AIDS Monitor 322
Scottish Development Department 300
Scottish Health Board, nursing certificate 163
Scottish Home and Health Department 300
Scottish Hospitals Endowment Research Trust 277
Scottish Lithotripter Centre 350
Scottish Mycobacteria Reference Laboratory 294, 344, 398, 399, 403
Scottish National Blood Transfusion Service 321
Scottish-Scandinavian Conferences on Infectious Diseases 240
Seaton, Dr Anthony, Professor of Environmental and Occupational Medicine, Aberdeen 182
sedan chairs 150
Seiler, Dr H.E., MOH 178, 180, 248, 253, 269
Selwyn, Sydney, Professor of Medical Microbiology, Westminster and Charing Cross Hospitals 278
sensitivity testing, tubercle bacilli 251
separation room 123
serum sickness 160
servants and quarantine, High School Yards building 62
service road holdups 110
sewer construction for RIE 53–4
Shandley, Mrs Kim, head medical social worker 373–5
Shaw, Mrs Sinclair, art therapy classes 371
Shiells, Miss, medical social worker 371
Shigella flexneri 248, 256
Shigella newcastle 256
Shigella sonnei 237, 248, 256, 261, 264

Simpson, Dr G.W. 193
Skeyne, Gilbert, *Ane Breve Descriptioun of the Pest* 1568 12
Slateford Fever Hospital 210
slates, specifications 105
smallpox 7
   1880–96 figures 76
   1942 outbreak 207–12, 213–15
   cases 1898–1904 145–47
   cases 1920 163
   epidemic 1871 51
   epidemic 1892–95 72, 74–81
   epidemics 13
   eradication 207–8, 215
   high mortality 11–13
   inoculation 13
   late nineteenth century 65
   notification 1879 31
   outbreak 1877 51
   rashes 79
   rise in 1890s 74
   treatment by Canongate Poorhouse 55
   vaccination 75, 148, 163, 207
Smallpox Accommodation of 1910, Report 147–8
smallpox cottages 126
smallpox hospital, total isolation necessary 147–8
Smith, Dr A. Brownlie, ENT Consultant 286–7
Smith, Dr C. Christopher, Senior Registrar 316, 317
Smith, Dr G.H. Sharwood 287
Smith, Dr Roger G., Senior Lecturer in Geriatric Medicine 291
Smith, Mr Jim, Operational Services Manager 313, 354
smoking 220
Smout, T.C. 11, 13
Snell, Mr Frank, Hon President of League of Friends 395
Society for the Destitute Sick, Visitors 44
Society for the Suppression of Begging 39
soiled-linen chute 125
Soluseptacide 202
Soutar, Dr Colin 337
South Bridge Primary School 58
South Eastern Regional Hospital Board 234

South Edinburgh School of Nursing 303
South-Eastern Regional Hospital Board 2, 310
Southfield Hospital 170, 236, 258
   geriatric patients 263, 290
   X-ray cover by City Hospital 347, 348
Southfield Hospital Research Laboratory, move to City Hospital 263
Spiers, Colin, Clinical Research Fellow with Eli Lilly 278
Spittal Street
   Royal Victoria Dispensary 169
   TB Clinic, social work 373
Springfield House, Polton, for convalescent tuberculosis patients 170
sputum mug routine 219
staff, infection 45–6, 158
Standing Conference on Drug Abuse (SCODA) 325
staphylococcal endocarditis 2, 319
staphylococci, hospital problem 269
State Enrolled Nurse posts 302
Stevenson, Dr David 284
Stewart, Dr Sheila 178, 293
Stirling, Mr, Hospital Steward 205
Stokes, Mr Mike, Practice Manager of Social Workers 375
stone
   delivery delays 111
   used for building 104
store block 127
Strang, Mr Bob, laundry manager 382
Streptococcus pyogenes 200, 201
streptomycin 179, 181, 243, 251, 261
sub-contractors' pay claims 113
Sudlow, Dr Michael F, Hon. Senior Lecturer 338
sulphaguanidine 222
sulphanilamide 202
sulphapyridine, in meningitis 201, 203
sulphonamide drugs 190, 200–3, 243
sunlight importance 100
sunrooms 100
Surgeons' Hall 47
Surgical Hospital, new, Adam gates 70
Surgical Hospitals, old, refitment for smallpox patients 1881 55
surgical trolley-top trays 383

Sutherland, Mr James, Senior Technician 292
Swainson, Dr Charles, RIE Medical Director 313
swimming baths 58
Syme, James, Consultant Paediatrician 278
syphilis 7, 9
syringe, sterile service 280

Tait, Dr W. Anne, Consultant Psychiatrist 323
Tayler, Mr Winston, Lothian Health Board General Manager 312
Taylor, Miss J.K., Matron 211, 222, 258, 302, 304–5, 351, 352
 with cerebro-spinal meningitis survivor 192
Taylor, Mr David MBE
 AIDS Co-ordinator for Lothian Region 375
 head medical social worker 375
telephone
 1958 improvement 262
 internal system 128
 link request 74–5
television sets 245
Telfer, Rev Harry, chaplain 392
tenders for building 106
Terry, Mr Nigel, portering supervisor 386
tetracycline 179, 261
Thin, Dr Robert 290
Thomas, Miss I., Lady Superintendent of Nurses 154, 351, 354
Thompson, Alison (Parker), Dietetic Manager 368
Thompson, Dr Carolyn 317
Thomson, Dr T. Lauder 149
Thomson, Dr Winifred 293
Thomson, Dr W. Norman, Consultant Radiologist 278, 349
Thomson, Nurse Diana, prizewinner 256
thoracic surgery 2
thoracic surgical team 178
thoracoplasty 179
timber specifications 105
Tinne, Dr John, bacteriologist 292
Tippethill Hospital closure 250
Todd, Dr W.T. Andrew, Registrar 317

tonsillitis 200
Town Council, fever patient responsibility 57
tracheotomy theatres 100
Trinity Church 10
Triple Antigen Investigation 253
tropical disease advice centre 329
tuberculosis
 1921 accommodation 164
 bovine 14
 notification 33, 168
 pulmonary, notifiable 160
 revolving wooden shelters 173–4
 streptomycin injections 357
 X-ray screening 1
tuberculosis dispensary, first, Bank Street 169
Tuberculosis Officer 167
Tuberculosis and Respiratory Diseases Unit 263
Tuberculosis Trust 236
tuberculous meningitis 149
Tulloch, Mr W. Selby 277, 349
Turner, Dr Logan 37–8, 40, 42, 46, 47
Tweeddale, Dr Patricia, Respiratory Function Laboratory 334
typhoid fever 14
 late nineteenth century 65
 notification 1879 31
 treatment by RIE 55
 ward plan 124
typhus fever 13–14
 1880–96 figures 76
 epidemics 47
 late nineteenth century 65
 notification 1879 31
 rise in 1890s 74
 single-storey blocks 122
 treatment by Canongate Poorhouse 55

United Hospitals Unit 312
urethritis 277
Usher Institute of Public Health, sputum analysis 32–3

vaccination 75, 148, 207
vaccination centres 207
Vaccination (Scotland) Act 1863 29

Index   467

vaccine associated deaths 207
vaccines, combined 253
vans, horse-drawn, for bedding 152-3
ventilation 127
Victoria Dispensary for Consumption 169
Victoria Hospital for Consumption, later Royal Victoria Hospital 169-70
Victoria Park House, smallpox contacts 209
viomycin 179
Vitamin D, for house-bound elderly 369
Voluntary Health Workers' Association 216

Wade, Mr David, Consultant Thoracic Surgeon 178, 246, 248, 289
wages 1894-95 72
Walbaum, Mr Philip R., Consultant Thoracic Surgeon 178, 246, 248, 289
  thoracic surgery development 338-9
Walker, James, surveyor, arbiter between client and builder 116, 119
Walker, Mr William (Bill) S., cardio-thoracic surgeon 339, 340
Wallace, Dr Archie 178, 238, 240, 254, 256, 292, 403
wards
  1893 65
  cubicle 199
  windows double-glazed 105
Warren, Dr Patricia, Rayne Laboratory 334, 335, 337
water supplies
  defects 26
  from Comiston Springs 22
  from Glencorse 22
  New Town 22
  Old Town 21
Waters, Mr Colin, buildings officer 387
Watson, Colin, voice analysis 342
Watt, Dr Brian, Director of Scottish Mycobacteria Reference Laboratory 294, 324, 403
Waverley Care Trust 327
Webber, William 358
  Chief Medical Laboratory Scientific Officer 238, 292
Weil's disease 255
Weir, Miss Mary, Personnel Officer 315

Wellcome Trust, funding for respiratory pathogen research 263
Wellcome Research Trust Virus Laboratory, later Regional Virus Laboratory 270, 292, 293, 356
Welsby, Dr Philip D., Consultant Physician 317-18
  with smallpox warning notice 213
Welsh, Dr Benjamin, superintendent of Queensberry House Fever Hospital 42
Welstead, Mr Alec, Hospital Group Secretary 126, 178, 179, 261, 269, 272, 274-5, 305, 308
Western General Hospital 51
Wheatley, Mr David, Senior Lecturer in cardiac surgery 338-9
White, Mr Peter, supervisor 387
Whiteheart, Andrea, domestic manager 386
Whiteoak, Ernie, Deputy Records Manager 378
Whitley Council Regulations 236
whole time equivalent staff (WTE) 314
whole time equivalent staff (WTE), in physiotherapy 363
whooping cough
  1904 mortality 149
  1925 mortality 166
  1956 epidemic 257
  1975 rise 315
  first-case notification 165
  late nineteenth century 65
  single-storey blocks 122
Whyte, Dr A., Senior Medical Assistant 205, 206, 230
Wightman, Dr A.J.A., Consultant Radiologist, *Clinical Radiology* 349
Wilks, Dr David, Consultant Physician 319
  Infectious Diseases Manual co-author 319
Will, Professor Robert, HIV neurological problems 323
Williams, Dilys, Superintendent of Physiotherapy 362
Williamson, Dr A. Maxwell 160, 161, 171-3
Williamson, Dr James, Professor of Geriatrics 178, 179, 261, 289, 290-2
  Care of the Elderly Unit 403

rehabilitation services 291
speech therapy requirement 366
Williamson, Mr Charlie, portering supervisor 386
Willox, Miss I.S., Matron 304, 351
Wilson, Dr Alistair M.M., Consultant Bacteriologist 293–4
Wilson, Jimmy, records office 377
Wilson, Miss Elizabeth, RIE Diabetic and Dietetic Outpatient Clinic 368
Wilson, Mr Tom, Catering Manager 379
Wilson, Ms Eileen, Catering Department 379
Wilson, Tracey, dietetic secretary 368
Wishart, Mrs Margaret, dining room servery 380
Women's Royal Voluntary Service (WRVS) 393
Wong, Roger 327
Wood, Miss Peggy, head social worker 371
Working for Patients (Scotland) 313
World Health Organisation (WHO) 181
Wright, Dr Frederick J., Consultant in Tropical Medicine 282, 283–4
Wright, Dr Helen 238
Wright, Mr Malcolm, Chief Executive of Royal Hospital for Sick Children 312
Wylis, Mrs, domestic manager 386
Wyllie, Dr John, Consulting Physician to City Hospital, 600 bed support 103

X-rays
  mass campaign 261
  for tuberculosis 241, 244

yellow fever vaccination 283

Zealley, Dr Helen E., Chief Administrative Medical Officer 293
  Director of Public Health 325
  Health in Lothian 1974–89 report 325
zidovudine (AZT) 324, 330
zinc, use in long-term care patients 369